An Introduction to the Psychology of Hearing

An Introduction to the Psychology of Hearing

Second Edition

Brian C. J. Moore
University Lecturer in Experimental Psychology
University of Cambridge

1988

ACADEMIC PRESS
Harcourt Brace Jovanovich, Publishers
London   San Diego   New York
Boston   Sydney   Tokyo   Toronto

ACADEMIC PRESS LIMITED
24–28 Oval Road,
London NW1 7DX

United States Edition published by
ACADEMIC PRESS INC.
San Diego, CA 92101

British Library Cataloguing in Publication Data
Moore, B. C. J.
    Introduction to the psychology of hearing.—2nd ed.
    1. Auditory perception
    I. Title
    152/1'2   BF251
    ISBN 0-12-505620-6 Hardback
    ISBN 0-12-505622-2 Paperback

    LCCN 81-69595

Typeset by Oxprint Limited, Oxford
Printed in Great Britain by St Edmundsbury Press Limited,
Bury St Edmunds, Suffolk

To Carol

Preface

In 1971 I gave my first course of lectures on auditory perception, as part of the psychology course at the University of Reading. Anyone who has attempted to give or attend lectures on auditory perception will be aware of two major problems which I encountered. Firstly, there is no textbook which is both up to date and at a level suitable for undergraduate use. Secondly, scientific papers on hearing in psychological and physiological journals are almost incomprehensible to the beginner in this area. I became increasingly frustrated at having to say to my students "I'm sorry, but there is no book I can recommend," and finally I decided that the only solution to the problem was to write such a book myself.

This book, then, is primarily intended as an undergraduate textbook to accompany courses in auditory perception or hearing. To this end it contains a chapter introducing the basic physics of sound and describing the most important anatomical and physiological features of the auditory system. Some very basic knowledge is assumed (for example, the terms 'neurone' and 'nerve firings' are not explained), but the approach is very much to start from first principles.

As it turned out, the book contains very much more material than I would normally get through in a single course of lectures, so that it could also serve as a text to accompany advanced undergraduate or graduate courses in auditory perception. The general approach throughout the book is to relate the psychological and perceptual aspects of sound to the underlying physiological mechanisms. Thus the book should also be of use and interest to sensory physiologists, physicians and audiologists.

Although the emphasis throughout the book is on laboratory experiments performed under carefully controlled conditions, I have been careful to point out, wherever possible, the real-life or applied relevance of the problems under discussion. Indeed the final chapter of the book is mainly concerned with practical applications. In addition, there is a chapter on speech perception in which links with psychoacoustic phenomena are emphasized. Thus the book should also have something of interest for phoneticians, speech researchers, speech pathologists, linguists, and engineers concerned with problems of the recording, transmission and reproduction of sound or with problems of automatic speech recognition and speaker identification.

Preface

My major aim in writing this book was that it should be reasonably up to date, but at the same time not too technical for the novice. Inevitably this has resulted in the omission of some details and the simplification of some concepts. I hope that I have managed to do this without too much distortion, and that the essential flavour of current trends in auditory research has been preserved. Many areas which are traditionally discussed in textbooks on hearing have been omitted entirely; for example, volume and density as attributes of pure tones are not mentioned, nor is the mel scale of pitch. This reflects my own prejudices to some extent, but the basis for omission has generally been the lack of use of these concepts in the last ten years or so.

Perhaps the hardest thing about writing this book was to stop writing it! Almost every day I came across new papers with exciting results which ought to have been mentioned. However, one has to draw the line somewhere, and the book was never intended to be a complete review. I apologize to those whose work has been omitted or mentioned too briefly. The balance of space has inevitably been influenced by my own interests, and I hope that I will be forgiven for devoting so much space to the role of 'timing' information in nerve impulses.

Auditory perception has been a sadly neglected area in British psychology, although this is much less true in the United States and Holland. I hope that this book will help to correct the balance, and that those who teach in this area will find the book of some use.

Finally, I would like to thank all those colleagues and friends who read parts of the manuscript and provided helpful comments. The manuscript was written while I was a lecturer in Psychology at the University of Reading. Thanks are due particularly to: Mark Haggard, Max Coltheart, Bernard Moulden, Alan Allport, David Raab, Roy Davis, Wynford Bellin, Mark Terry, Peter Bailey, Arthur Summerfield, Dave Martin, John Gundry, Carol Moore and Pat Sheldon. The responsibility for mistakes is of course mine. Mrs P. Williams typed the manuscript accurately and quickly through many drafts to its final form; I am very grateful to her. Susan and Paul Scott, and my wife Carol, provided valuable help in sorting out the references.

Reading, 1977   B. C. J. M.

Preface to the Second Edition

I have had three main aims in writing the second edition of this book: firstly to clarify certain sections which students and colleagues have told me were difficult to follow in the first edition; secondly to describe some of the most important experimental results which have appeared since the first edition was completed; finally to introduce new material in areas which were thought by colleagues to be important, but which were not covered in the first edition. In this final category, the most important change is a new chapter on 'Auditory pattern and object perception'. I hope that this chapter will go some way towards answering the complaints of those who thought that the first edition did not contain enough on 'perception' or 'psychology'. I have been careful, in this chapter, to emphasize links with other areas of psychology, and particularly that of selective attention.

I wish to clarify which students the book is appropriate for. In the UK the book is suitable for advanced undergraduate, and Master's level courses in psychology, speech and hearing sciences, and audiology. In the USA the book might be found a little difficult for undergraduate psychologists, but it would be well suited to graduate courses in perception. The book is suitable for those in the USA taking undergraduate *and* graduate level courses in subjects with a greater emphasis on hearing, such as audiology, and speech and hearing science.

Finally, I wish to thank all those who helped in the preparation of the second edition. The following people provided valuable comments, criticisms and suggestions: Bernard O'Loughlin, Robert Milroy, Brian Glasberg, Michael Shailer, Roy Patterson, Robert Peters, Paul Whittle and Tony Marcel. Kay Knights quickly and patiently typed many drafts of the revised manuscript, and Roy Hammans helped in the preparation of new figures.

Cambridge, 1982   B. C. J. M.

Contents

1 The nature of sound and the structure of the auditory system

1 INTRODUCTION

One of the general aims of this book is to specify, as far as possible, the relationships between the characteristics of the sounds which enter the ear and the sensations which they produce. Wherever possible these relationships will be specified in terms of the underlying mechanisms. In other words, we will be trying to understand how the auditory system works, as well as to look at what it does. It is not always possible to fulfil both of these objectives. While some aspects of auditory perception can be explained by reference to the anatomy or physiology of the auditory system, our knowledge in this respect is not usually as precise or as far reaching as we would like. Often the results of behavioural studies (generally psychophysical experiments) provide us with evidence as to the kinds of things which are occurring in the auditory system, but we may not be able to specify the detailed physiological mechanisms which are involved. Sometimes we can use the results of psychophysical experiments to determine whether a particular type of neural coding (see later), which in principle could convey information about a sound, is actually involved in the perception or discrimination of that sound. Before we can begin to specify underlying mechanisms, however, we must know something of the physical nature of sounds, and of the basic anatomy and physiology of the auditory system. That is the purpose of this chapter.

2 THE PHYSICAL CHARACTERISTICS OF SOUNDS

Sound originates from the motion or vibration of an object. This motion is impressed upon the surrounding medium (usually air) as a pattern of changes in pressure. What actually happens is that the atmospheric particles, or molecules, are squeezed closer together than normal, and then pulled farther apart than normal. The sound wave moves outwards from the vibrating body, but the molecules do not advance with the wave: they vibrate about an average resting place. The sound wave generally weakens

1

as it moves away from the source, and also may be subject to reflections and refractions caused by walls or objects in its path. Thus the sound 'image' reaching the ear will differ somewhat from that initially generated.

One of the simplest type of sound is the sine wave, also known as a sinusoidal vibration, which has the waveform (pressure variation plotted against time) shown in Fig. 1.1. This wave is simple both from the physical

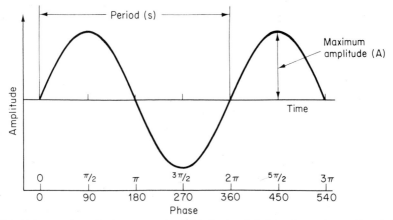

FIG. 1.1 The waveform of a sine wave or sinusoidal vibration. Only 1.5 cycles are shown, although the waveform should be pictured as repeating indefinitely. The instantaneous amplitude is given by the expression $A \sin (2\pi ft)$, where t = time, f = frequency and A = maximum amplitude. Phase is indicated along the bottom, using as a reference point the first zero-crossing of the wave. Phase may be measured in degrees or in radians. One complete cycle corresponds to 360° or 2π radians.

and mathematical point of view and from the point of view of the auditory system. It happens that sine waves produce particularly simple responses in the auditory system, and that they have a very 'clean' or 'pure' sound, like that of a tuning fork. Thus they are also called simple tones or pure tones. To describe a sine wave we need to specify three things: the *frequency*, or the number of times per second the waveform repeats itself (specified in hertz, where 1 hertz (Hz) = 1 cycle/s); the *amplitude*, or the amount of pressure variation about the mean or normal; the *phase*, or the portion of the cycle through which the wave has advanced in relation to some fixed point in time. For continuous sinusoids phase is only important when we are interested in the relationship between two or more different waves. The time taken for one complete cycle of the waveform is called the period, which is the reciprocal of the frequency.

A sine wave is not the only kind of sound which repeats regularly. Many of the sounds which we encounter in everyday life, such as those produced by musical instruments, and certain speech sounds, also show such regularity, and hence are called periodic sounds. Although these sounds are generally more complex than sine waves, they share a common subjective characteristic with sine waves in that they have pitches. Pitch may be defined as that attribute of auditory sensation in terms of which sounds may be ordered on a musical scale. In other words, pitch is that attribute the variation of which constitutes melody. Any sound which produces pitch may be called a tone. In general, tones are periodic, but as we shall see later, this is not always the case.

The pitch of a sound is related to its repetition rate and, hence, in the case of a sine wave, to frequency. It should be emphasized that pitch is a subjective attribute of a stimulus, and as such cannot be measured directly. However, for a sine wave the pitch is closely related to the frequency; the higher the frequency, the higher the pitch. For a more complex sound the pitch is often investigated by asking the subject to adjust a sine wave so that it has the same pitch as the complex sound. The frequency of the sine wave is then taken as a measure of the pitch of the complex sound.

Although all sounds can be specified in terms of variations in sound pressure occurring over time, it is often more convenient, and more meaningful, to specify them in a different way when the sounds are complex. This method is based on a theorem by Fourier, who proved that any complex waveform (with certain restrictions) can be analysed, or broken down, into a series of sine waves with specific frequencies, amplitudes and phases. Such an analysis is called Fourier analysis, and each sine wave is called a frequency (or Fourier) component of the complex sound. The frequency components are also sometimes called partials. We may thus define a complex tone as a tone composed of a number of simple tones, or sine waves.

The simplest type of complex tone to which Fourier analysis can be applied is one which is *periodic*. Such a tone is composed of a number of simple tones each of which has a frequency which is an integral multiple of some common (not necessarily present) fundamental component. The fundamental component thus has the lowest frequency of any of the components in the complex tone, and it may be said to form the 'foundation' for the other components. The fundamental component has a frequency equal to the repetition rate of the complex waveform as a whole. The frequency components, or partials, of the complex tone are known as harmonics, and are numbered, the fundamental being given harmonic number 1. Thus, for example, a note of middle C played on the piano would have a fundamental component or first harmonic of frequency 256 Hz, a second harmonic of frequency 512 Hz, a third harmonic of frequency 768 Hz, etc. The nth harmonic has a frequency which is n times that of the fundamental. An illustration of how a complex tone can be built up from a series of sine waves is given in Fig. 1.2.

One of the reasons for representing sounds in this way is that humans do seem to be able to hear the harmonics of a periodic sound wave individually

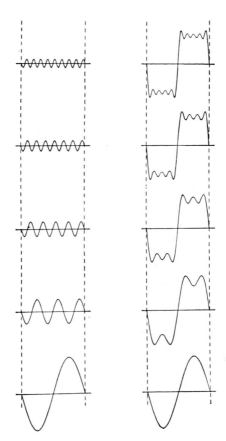

FIG. 1.2 An illustration of how a complex waveform (a square wave) can be built up from a series of sinusoidal components. The square wave is composed of odd harmonics only, and the 1st, 3rd, 5th, 7th and 9th harmonics are shown on the left. The series on the right shows progressive changes from a simple sine wave as each component is added. If enough additional harmonics, with appropriate amplitudes and phases, were added, the composite wave would approach a perfectly square shape. From Newman (1948), by permission of John Wiley, New York.

to a limited extent. For example, Mersenne (1636) stated that "the string struck and sounded freely makes at least five sounds at the same time, the first of which is the natural sound of the string and serves as the foundation for the rest . . ." The phenomenon that humans can hear out the sinusoidal components of a complex tone is known as Ohm's Acoustical Law, after the German physicist Georg Ohm. Normally, when we are presented with a complex tone, we do not listen in this way, but nevertheless we do appear to be *able* to hear out the lower harmonics of a complex sound to some extent (see Chapters 3 and 4 for further discussion of this). When we are presented with two simultaneous pure tones, whose frequencies are not too similar, then these will often be heard as two separate sounds rather than as a single complex sound. Thus our perception corresponds to the analysis of the sound in terms of its Fourier components. Notice that our perception of colour is quite different; if lights of two different frequencies (or wavelengths) are mixed, we see a single colour corresponding to the mixture, rather than seeing two component hues.

The structure of a sound, in terms of its frequency components, is often represented by its spectrum—a plot of sound amplitude (or energy) against frequency. Examples of spectra are given in Fig. 1.3. For periodic sounds of

FIG. 1.3 On the left are shown the waveforms of some common auditory stimuli, and on the right are the corresponding spectra. The periodic stimuli (pure tone, square wave and train of pulses) have line spectra, while the nonperiodic stimuli (single pulse, white noise and short tone burst) have continuous spectra.

long duration, the energy falls at specific discrete frequencies and the spectrum is known as a line spectrum. The first three examples are of this type. The sinusoid, by definition, consists of a single frequency component. The square wave, as shown in Fig. 1.2, consists of the odd harmonics of the fundamental component (1 kHz in our example), and the amplitudes of the harmonics decrease with increasing harmonic number. The train of brief pulses, or clicks, contains all the harmonics of the fundamental at equal amplitude. However, since each pulse contains only a small amount of energy, and since there are many harmonics, each harmonic has a low amplitude.

For sounds which are not periodic, such as white noise (a hissing sound), the spectrum tends to be more complex, and is obtained by use of a mathematical device known as the Fourier transform. Our last three examples are of this type. The spectra of such sounds are known as continuous spectra; the energy is spread over certain frequency bands, rather than being concentrated at particular frequencies. The single pulse, or click, and the white noise both have flat spectra; the amplitude does not vary as a function of frequency. We should remember, however, that any particular sample of 'white' noise may not have a flat spectrum. It is only when the spectrum is averaged over a long period of time that it becomes flat. Although the pulse and the noise have spectra of the same shape, the amplitude of the spectrum of the pulse is lower, since it contains much less energy than the noise. The pulse and the noise differ in their phase spectra, the distributions of phase as a function of frequency (not shown in the figure). For the noise the phases of the components are randomly distributed. For the pulse the components have a phase of 90° or $\pi/2$ radians at time zero. This is known as cosine phase, and it means that each component is at its peak amplitude at time zero. The result is that at this time the components all add, whereas at other times they cancel.

The final example shows a short burst of a sinusoid, often called a tone pulse or tone burst. The spectrum of a sinusoid is only a line if the sinusoid lasts an indefinite time. For tone pulses of short duration the frequency spectrum contains energy over a wide range of frequencies. Although the peak in the spectrum occurs at the nominal frequency of the tone pulse, there is considerable energy at other frequencies. This spread of energy increases as the duration of the tone pulse is shortened. Corresponding changes occur in our perception of such tone pulses; as a tone pulse is shortened in duration, it becomes less tonelike and more clicklike.

In general, whenever a stimulus is changed abruptly (e.g. by a change in level or a change in frequency), a spread in spectral energy occurs. This spreading of spectral energy over frequency is often called 'energy splatter'. Energy splatter can be reduced by slowing down the changes (e.g. by switching tones on and off gradually), but it cannot be completely eliminated. We shall see later that energy splatter may play an important role in studies of masking and of pitch discrimination.

Let us now turn to the measurement of sound levels. The instruments used to measure these, such as microphones, normally respond to changes in air pressure, and thus give an output proportional to the amplitude of the sound. We use the term 'amplitude' here to refer to deviations in pressure from the mean value (normal atmospheric pressure). However, it is more usual to specify sound levels in terms of intensity, which is the sound power transmitted through a given area in a sound field. For a medium such as air there is a simple relationship between the amplitude of a plane (flat-fronted) sound wave in a free field (i.e. in the absence of reflected sound) and the acoustic intensity; intensity is proportional to the square of amplitude.

It turns out that the auditory system can deal with a huge range of sound intensities (see Chapter 2). This makes it inconvenient to deal with sound intensities or powers directly. Instead a logarithmic scale expressing the *ratio* of two intensities is used. One intensity is chosen as a reference level, I_0, and the other intensity, I_1, is expressed relative to this. One bel corresponds to a ratio of intensities of 10:1. Thus the number of bels corresponding to a given intensity ratio is obtained by taking the logarithm to the base 10 of the intensity ratio. For example, an intensity ratio of 100:1 corresponds to 2 bels. Unfortunately, the bel is a rather large unit for everyday use, and to obtain units of convenient size the bel is divided into 10 decibels (dB). Thus the number of decibels corresponding to a given ratio of acoustic intensity is

$$\text{number of decibels} = 10 \log_{10} (I_1/I_0).$$

Notice that a given number of decibels represents an intensity or power ratio, not an absolute intensity. In order to specify the absolute intensity of a sound it is necessary to state that the intensity (or power) of the sound, I_1, is n dB above or below some reference level I_0. The reference level most commonly used is an intensity of 10^{-16} watts per square centimetre (W/cm²), which is equivalent to a pressure of 2×10^{-5} N/m² or 20 μPa (micropascal). A sound level specified using this reference level is referred to as a sound pressure level (SPL). Thus a sound at 60 dB SPL is 60 dB higher in level than the reference level of 0 dB (10^{-10} W/cm²), and has an intensity of 10^{-10} W/cm². Notice that multiplying (or dividing) the ratio of intensities by 10 increases (or decreases) the number of decibels by 10. It is also convenient to remember that a two-fold change in intensity corresponds to a change in level of 3 dB.

The reference sound level, 0 dB SPL, is a low sound level which was chosen to be close to the average human absolute threshold for a 1000 Hz pure tone. The absolute threshold is the minimum detectable level of a sound in the absence of any other external sounds (the manner of presentation of the sound and method of determining detectability must be specified). In fact the average human absolute threshold at 1000 Hz is about 6.5 dB SPL. Sometimes it is convenient to choose as a reference level the threshold of a subject for the sound being used. A sound level specified in this way is referred to as a sensation level (SL). Thus, for a given subject, a sound at 60 dB SL will be 60 dB above the absolute threshold of that subject for that sound. The physical intensity corresponding to a given sensation level will, of course, differ from subject to subject, and from sound to sound.

Finally, it is useful to adapt the decibel notation so that it expresses ratios of pressure as well as ratios of intensity. This may be done by recalling that intensity is proportional to the square of pressure. If one sound has an intensity of I_1 and an amplitude (pressure) A_1, and a second sound has an intensity I_2 and amplitude A_2, then the difference in level between them is

number of decibels $= 10 \log_{10}(I_1/I_2) = 10 \log_{10}(A_1/A_2)^2 = 20 \log_{10}(A_1/A_2)$.

Thus a 10-fold increase in amplitude (pressure) corresponds to a 100-fold increase in intensity and is represented by $+ 20$ dB. Table I gives some examples of intensity and pressure ratios expressed in decibels, and also indicates sound levels, in dB SPL, corresponding to various common sounds.

TABLE I

The relationship between decibels, intensity ratios and amplitude ratios. Sound levels in dB SPL are expressed relative to a level I_0 of 10^{-16} W/cm². This is equivalent to 2×10^{-5} N/m². 10^n means 1 followed by n zeros.

Sound level, dB SPL	Intensity ratio, I/I_0	Amplitude ratio, A/A_0	Typical example
180	10^{18}	10^9	Saturn rocket from 45 m
140	10^{14}	10^7	Loud rock group
100	10^{10}	10^5	Shouting at close range
80	10^8	10^4	Busy street
70	10^7	3.2×10^3	Normal conversation
50	10^5	316	Quiet conversation
30	10^3	31.6	Soft whisper
20	100	10	Country area at night
6.5	4.5	2.1	Mean threshold at 1 kHz
3	2	1.4	
0	1	1	Reference level I_0
−10	0.1	0.32	
−60	10^{-6}	10^{-3}	

For sounds with discrete spectra, or line spectra, the sound level can be specified either as the over-all (total) level, or in terms of the levels of the individual components. The total level can be calculated from the total power of the sound, which in turn is proportional to the mean square pressure (measured as the deviation from normal atmospheric pressure). If we wish to calculate levels in terms of pressure, then we have to express the pressure of the sound as its root-mean-square (RMS) value.

For sounds with continuous spectra we can also specify the over-all level, but if we wish to indicate how the energy is distributed over frequency, we need some other measure. This measure is obtained by specifying the total energy or power between certain frequency limits, i.e. over a certain band of frequencies. Conventionally, a bandwidth of 1 Hz is chosen, and the energy in this one-cycle band, at a given frequency, is known as the energy density. For a continuous noise we may also specify the energy per unit time (i.e. the power or intensity) in this one-cycle band, and this is known as the noise power density. When the noise power density is expressed relative to the standard reference intensity of 10^{-16} W/cm^2 (equivalent to 2×10^{-5}N/m^2), it is known as the *spectrum level*, and has units dB SPL/Hz. Thus a noise may be characterized by its spectrum level as a function of frequency. A white noise has a uniform spectrum level.

3   THE CONCEPT OF LINEARITY

One concept which is widely used in auditory research is that of *linearity*. The auditory system is often conceived as being made up of successive stages, the output of a given stage forming the input to the next. Each of these stages can be considered as a device or system, with an input and an output. For a system to be linear certain relationships between the input and output must hold true. The following two conditions must be satisfied. Firstly, the output of the system in response to a number of independent inputs presented simultaneously should be equal to the sum of the outputs that would have been obtained if each input were presented alone. Secondly, if the input to the system is changed in magnitude by a factor k, then the output should also change in magnitude by a factor k, but be otherwise unaltered. These two conditions are known as superposition and homogeneity, respectively. In a linear system, if the input is doubled, then the output is doubled, but without any change in the form of the output. Further, the output of a linear system *never* contains frequency components that were not present in the input signal. Thus a sinusoidal input gives rise to a sinusoidal output. This is not necessarily true for other types of waveforms.

If a system is linear, then its analysis and characterization become relatively simple. If we measure its response to a sinusoidal input, as a function of frequency, then that response tells us all that we need to know about the system. To predict the response to any arbitrary complex input, we first need to perform a Fourier analysis of the input. We already have the information to calculate the response to each of the sinusoidal components comprising the input. The response to the whole complex can then be calculated as the sum of the responses to its individual sinusoidal components. This is a powerful method, and it gives another reason for using sinusoids as stimuli. We shall see later that some parts of the auditory system behave as though they were approximately linear, while others behave in a grossly nonlinear way. When a system is nonlinear, the response to complex inputs cannot generally be predicted from the responses to the sinusoidal components

comprising the inputs. Thus the characteristics of the system must be investigated using both sinusoidal and complex inputs.

4   FILTERS AND THEIR PROPERTIES

In many psychoacoustic experiments the experimenter may desire to
manipulate the spectra of the stimuli in some way. For example, he may wish
to remove certain frequency components from a complex stimulus, while
leaving other components unchanged. In practice this is usually achieved by
altering the electrical signal before it is converted into sound by a loudspeaker or headphone. The electronic devices which may be used to
manipulate the spectrum of a signal are known as filters. They are generally
linear devices, so that, in response to a sinusoidal input, the output is a
sinusoid of the same frequency. However, they are designed so that at their
outputs some frequencies are attenuated more than others. A high-pass
filter removes all frequency components below a certain cutoff frequency,
but does not affect components above this frequency. A low-pass filter does
the reverse. A bandpass filter has two cutoff frequencies, passing components between those two frequencies, and removing components outside
this range. A bandstop filter also has two cutoff frequencies, but it removes
components between these two frequencies, leaving other components intact. Such filters may be used not only for manipulating simuli, but also for
analysing them.
   Bandpass filters will be of particular interest to us, not only because of
their widespread use for analysis, but also because the peripheral auditory
system is often likened to a bank of bandpass filters, each of which has a
different centre frequency, so that the whole range of audible frequencies is
covered. This concept will be used extensively later in the book, so it is
instructive to consider the properties of filters in some detail.
   In practice it is not possible to design filters with perfectly sharp cutoffs.
Instead there will be a range of frequencies over which some components
will be reduced in level, but not entirely removed. Thus in order to specify a
filter we have to define both the cutoff frequency (or frequencies) and the
slope of the filter. Some typical filter characteristics are illustrated in Fig.
1.4. The cutoff frequency is usually defined as the frequency at which the
output of the filter has fallen by 3 dB, relative to the output in the passband.
This corresponds to a reduction in power or intensity by a factor of two, and
a reduction in amplitude by a factor of $\sqrt{2}$ (see Table I). For a bandpass
filter the range of frequencies between the two cutoffs defines the bandwidth
of the filter. This bandwidth is called the 3 dB bandwidth, or (equivalently)
the half-power bandwidth.
   The response characteristics of electronic filters outside their passbands

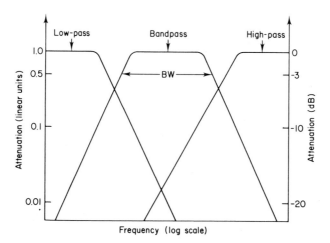

FIG. 1.4 Typical characteristics for three types of filters: low-pass, bandpass and high-pass. The input to each filter is a sinusoid of variable frequency. The output of each filter is plotted relative to the input, as a function of frequency. The left ordinate gives the ratio of the output to the input in linear units. The right ordinate gives that ratio in dB.

can often be approximated as straight lines when they are plotted in dB versus log frequency coordinates. Thus it is useful to express the slopes of filters in units such that equal frequency *ratios* represent equal amounts. One unit which does this is the *octave*. An octave corresponds to a frequency ratio of 2:1. Thus if we say that a low-pass filter has a slope of 24 dB/octave, this means that the output outside the passband decreases by 24 dB each time the frequency is doubled. Sometimes it is not possible to measure the response of a filter over a frequency range as large as an octave. Thus we need to be able to work out the proportion of an octave corresponding to any given frequency ratio. Consider two frequencies, f_1 and f_2. Their relative frequency, expressed as a certain number of octaves, n, is given by the relation:

$$f_1/f_2 = 2^n$$

where n may be positive, negative, a fraction or a number of octaves. Taking the logarithm on both sides of this equation, we get:

$$\log_{10} (f_1/f_2) = n \times 0.301$$

from which it is possible to calculate n given f_1/f_2, and vice versa.

Sometimes the bandwidths of bandpass filters are expressed in octaves. In this case the two frequencies involved are the upper and lower cutoffs of the filter, i.e. the 3-dB down points. One type of filter in common use has a bandwidth of 1/3 octave. For such a filter the upper cutoff has a frequency 1.26 times that of the lower cutoff.

If a signal with a 'flat' spectrum, such as a white noise or a single brief click, is passed through a filter, the spectrum of the output of the filter will have the same shape (i.e. be the same function of frequency) as the filter characteristic. Thus we can also talk about a high-pass noise, a bandpass click, and so on. Any alteration of the spectrum of a signal by filtering also produces a corresponding alteration in the waveform of the signal, and usually an alteration in the way it is perceived. For example, if white noise is passed through a narrow bandpass filter, the waveform at the output of the filter resembles a sinusoid which is fluctuating in amplitude from moment to moment. This narrowband noise has a pitchlike quality, the pitch corresponding to the centre frequency of the filter.

The response of a filter to a single brief click, or impulse, can be very informative. In fact this response, known as the impulse response, completely defines the filter characteristic. Since a click has a flat spectrum, the spectrum of the output of the filter, namely the impulse response, will have the same shape as the filter characteristic. Hence the filter characteristic, or shape, can be obtained by calculating the Fourier transform of the impulse response.

Figure 1.5 shows a series of impulse responses from filters having passbands centred at 1 kHz, but with various bandwidths. At the bottom right (f) is shown a sinusoid of 1 kHz, which should be imagined as continuing indefinitely in time. This is the response which would be obtained if it were possible to build a filter with zero bandwidth, and excite it with an infinitely intense impulse. All of the other sections of the figure show impulse responses from real filters. For the narrowest filter (top, left) the response looks like a sinusoid which builds up and decays smoothly, and which has a frequency close to 1 kHz. This is described as a 'ringing' response, and it is similar to what is heard when a wine glass is tapped with a spoon. The filter 'rings' at its own preferred frequency. As the filter bandwidth increases, the frequency of the ringing becomes less regular, and the duration of the response tends to decrease. For the widest filter bandwidth the impulse response has a waveform resembling that of the input impulse. For an infinitely wide filter the output would exactly match the input. This figure illustrates a general limitation of analysing sounds with filters. The narrower the bandwidth of a filter, and the steeper its slopes, the longer is its response time. Thus an increase in frequency selectivity can only be obtained at the expense of a loss of resolution in time.

If a filter with a narrow bandwidth is excited with a series of impulses, then the response to one impulse may not have died away before the next impulse occurs. Thus the impulse responses will merge together. If, for example, an impulse occurs every 2 ms (repetition rate 500 pulses/s), then for the narrowest filter in Fig. 1.5, the merged impulse responses will form a continuous sinusoid with a frequency of 1 kHz. In effect the filter has 'picked

FIG. 1.5 Section (f) shows a sinusoid with a frequency of 1 kHz. The other sections show the responses of filters to brief impulses. For (a) to (d) the filters had a centre frequency of 1 kHz, and bandwidths as indicated in the figure. For (e) the filter passed all frequencies in the audible range. The sections are not drawn to scale: the amplitude of response increases as filter bandwidth increases.

out' the second harmonic of the pulse train, and is responding only to that harmonic. Filters with different centre frequencies will respond to different harmonics in the pulse train. However, if the bandwidth of the filter is not sufficiently narrow, it will respond to more than one harmonic. The waveform at the output will not be sinusoidal, but will fluctuate at a rate equal to the repetition rate of the pulse train. When the filter bandwidth is very wide then a series of isolated impulse responses will be observed. These phenomena are illustrated in Figs 1.10 and 4.5, and we will discuss them more fully later in this chapter and in Chapter 4.

5   BASIC STRUCTURE OF THE AUDITORY SYSTEM

Figure 1.6 shows the structure of the peripheral part of the human auditory system. The outer ear is composed of the pinna (the part we actually see) and the auditory canal or meatus. The pinna has generally been considered a rather unimportant part of the auditory system, but it does in fact significantly modify the incoming sound, particularly at high frequencies, and this

Semicircular
canals

Cochlea

Auditory nerve

Oval
window

Round window

Incus

Stapes

Malleus

Eardrum

Auditory canal

FIG. 1.6 Illustration of the structure of the peripheral auditory system showing the outer, middle and inner ear. From *Human Information Processing*, by Lindsey, P. H. and Norman, D. A. (1972), by permission of the authors.

is important in our ability to localize sounds (see Chapter 5). Sound travels down the meatus and causes the eardrum, or tympanic membrane, to vibrate. These vibrations are transmitted through the middle ear by three small bones, the ossicles, to a membrane-covered opening in the bony wall of the spiral-shaped structure of the inner ear—the cochlea. This opening is called the oval window. The three bones are called the malleus, incus and stapes, the stapes being the lightest and smallest of these, and the one which actually makes contact with the oval window. The major function of the middle ear is to ensure the efficient transfer of sound from the air to the fluids in the cochlea. If the sound were to impinge directly onto the oval window, most of it would simply be reflected back, rather than entering the cochlea. The middle ear acts as an impedance-matching device or transformer to improve sound transmission. This is accomplished mainly by the difference in effective areas of the eardrum and the oval window, and to a small extent by the lever action of the ossicles.

The ossicles have minute muscles attached to them which contract when we are exposed to intense sounds. This contraction, known as the middle ear reflex, is probably mediated by neural centres in the brain stem, but its anatomical basis is not fully known. The reflex reduces the transmission of sound through the middle ear, particularly at low frequencies, and it may help to prevent damage to the delicate structures of the cochlea. However, the activation of the reflex is too slow to provide any protection against impulsive sounds, such as gun shots or hammer blows. Two other functions have been suggested for the reflex. The first is the reduction of the audibility of self-generated sounds, particularly speech. It has been shown that the reflex is activated just before vocalization. The second is a reduction of the masking of middle and high frequencies by lower ones, a function which is particularly important at high sound levels (see Fig. 3.1, and the discussion of the 'upward spread of masking' in Chapter 3, section 2).

The cochlea is the most important part of the ear from our point of view, and an understanding of what goes on in the cochlea can provide a key to many aspects of auditory perception. The cochlea is filled with incompressible fluids, and it also has bony rigid walls. It is divided along its length by two membranes, Reissner's membrane and the basilar membrane (see Fig. 1.12). It is the motion of the basilar membrane in response to sound which is of primary interest to us. The start of the cochlea, where the oval window is situated, is known as the base, while the other end, the inner tip, is known as the apex. At the apex there is a small opening (the helicotrema) between the basilar membrane and the walls of the cochlea, so that fluid can flow between the two main chambers of the cochlea, the scala vestibuli and the scala tympani. Inward movement of the oval window results in a flow of fluid around the helicotrema and a corresponding outward movement in a membrane covering a second opening in the cochlea—the round window.

When the oval window is set in motion by an incoming sound, a pressure is applied by the fluids in the cochlea essentially simultaneously along the whole length of the basilar membrane. The pattern of motion on the basilar membrane, however, takes some time to develop. The pattern which occurs does not depend on which end of the cochlea is stimulated. Sounds which reach the cochlea via the bones of the head rather than through the air (e.g. our own voices) do not produce atypical responses.

The response of the basilar membrane to sinusoidal stimulation begins as a bulge at the basal end. This bulge takes the form of a travelling wave which moves along the basilar membrane towards the apex. The amplitude of the wave increases slowly at first and then decreases rather abruptly. This is illustrated in Fig. 1.7, which shows the instantaneous displacement of the

Distance from stapes in mm

FIG. 1.7   The instantaneous displacement of the cochlear partition at two successive instants in time, derived from a cochlear model. The pattern moves from left to right, building up gradually with distance, and decaying rapidly beyond the point of maximal displacement. The dotted line represents the envelope traced out by the amplitude peaks in the waveform. From von Békésy (1947), by permission of *J. Acoust. Soc. Am.*

basilar membrane (derived from a cochlear model) for two successive instants in time, in response to a 200 Hz sinusoid. This figure also shows the line joining the amplitude peaks, which is called the envelope. The distance between peaks or zero-crossings in the wave decreases as the wave travels along, and the envelope shows a peak at a particular position on the basilar membrane.

The response of the basilar membrane to sounds of different frequencies is strongly affected by its mechanical properties, which vary considerably from base to apex. At the base it is relatively narrow and stiff, while at the apex it is wider and much less stiff. The position of the peak in the pattern of vibration thus differs according to the frequency of stimulation. High frequency sounds produce a maximum displacement of the basilar membrane near the oval window, so that there is little activity on the remainder of the membrane. Low frequency sounds produce a pattern of vibration which extends all the way along the basilar membrane, but which reaches a maximum before the end of the membrane. Figure 1.8 shows the envelopes of the patterns of vibration for several different low frequency sinusoids (from von Békésy, 1960). It is clear that sounds of different frequencies produce maximum activity at different places along the basilar membrane. In effect the ear is behaving like a Fourier analyser, although with a much less than perfect frequency analysing power.

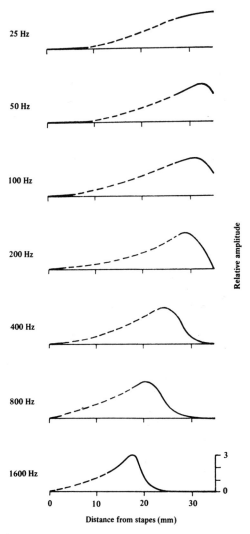

FIG. 1.8 Envelopes of patterns of vibration on the basilar membrane for a number of low frequency sounds. Solid lines indicate the results of actual measurements, while the dashed lines are von Békésy's extrapolations. From *Experiments in Hearing* by von Békésy, G. (1960), used with the permission of McGraw-Hill.

It is worth noting that in response to steady sinusoidal stimulation each point on the basilar membrane vibrates in a sinusoidal manner with a frequency equal to that of the input waveform. For example, if we apply a 1000 Hz pure tone, each point on the basilar membrane for which there is a detectable amount of vibration will be vibrating at that frequency. Some parts of the basilar membrane will be vibrating with a greater amplitude than others, and there will be differences in the phase of the vibration at different points along the membrane, but the frequency of vibration of each point will be the same. This is true whatever the frequency of the input waveform, provided it is a single sinusoid within the audible range of frequencies.

A number of different methods may be used to specify the 'sharpness' of tuning of the patterns of vibration on the basilar membrane. These methods allow us to describe quantitatively the frequency resolution of the basilar membrane, i.e. its ability to separate sounds of differing frequencies. Most of the measures are analogous to those used with electronic filters, which we discussed in section 4. Each point on the basilar membrane can be considered as a bandpass filter with a certain centre frequency and bandwidth, and with slopes outside the passband. Thus measures such as the 3 dB bandwidth, and slopes in dB/octave, can be applied to the basilar membrane. Often it is difficult to measure the 3 dB bandwidth accurately, and a measure taken further down from the passband is used. The commonest measure is the 10 dB bandwidth, which is the difference between the two frequencies at which the response has fallen by 10 dB. For many types of filters, and for the response of the basilar membrane, the bandwidth is not constant, but increases in proportion with centre frequency. Thus it is sometimes useful to use the relative bandwidth, which is the bandwidth divided by the centre frequency. The reciprocal of the relative bandwidth gives a measure of the sharpness of tuning, known as Q. Normally it is assumed that the 3 dB bandwidth is used to define Q. However, it is quite common in measurements of basilar membrane responses, and neural responses (see later), to use the 10 dB bandwidth. In this case the measure of sharpness of tuning is described as $Q_{10\,dB}$.

Most of the pioneering work on patterns of vibration along the basilar membrane was done by von Békésy (1928, 1942). His technique involved the use of a light microscope and stroboscopic illumination to measure the vibration amplitude at many points along the basilar membrane in human cadaver ears. For practical reasons his measurements were limited to the apical end of the basilar membrane, so that he measured mainly low frequency responses. The 'tuning curves' found by von Békésy were rather broad. The relative bandwidth was about 0.6 in the frequency range observed. This has presented a considerable problem for auditory theorists, since the observed frequency selectivity appears to be insufficient to explain either our psychoacoustically observed frequency resolving power (e.g. the ability to 'hear out' partials in a complex tone or to detect a small change in frequency), or the selectivity observed in individual neurones in the auditory nerve (see later on in this chapter). This problem will be discussed more fully in Chapters 3 and 4.

There are a number of difficulties associated with the technique used by von Békésy. Firstly, the vibration amplitudes had to be at least of the order of one wavelength of visible light, which required very high sound levels— about 140 dB SPL. It may be that the vibration of the basilar membrane is nonlinear, so that it is not valid to extrapolate from these high levels to more normal sound levels. Secondly, the frequency analysing mechanism may be physiologically vulnerable, so that the use of cadaver ears is questionable. Recent measurements of basilar membrane vibration, using different techniques, have shown that these difficulties are of considerable importance. One technique which has been extensively exploited uses an effect discovered by Mössbauer. A radioactive source of gamma rays, of very small mass and physical dimensions, is placed upon the basilar membrane. Changes in the velocity of this source, produced by motion of the basilar membrane, can be detected as a change in the wavelength of the emitted radiation. For the technically minded, this is an example of a Doppler shift. The sensitivity of this method increases with increasing frequency; at 1000 Hz a peak deflection of about 20 nanometres (nm) (1 nm is a ten-millionth of a centimetre) can be measured, while at 10 kHz the limit is about 2 nm. This corresponds to a SPL of 70–80 dB. Thus this method has been used mainly at high frequencies, where sound levels much lower than those used by von Békésy can be utilized.

Results using this technique in live animals were reported by Johnstone and Boyle (1967), and these results have been confirmed and extended by more recent work (e.g. Johnstone *et al.* 1970; Rhode, 1971). Figure 1.9 compares data from Rhode and Johnstone *et al.* with those of von Békésy. It

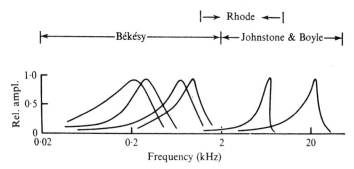

FIG. 1.9 A comparison of the shapes of 'tuning curves' on the basilar membrane obtained by three different sets of workers. Each curve was obtained by measuring the amplitude of vibration at a particular point on the basilar membrane as a function of the frequency of stimulation. From Johnstone and Sellick (1972), by permission of the authors.

is apparent that the 'tuning curves' obtained using the Mössbauer technique are much sharper than those of von Békésy. The slopes of his curves were 6 dB/octave on the low frequency side and 20 dB/octave on the high frequency side. The corresponding slopes reported by Johnstone *et al.* were 13 dB/octave and 105 dB/octave, while Rhode reported slopes of up to 200 dB/octave on the high frequency side. It should be emphasized that these steep slopes were obtained in animals (guinea-pig and squirrel monkey) and were made in regions of the basilar membrane different from those used by von Békésy, so that direct comparison is difficult. However, the discrepancy does seem great enough to cast some doubt on von Békésy's quantitative measurements.

We mentioned above two possible difficulties associated with von Békésy's method. The first, that basilar membrane vibration may be non-linear, has been confirmed by Rhode (1971) and Rhode and Robles (1974). The nonlinearity causes the peak in the pattern of vibration to flatten out at high intensities, so that a broader tuning would have been observed at the high sound levels used by von Békésy. The second, that basilar membrane responses may change after death, has been confirmed by Kohllöffel (1972) using a technique based on laser illumination of the basilar membrane, and by Rhode and Rhodes (1974). Not only do basilar membrane responses broaden after death, but also the nonlinearity reported by Rhode disappears. Thus it appears that some aspect of the filtering action of the basilar membrane is physiologically vulnerable.

The nonlinearity reported by Rhode (1971) using the Mössbauer technique is still the subject of some controversy. Rhode found that at high sound levels the peak of the 'tuning curve' increased by only 10 dB when the sound level was increased by 20 dB. Wilson and Johnstone (1972), using a method involving a capacitive probe, found that basilar membrane responses were essentially linear for sound levels up to 110 dB SPL. Unfortunately, the capacitive probe method requires the basilar membrane to be dry at the point of measurement, so that some of the fluids in the cochlea had to be drained. At the present time it is not clear whether this draining of the fluids would have been sufficient to produce the difference in results. Kohllöffel maintained a constant fluid level above the basilar membrane, in his measurements using laser light, and reported that the fluid level itself had no influence on the frequency response curves. Kohllöffel also reported that basilar membrane vibration was linear. One possible explanation for the discrepancies between the different methods is a species-specific difference; Rhode worked with the squirrel monkey, whereas Wilson and Johnstone, and Kohllöffel, used guinea-pigs. It is to be hoped that this question will soon be resolved, since the report of nonlinearities has aroused considerable theoretical interest and may provide a key to the understanding of certain combination tones which occur in the auditory system (see Chapter 4).

So far we have described the responses of the basilar membrane to steady sinusoidal stimulation. While there are some disagreements about the details of patterns of vibration, it is now beyond doubt that pure tones produce patterns with single maxima, whose positions depend upon frequency. In other words, there is a frequency-to-place conversion. The situation with other types of sounds is somewhat more complex. Consider first the case of two sinusoids, of different frequencies, presented simultaneously. The kind of pattern that will occur depends on the frequency separation of the two tones. If this is very large, then the two tones will produce two, effectively separate, patterns of vibration. Each will produce a maximum at the place on the basilar membrane which would have been excited most had that tone been presented alone. Thus the response of the basilar membrane to a low frequency tone will be essentially unaffected by a high frequency tone, and vice versa. In this kind of situation the basilar membrane behaves like a Fourier analyser, breaking down the complex sound into its sinusoidal components. When the two tones are relatively closer together in frequency, however, the patterns of vibration on the basilar membrane will interact, so that some points on the basilar membrane will be responding to both of the component tones. At those points the displacement of the basilar membrane as a function of time will not be sinusoidal, but will be a complex waveform resulting from the interference of the two tones. When the two tones are sufficiently close in frequency, there will no longer be a separate maximum in the pattern of vibration for each of the component tones; instead there will be a single, broader, maximum. Thus, in a sense, the basilar membrane has failed to resolve the individual frequency components. We shall see, in Chapter 3, that the frequency resolving power of the auditory system, as observed psychoacoustically, is greater than would be expected from the patterns of vibration on the basilar membrane. Two tones an octave apart overlap considerably on the basilar membrane but are easily 'heard out' as two separate tones.

The position of the basilar membrane which is excited most by a given frequency varies approximately with the logarithm of frequency, for frequencies above 500 Hz. Further, the relative bandwidths of the patterns of vibration on the basilar membrane in response to sinusoidal stimulation are approximately constant in this frequency range. This means that the frequency separation necessary for the resolution of two tones is proportional to centre frequency. Consider how this applies to the kind of complex sound which might be produced by a musical instrument, namely a harmonic complex tone. The frequency separation between adjacent harmonics is constant (and equal to the fundamental frequency). Thus the patterns of vibration for the higher harmonics will overlap much more than those for the lower harmonics. This is illustrated schematically in Fig. 1.10, which shows

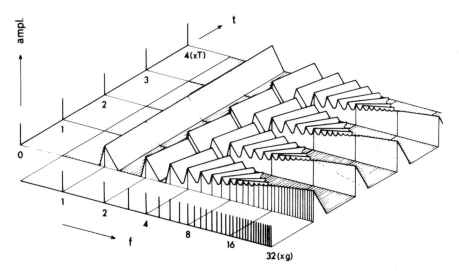

FIG. 1.10 Schematic representation of the response of the basilar membrane to a series of periodic impulses. Time is plotted along the *t* axis on a linear scale; frequency (*f*) and amplitude (ampl.) scales are logarithmic. The waveform of the stimulus is indicated on the left and its spectrum is at the bottom. For the central part of the figure the frequency axis may be considered as equivalent to a position axis, indicating distance along the basilar membrane. This part of the figure shows the envelopes of the travelling wave patterns as a function of time and position. From Duifhuis (1972), by permission of the author.

responses to a periodic pulse train; this stimulus is composed of harmonics which all have the same amplitude (Fig. 1.3). The figure shows idealized envelopes of the patterns of vibration as a function of time (linear scale) and frequency (logarithmic scale). The lower harmonics are separated out to some extent, while at the same time the patterns of vibration corresponding to those harmonics fluctuate relatively little as a function of time. The response as a function of time to a single low harmonic is similar to the response which would have been observed if the harmonic had been presented alone. For the higher harmonics the patterns of vibration overlap to a considerable extent. The individual harmonics are no longer resolved, but the amplitude of their joint excitation pattern fluctuates strongly as a function of time. For the higher harmonics the time pattern of the response on the basilar membrane closely resembles that of the stimulus as a whole. We shall see in Chapters 3 and 4 that these factors play a crucial role in our perception of complex tones.

The response of the basilar membrane to a sudden change in sound pressure (a step function) or to a short impulse (a single click) is somewhat different. The spectra of these stimuli contain a wide range of frequencies, so that we can expect to see responses all along the basilar membrane. What happens is that a 'travelling bulge', looking like a short decaying wave train, is set up on the basilar membrane, and travels all the way along it. A number of workers have investigated the response of a single point on the basilar membrane in response to a brief click; this is called the impulse response function of that point. Figure 1.11 shows an impulse response function

FIG. 1.11 The response at a particular point on the basilar membrane to a short impulse. From Wilson & Johnstone (1972), by permission of the authors.

computed from the data of Wilson and Johnstone (1972). It looks like a damped, or decaying, sinusoidal oscillation. The frequency of this oscillation depends on which part of the basilar membrane is being studied. The basal end of the basilar membrane, which responds best to high frequencies, will show a high frequency oscillation, while the apical end, which responds best to low frequencies, will show a low frequency oscillation. Thus the waveform as a function of time will vary continuously with position along the basilar membrane, according to the frequency which excites that position most. We shall see in Chapter 5 that this pattern of responses affects our ability to localize sounds of a transient character.

So far we have been concerned with the mechanical responses of the basilar membrane to sound stimulation. We have seen that the basilar membrane acts as a kind of spectrum analyser, or Fourier analyser, but with a limited resolving power. Let us consider how the information about frequency, amplitude and time, which is carried in the vibration patterns of the basilar membrane, is converted or coded into neural signals in the auditory nervous system. Attached to the basilar membrane are hair cells, which form part of a structure called the organ of Corti (see Fig. 1.12). The hair cells are divided into two groups by an arch known as the tunnel of Corti. Those on the side of the arch closest to the outside of the cochlea are

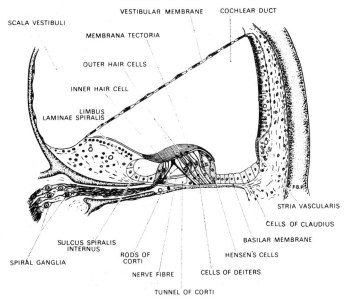

FIG. 1.12 Cross-section of the cochlea, showing the organ of Corti. The actual receptors are the hair cells lying on either side of the tunnel of Corti. From Hamilton, *Textbook of Human Anatomy*, Macmillan (1976).

known as outer hair cells, and are arranged in three rows. The hair cells on the other side of the arch form a single row, and are known as inner hair cells. There are about 25 000 outer hair cells, each with about 140 hairs protruding from it, while there are about 3500 inner hair cells, each with about 40 hairs. The tectorial membrane, which has a gelatinous structure, lies above the hairs. It appears that the hairs of the outer hair cells actually make contact with the tectorial membrane, but this may not be true for the inner hair cells. The tectorial membrane appears to be effectively hinged at one side (the left in Fig. 1.12), so that when the basilar membrane moves up and down, a shearing motion is created between the basilar membrane and the tectorial membrane. As a result the hairs at the tops of the hair cells are bent, and it is thought that this bending is the mode of excitation of the hair cells, which leads to the generation of action potentials in the neurones of the auditory nerve. Thus the hair cells act to transduce mechanical movements into neural activity.

There are many details of the transduction process which remain poorly understood. It has been suggested that the two types of hair cells respond differently to different types of shearing motions between the basilar membrane and the tectorial membrane (see Tonndorf, 1970). More recently it has been suggested (Dallos *et al.*, 1972; Billone and Raynor, 1973) that the electrical potentials produced by the outer hair cells are proportional to the displacement of the basilar membrane, while the potentials produced by the inner hair cells are proportional to the velocity of the basilar membrane. There is general agreement that the outer hair cells have greater sensitivities than the inner hair cells (i.e. that they respond at lower sound levels), and that they are more easily damaged by intense sounds. It is also possible that, because of their different modes of responding, the frequency selectivities of the inner and outer hair cells may differ (Billone and Raynor, 1973). The way in which the inner and outer hair cells are innervated is also a subject of debate. According to Spoendlin (1970), 10% of auditory nerve fibres originate from outer hair cells and 90% from inner hair cells. If this were the case, we might expect that there would be two distinct sets of auditory neurones with differing properties. The majority of neurones should have 'high' thresholds, but a few, deriving their activity from the outer hair cells, should have 'low' thresholds. In fact the evidence as to whether there is a bimodal distribution of thresholds is controversial (Tasaki, 1954; Kiang, 1968). The majority of neurones seem to have 'low' thresholds, but a small group can be identified with very high thresholds (Liberman, 1978), a result opposite from that predicted. Recordings from single inner hair cells (Russell and Sellick, 1978) indicate that they are more sharply tuned than the patterns of displacement on the basilar membrane. Indeed they appear to be as sharply tuned as the nerve fibres in the auditory nerve (see the following section). The role of the outer hair cells in influencing the activity in auditory nerve fibres is still uncertain, and research in this area is actively continuing.

6   NEURAL RESPONSES IN THE AUDITORY NERVE

Most of the recent studies of activity in the auditory nerve have used electrodes with very fine tips, known as microelectrodes. These record the nerve impulses, or spikes, in single auditory nerve fibres (often called single units). Three general results have emerged, which seem to hold for most mammals. Firstly, the fibres show background or spontaneous firing in the absence of sound stimulation. Spontaneous firing rates range from close to 0 per second up to about 150 per second. Secondly, the fibres respond better to some frequencies than to others; they show frequency selectivity. Finally, the fibres show phase-locking; neural firings tend to occur at a particular phase of the stimulating waveform, so that there is a temporal regularity in the firing pattern of a neurone in response to a periodic stimulus. We will consider the last two factors in more detail.

The frequency selectivity of a single nerve fibre is often illustrated by a tuning curve, which shows the cell's threshold as a function of frequency. The curve is obtained by determining the lowest level of a sinusoid for which the experimenter, by auditory and visual monitoring of the activity in the fibre, can detect a change in activity of the fibre. The stimuli are usually tone bursts, rather than continuous tones, so that changes in activity are more easily detected. The frequency at which the threshold of the fibre is lowest is called the characteristic frequency (CF). Some typical tuning curves are presented in Fig. 1.13. It may be seen that, on the logarithmic frequency

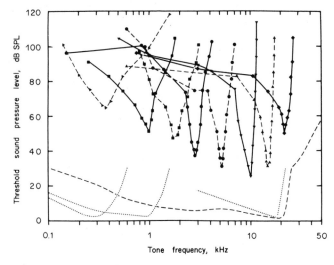

FIG. 1.13 A sample of tuning curves (frequency threshold curves) of single fibres in the auditory nerve of anaesthetized cats. For each fibre the threshold is plotted as a function of stimulating frequency (logarithmic scale). The dotted and dashed curves at the bottom show corresponding measurements from the basilar membrane. The sound level required to produce a constant amplitude of vibration at a particular point on the basilar membrane is plotted as a function of frequency. The position of these curves on the ordinate is arbitrary; they have been shifted downwards for clarity. From Evans (1975), by permission of the author.

scale used, the tuning curves are generally steeper on the high frequency side than on the low frequency one. It is generally assumed that the frequency selectivity in single auditory nerve fibres occurs because those fibres are responding to activity in restricted regions of the basilar membrane. In other words, a single nerve fibre is assumed to derive its output from a particular part of the basilar membrane. This supposition is supported by the finding that CFs are distributed in an orderly manner in the auditory nerve. Fibres with high CFs are found in the periphery of the nerve bundle, and there is an orderly decrease in CF towards the centre of the nerve bundle (Kiang *et al.*,

1965). This kind of organization is known as tonotopic organization, and indicates that the place representation of frequency along the basilar membrane is preserved as a place representation in the auditory nerve. One problem in interpreting tuning curves is that their slopes are generally steeper than the corresponding slopes for patterns of vibration on the basilar membrane. This problem is discussed more fully in Chapter 3.

In order to provide a description of the characteristics of single fibres at levels above threshold, iso-rate contours can be plotted. To determine an iso-rate contour, the intensity of sinusoidal stimulation required to produce a predetermined firing rate in the neurone is plotted as a function of frequency. The resulting curves are generally similar in shape to tuning curves. An alternative method is to record firing rates at equal sound levels as a function of tone frequency. The resulting curves (iso-intensity contours) generally vary in shape according to the sound level chosen, and differ considerably from tuning curves (see Fig. 1.14). The interpretation of iso-

FIG. 1.14 Iso-intensity contours for a single fibre in the auditory nerve of an anaesthetized squirrel monkey. Note that the frequency producing maximal firing varies as a function of level. From Rose *et al.* (1971), by permission of the authors.

intensity contours is difficult, because their shape will depend upon how the rate of firing of the nerve fibre varies with intensity; this is not usually a linear function (see later). However, it is of interest that for some fibres that frequency producing maximal firing varies as a function of level. This poses some problems for one of the theories of pitch perception which will be discussed in Chapter 4.

Figure 1.15 shows how the rate of discharge of an auditory nerve fibre changes as a function of stimulus level. The stimulus was a continuous tone at the CF of the unit. The general shape of the curve is typical of most auditory nerve fibres, although there is considerable variability in both the

FIG. 1.15 An example of how the discharge rate of a single auditory nerve fibre varies as a function of stimulus level, for a continuous stimulating tone at the CF of the neurone. The threshold of the neurone is the lowest sound level at which there is a detectable change in firing rate and is indicated by the letters AVDL (audiovisual detection level). Above a certain sound level increases in level do not produce increases in firing rate; the neurone is saturated. The range of levels between threshold and saturation is known as the 'dynamic range' and is typically 30–40 dB. The sound level is specified in dB with an arbitrary reference level. The level at the point marked AVDL corresponds to about 2 dB SPL. From Kiang (1968), by permission of the author.

spontaneous firing rate and the maximum firing rate. Notice that above a certain sound level the neurone no longer responds to increases in sound level with an increase in firing rate; the neurone is said to be saturated. For the cat the saturation level is within about 40 dB of threshold. This dynamic range varies somewhat from neurone to neurone and species to species, but in the majority of cases the dynamic range is between 20 and 50 dB. This poses a difficulty for theories of how intensity is coded in the auditory nerve, since we are capable of dealing with a very much larger range than this. The difficulty is compounded by the fact that for the majority of neurones the range of thresholds at a given CF is quite narrow (Kiang, 1968). This problem is discussed more fully in Chapter 2.

Although the technique of recording from single auditory neurones has provided very valuable evidence about the coding of sounds in the auditory system, it is lacking in one very fundamental respect: it does not tell us anything about the pattern of neural responses over different auditory neurones, or about possible interactions or mutual dependencies in the firing patterns of different auditory neurones. A considerable advance has come recently from studies of the responses of a great many single neurones within one experimental animal to a limited set of stimuli (Pfeiffer and Kim, 1975; Kim and Molnar, 1979; Sachs and Young, 1980). These studies have shown, as we would expect, that in response to a single, low level, pure tone there is a high level of activity in neurones with CFs close to the tone frequency, with activity dropping off for CFs on either side of this. However at higher sound levels the picture is more complicated. As a result of neural saturation there may be a more-or-less uniform high level of activity over a wide range of CFs, with activity only falling off at CFs far removed from the stimulus frequency. We will discuss some of the implications of this in Chapters 2, 3 and 4.

The distribution of neural activity as a function of CF is sometimes called the 'excitation pattern'. However, the definition of an appropriate measure of 'activity' is difficult, since both spontaneous and maximum firing rates vary considerably, even in neurones with similar CFs. Thus at best we could only represent what was happening in an 'average' neurone at a given CF. This last problem can be partially overcome by representing excitation patterns in a different way; instead of determining the amount of neural activity at each CF, we determine what the level of a pure tone with frequency equal to that CF would have to be in order to produce an equal amount of neural activity. Thus the excitation pattern becomes a representation of the effective amount of excitation produced by a stimulus as a function of CF, and is plotted as effective level (in dB) against CF. Normally the CF is plotted on a logarithmic scale, roughly in accord with the way that frequency appears to be represented on the basilar membrane. An idealized excitation pattern is shown in Fig. 1.16. We shall see in Chapter 3 that

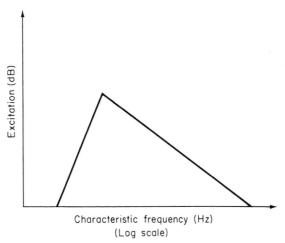

FIG. 1.16 A schematic and idealized representation of the 'excitation pattern' evoked by a pure tone. The pattern represents the effective level of the stimulus in dB at each characteristic frequency.

psychoacoustic techniques have been developed which, given certain assumptions, allow the determination of excitation patterns represented in this way, and that such excitation patterns can be considered as an internal representation of the spectrum of the stimulus.

So far we have described only the changes in *rate* of firing which occur in response to a given stimulus. However, information about the stimulus is also carried in the temporal patterning of the neural firings. In response to a pure tone the nerve firings tend to be phase-locked or synchronized to the stimulating waveform. A given nerve fibre does not necessarily fire on every cycle of the stimulus, but when firings do occur, they occur at the same phase of the waveform each time. Thus the time intervals between firings will be (approximately) integral multiples of the period of the stimulating wave-form. For example, a 500 Hz tone will have a period of 2 milliseconds (2 ms), so that the intervals between nerve firings might be 2 ms, or 4 ms, or 6 ms, or 8 ms, etc. In general, the nerve does not fire in a completely regular manner, so that there will not be exactly 500, or 250 or 125 spikes/s. However, information about the period of the stimulating waveform is carried un-ambiguously in the temporal pattern of firing of a single neurone, and if we consider the responses over an ensemble of fibres, then there will be some nerve spikes on every cycle of the stimulus. Phase-locking is just what we would expect to occur as a result of the transduction process; when the basilar membrane moves upwards, towards the tectorial membrane, the hair cells are bent and a neural response is initiated. No response will occur when the basilar membrane moves downwards. Thus nerve firings tend to occur on a positive deflection of the basilar membrane produced by the rarefaction phase of the signal.

One way to demonstrate phase-locking in a single auditory nerve fibre is to plot a histogram of the time intervals between successive nerve firings. Several such interspike interval histograms are shown in Fig. 1.17, for a neurone with a characteristic frequency (CF) of 1.6 kHz. For each of the different stimulating frequencies (from 0.408 to 2.3 kHz in this case) the intervals between nerve spikes lie predominantly at integral multiples of the period of the stimulating tone. These intervals are indicated by dots below each abscissa. Thus, although the neurone does not fire on every cycle of the stimulus, the distribution of time intervals between nerve firings depends closely on the frequency of the stimulating waveform.

Phase-locking does not occur over the whole range of audible frequencies. The upper frequency limit seems to lie at about 4–5 kHz (Rose *et al.*, 1967). This upper limit is not determined by the refractory periods of neurones or by their maximum firing rates. Rather it is determined by the precision with which the initiation of a nerve impulse is linked to a particular phase of the stimulus. It turns out that there is a certain 'jitter' in the exact instant of initiation of a nerve impulse. At high frequencies this jitter becomes com-

FIG. 1.17 Interspike interval histograms for a single auditory neurone (in the squirrel monkey) with a CF of 1.6 kHz. Tone frequency and mean response rate in spikes per second are indicated above each histogram. All tones were at 80 db SPL and of duration 1 s. Notice that the time scales in E and F differ from those in A to D. From Rose *et al.* (1968), by permission of the authors.

parable with the period of the waveform, so that above a certain frequency the spikes will be 'smeared out' over the whole period of the waveform, instead of occurring primarily at a particular phase. It is this smearing which is responsible for the loss of phase-locking above 4–5 kHz.

There is still considerable controversy over the extent to which information carried in the timing of neural impulses is actually used in perceptual processes. Most workers accept that our ability to localize sounds depends in part on a comparison of the temporal information from the two ears, but the relevance of temporal information in masking and in pitch perception is still hotly debated. These problems will be discussed more fully in Chapters 3 and 4.

So far we have discussed the responses of auditory neurones to single pure tones. One of the reasons for using pure tones as stimuli is that, in many physical systems, the response to complex stimuli may be predicted from the responses to pure tones. Such systems are said to be linear; the response to a complex stimulus is the linear sum of the responses to the sinusoidal (Fourier) components of the stimulus (see section 3). Although neural responses themselves are clearly nonlinear (showing, for example, thresholds and saturation), they sometimes behave as though the driving system were linear. In other situations the behaviour is clearly nonlinear, so that it is necessary to investigate directly the neural responses to complex stimuli, if we are to understand how the properties of these complex stimuli are coded in the auditory system.

Auditory nerve responses to two tones have been investigated by a number of workers. One striking finding which has emerged is that the tone-driven activity of a single fibre in response to one tone can be suppressed by the presence of a second tone. This has been called two-tone inhibition (Sachs and Kiang, 1968), although the term 'two-tone suppression' is now generally preferred. Typically the phenomenon is investigated by presenting a tone at, or close to, the CF of a neurone. A second tone is then presented, its frequency and intensity are varied, and the effects of this on the response of the neurone are noted. The suppressing tone usually has its greatest effect at frequencies slightly above or below the area of the unit's excitatory response to a single tone (see Fig. 1.18). The suppression effects begin and cease very rapidly, within a few milliseconds of the onset and termination of the second tone (Arthur *et al.*, 1971). Thus it is unlikely that the suppression is established through any elaborate neural interconnections. It is possible that it is related to nonlinear mechanical events on the basilar membrane (Legouix *et al.*, 1973; Rhode and Robles, 1974).

The effects of two-tone stimulation on temporal patterns of neural firing have also been studied. For tones which are nonharmonically related Hind *et al.* (1967) found that discharges may be phase-locked to one tone, or the other, or to both tones simultaneously. Which of these occurs is determined

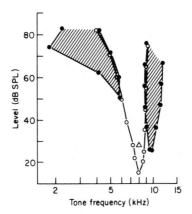

FIG. 1.18 The open circles show the tuning curve (threshold versus frequency) of a single neurone with a CF at 8 kHz. The neurone was stimulated with a tone at CF, and just above threshold (indicated by the open triangle). A second tone was then added and its frequency and intensity varied. Any tone within the shaded areas bounded by the solid circles would reduce the response to the tone at CF by 20% or more. These are the suppression areas.

by the intensities of the two tones and their frequencies in relation to the 'response area' of the fibre. When phase-locking occurs to only one tone of a pair, each of which is effective when acting alone, the temporal structure of the response may be indistinguishable from that which occurs when that tone is presented alone. Further, the discharge rate may be similar to the value produced by that tone alone. Thus the dominant tone appears to 'capture' the response of the neurone. We will discuss in Chapter 3 the possibility that this 'capture effect' underlies the masking of one sound by another. Notice that the 'capture effect' is probably another manifestation of two-tone suppression. The tone which is suppressed ceases to contribute to the pattern of phase-locking, and the neurone responds as if only the suppressing tone were present. Suppression measured by phase-locking can be shown even if the suppressor is within the excitatory response area of the neurone. However suppression of response *rate* is normally seen only when the suppressor is outside or at the edges of the response area. Otherwise the suppressor itself will evoke an excitatory response, and produce an increase in firing rate which 'hides' the suppression.

Brugge *et al.* (1969) investigated auditory nerve responses to pairs of tones with simple frequency ratios (i.e. harmonically related tones). They drew the following conclusions: (1) auditory nerve fibres are excited by deflections of the cochlear partition (basilar membrane) in only one direction; (2) the discharges occur at times which correspond to the elevations of the stimulating waveform; (3) the effective stimulating waveform can be approximated by addition of the component sinusoids, although the required amplitude and phase relations usually cannot be taken directly from the actual stimulus parameters. The results of Brugge *et al.* indicate that interactions between two tones may take place even when their frequencies are quite widely separated (frequency ratios between the two tones of up to 7:1 were used).

Javel (1980) investigated the responses in single auditory neurones to stimuli consisting of three successive high harmonics of a complex tone. He showed that a portion of the neural activity in the neurones responding to the component frequencies was phase-locked to the overall repetition rate of the stimulus (equal to the absent fundamental frequency). We will discuss in Chapter 4 the possibility that such temporal coding is responsible for the pitch of complex tones.

The responses of auditory neurones to clicks are closely related to the corresponding patterns of vibration which occur on the basilar membrane (see section 5). Such responses are often plotted in the form of poststimulus time (PST) histograms. To determine a PST histogram the click is presented many times, and the numbers of neural impulses occurring at various times after the instant of click presentation are counted. These are then plotted in the form of a histogram, with the instant of click presentation being taken as time zero (see Fig. 1.19). It may be seen that spikes tend to occur at certain

FIG. 1.19 A poststimulus time (PST) histogram showing the number of nerve spikes occurring in response to a click, presented repeatedly, as a function of the time delay from the instant of presentation of the click. The time interval between peaks in the histogram corresponds to the reciprocal of the CF of the neurone (540 Hz). From Kiang *et al.* (1965), by permission of the author and MIT Press.

preferred intervals after the presentation of the click, as indicated by the peaks in the histogram. The multiple peaks presumably occur because the response of the basilar membrane to a click is a damped or decaying oscillation (see Fig. 1.11). Nerve firings will tend to occur at a particular phase of this damped oscillation. The time intervals between the peaks correspond to the CF of the neurone. If the polarity of the click is reversed (e.g. from rarefaction to condensation) the pattern is shifted in time, so that peaks now appear where dips were located. The latency of the first peak is shortest for rarefaction clicks, again indicating that the excitation of hair cells occurs when the basilar membrane is deflected towards the tectorial membrane. These factors are particularly relevant to our ability to locate sounds of a transient character (see Chapter 5).

7   NEURAL RESPONSES AT HIGHER LEVELS IN THE AUDITORY SYSTEM

In the visual system it is known that neurones respond preferentially to certain features of the stimulus, such as lines of particular orientation, movement, colour, etc. There seems to be a hierarchy of specialized neural detectors (sometimes called feature detectors), ranging from centre-surround units to hypercomplex cells (Hubel and Wiesel, 1968). The information in the optic nerve is recoded and processed at different points in the visual system, so that the responses of cortical units are very different from those in the optic nerve.

Much the same thing seems to happen in the auditory system, except that it is much less clear what the crucial features of the stimulus are which will produce responses from a given neurone, or set of neurones. In addition, the anatomy of the auditory system is exceedingly complex, so that many of the neural pathways within and between the various nuclei in the auditory system have yet to be investigated in detail. It is beyond the scope of this book to give more than the briefest description of recent research on the neurophysiology of higher centres in the auditory system. We will content ourselves with describing some properties of cortical neurones, and will introduce other data later in the book, when they have some relevance to the mechanism or process under discussion. Some of the more important neural centres, or nuclei, in the auditory pathway are illustrated in Fig. 1.20.

It is likely that the cortex is concerned with analysing more complex aspects of stimuli than simple pitch or loudness. Many cortical neurones will not respond to steady pure tones at all, and the tuning properties of those which do respond to pure tones tend to differ from those found in primary auditory neurones. Abeles and Goldstein (1972) found three different types of tuning properties: narrow, broad and multirange (responding to a number of preferred frequencies). They considered that this suggested a hierarchical organization, with several narrow range units converging on one multirange unit. There is some dispute whether the tonotopic organization which is found at lower levels in the auditory system persists at the cortex. Merzenich *et al.* (1973a), using characteristic frequency determinations in the anaesthetized cat, reported a highly ordered tonotopic organiza-

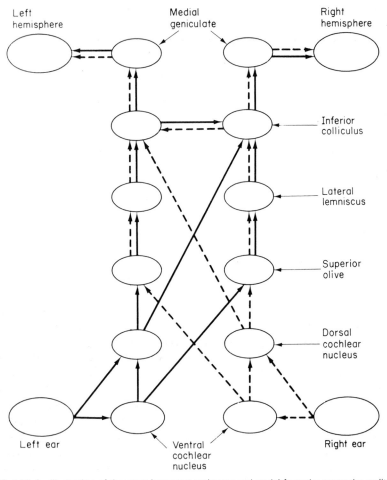

FIG. 1.20 An illustration of the most important pathways and nuclei from the ear to the auditory cortex. The nuclei illustrated are located in the brain stem.

tion; the CF changes in an orderly way according to the place of penetration of the electrode. On the other hand, Evans (1968), using unanaesthetized, unrestrained cats, found only a very general trend in the location of unit CFs. He considered that what little trend there was represented a residuum of anatomical arrangement from subcortical levels, rather than a property which had a functional significance for frequency analysis. A number of studies have indicated that anaesthetics do considerably alter the responses of cortical neurones, so that data obtained using anaesthetics must be interpreted with considerable caution.

Evans (1968), using mostly unanaesthetized cats, has reported that 20% of cortical neurones respond only to complex stimuli such as clicks, bursts of noise or 'kissing' sounds. Ten per cent of those neurones which would respond to tonal stimuli would only do so if the tone frequency was changing. Whitfield and Evans (1965) reported that frequency-modulated tones were very effective stimuli for the majority of neurones responding to tones. Many neurones exhibited responses which were preferential to certain directions of frequency change. These neurones have been called 'frequency sweep detectors'. Some neurones respond preferentially to particular rates of modulation or to particular rates of frequency sweep.

For other neurones repetition rate and duration of tonal stimuli were critical parameters. Seventeen per cent of all units studied responded only to the onset of a tonal simulus, while 10% responded only to the termination and 2% responded to both onset and termination. Over 50% of neurones were preferentially or specifically sensitive to particular locations of the sound source. This general finding has been confirmed and extended by Brugge and Merzenich (1973) for restrained, unanaesthetized monkeys. They found that many units were sensitive to interaural (between the ears) time or intensity differences. At low frequencies spike count was a periodic function of interaural time delay. In several penetrations neighbouring cells were most sensitive to the same interaural delay. Some cells were sensitive to small interaural shifts in sound pressure levels over a range of about 20 dB. We shall see in Chapter 5 that the features of the stimuli to which these cells are responsive are crucial in our ability to localize sounds.

Wollberg and Newman (1972) investigated the responses of cortical neurones in awake squirrel monkeys to recorded species-specific vocalizations. They found some cells which responded with temporally complex patterns of neural firing to many different vocalizations. Other cells responded to only one call, with simpler patterns of firing. Deletion of short segments of the calls revealed that specific segments of the calls are responded to by different cells, but that the relationship between the response and the temporal characteristics of the call is a complex one, involving preceding portions of the call. The results suggest that cortical cells are specialized for the detection of certain acoustic features which occur in monkey calls. At the present time we have no way of knowing whether there are similar neurones in humans which are specialized for the detection and analysis of specific speech sounds, although there do appear to be areas in the human brain which are specialized for the perception of speech (see Chapter 7).

8   GENERAL CONCLUSIONS

Sound consists of variations in pressure as a function of time. It is often convenient to analyse a complex pattern of pressure variation into its sinusoidal frequency components. Periodic sounds can be shown by Fourier analysis to have line spectra containing harmonics of the fundamental component. This component has a frequency equal to the repetition rate of the whole complex. Nonperiodic sounds can be analysed using the Fourier transform. They have continuous spectra, in which the energy is distributed over frequency, rather than being concentrated at discrete frequencies.

Sound levels are usually measured using the decibel (dB) scale. This is a logarithmic measure which expresses the ratio of two intensities. When the reference intensity is chosen to be 10^{-16} W/cm^2, the level has units of dB sound pressure level (dB SPL). When the reference intensity is the absolute threshold for a given sound and a given subject, the units are dB sensation level (dB SL).

The auditory system is often conceived as being composed of a series of successive stages. A stage is linear if it satisfies the conditions of superposition and homogeneity. The response of a linear system to a complex input can be calculated as the sum of the responses to the sinusoidal components of that input.

A filter is a device which passes certain frequency components, but attenuates others. Filters can be used both for the manipulation of stimuli, and for their analysis. Filters can be characterized by their cutoff frequencies, usually measured at the 3 dB down points, and by their slopes in dB/octave. The bandwidth of a bandpass filter is equal to the frequency range between the two 3 dB down points.

The peripheral auditory system is composed of the outer, middle and inner ear. The middle ear acts as an impedance-matching transformer, to improve the efficiency of the transfer of energy between the air and the fluid-filled cochlea. A membrane called the basilar membrane runs along the length of the cochlea, dividing it into two chambers. Sounds produce travelling waves along the basilar membrane, and for each frequency there is a maximum in the pattern of vibration at a different place. The basilar membrane thus acts as a crude Fourier analyser, or filter bank, splitting complex sounds into their component frequencies.

Movement of the basilar membrane causes a deformation of the hair cells which lie within the organ of Corti on the basilar membrane, and this leads to action potentials within the nerve fibres of the auditory nerve. The nerve fibres show spontaneous activity in the absence of sound, and each nerve fibre has a threshold and a saturation level, above which increases in intensity produce no change in response. The threshold of a given fibre is lowest for one frequency, called the characteristic frequency (CF), and increases for frequencies on either side of this. The plot of threshold versus frequency is called the frequency-threshold curve or tuning curve. Single nerve fibres appear to be more sharply tuned than the basilar membrane.

The temporal pattern of the firing within a given neurone can also carry information about the stimulus. Nerve firings tend to occur at a particular phase of the stimulating waveform, a process known as phase-locking. Phase-locking breaks down above 4–5 kHz.

Sometimes the response of a single neurone to a sinusoidal tone may be reduced by a second tone, even when the second tone alone produces no response in the neurone. This is known as two-tone suppression, and it is an example of a nonlinear process in the peripheral auditory system.

The responses of neurones at higher levels of the auditory system have not been studied as thoroughly as responses in the auditory nerve. Some neurones in the auditory cortex appear to respond only to complex stimuli, or stimuli with time-varying characteristics.

FURTHER READING

The following books contain useful chapters on the physics of sound as related to hearing:

Green, D. M. (1976). *An Introduction to Hearing.* Lawrence Erlbaum, New Jersey.

Van Bergeijk, W. A., Pierce, J. R. and David E. E. (1961). *Waves and the Ear.* Heinemann, London.

The physiology of the peripheral auditory system is covered fully in:

Dallos, P. (1973). *The Auditory Periphery.* Academic Press, New York.

The physiology of the whole auditory system is covered in the following:

Pickles, J. O. (1982). *An Introduction to the Physiology of Hearing.* Academic Press, London and New York.

2 Loudness, adaptation and fatigue

1 INTRODUCTION

The human ear is remarkable both in terms of its absolute sensitivity and in terms of the range of intensities to which it can respond. The loudest sound we can hear without damaging our ears has a level about 120 dB above the faintest sound we can detect. This corresponds to a ratio of powers of 1 000 000 000 000:1. One aim of this chapter is to discuss the possible ways in which such a range could be coded. A second aim is to discuss how the loudness of sounds depends upon frequency and intensity, and to relate this to the way in which these sounds are processed.

A problem which arises in studying the loudness of sounds, particularly when these are complex or of a transient nature, is that loudness is a subjective quantity, and as such cannot be measured directly. This problem has been tackled in a number of different ways: sometimes subjects are asked to match the loudness of a sound to some standard comparison stimulus (often a 1000 Hz tone); in other experiments subjects are asked to rate loudness on a numerical scale, a technique known as magnitude estimation. As we shall see, there are problems associated with each of these methods.

A third area of discussion will be that of loudness adaptation, fatigue and damage risk. In general, adaptation and fatigue in the auditory system are much less marked than in the visual system, and the effects also have different time courses. In certain types of deafness adaptation effects become more marked. We will discuss how this, and the phenomenon of recruitment (see below), can be used in the differential diagnosis of hearing disorders.

2 ABSOLUTE THRESHOLDS

A large number of workers have determined absolute thresholds as a function of frequency. It is important to define very carefully the way in which the physical intensity of the threshold stimulus is measured, and two methods have been in common use. One method requires the measurement of the sound pressure actually present at some point close to the entrance of the ear canal or inside the ear canal. The threshold so determined is called the minimum audible pressure (MAP). The measurement is usually made using miniature microphones, or microphones with thin probe tubes attached, and the sounds are usually delivered by headphone. The other method uses tones delivered by loudspeaker, usually in a large anechoic chamber. The measurement of sound level is made after the listener is removed from the sound field, at the point which had been occupied by the centre of the listener's head. The threshold determined in this way is called the minimum audible field (MAF). The two methods give somewhat different results since the head, the pinna and the meatus do have an influence on the sound field.

A typical set of results for MAP is shown in Fig. 2.1. These were obtained by Dadson and King (1952), using a sample of 198 ears, with sound pressures

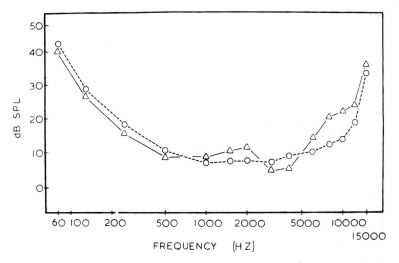

FIG. 2.1 The minimum audible sound level as a function of frequency for two positions close to the entrance of the ear canal (meatus). The solid curve gives sound levels measured 0.3 cm inside the entrance to the meatus, and the dashed curve levels measured 0.7 cm outside the entrance to the meatus. Redrawn from Dadson and King (1952), by permission of the authors and the Director of the National Physical Laboratory, UK.

measured at two positions close to the entrance to the meatus. The distribution of thresholds for the same group of listeners at four different frequencies is shown in Fig. 2.2. Although the subjects were 'otologically normal', with ages between 18 and 25 years, it is clear that there is a large variability among different observers. Part of this may be attributable to criterion differences; the proportion of 'yes' responses by the subject will be affected by his willingness to respond to minimal sensory evidence (see

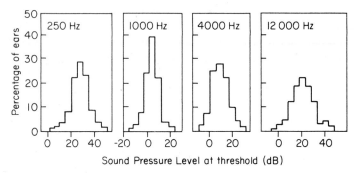

FIG. 2.2 The distribution of sound levels at threshold for 198 ears at four frequencies. Redrawn from Dadson and King (1952), by permission of the authors and the Director of the National Physical Laboratory, UK.

Chapter 3, section 9). However, the range of thresholds is probably much too large to be explained in this way. Tumarkin (1972) has suggested that the majority of the ears tested in this sample may have been biologically subnormal, and he cites evidence from Bredberg (1968) showing that the number of hair cells in the inner ear is diminishing almost from the day we are born. It is certainly puzzling that a considerable number of subjects had thresholds 20 dB or more below the mean.

The general shape of the frequency–threshold curve (often called the audiogram) is now well established. We are most sensitive to frequencies in the range 1000–5000 Hz, while thresholds increase rapidly at very high and very low frequencies. At least part of our sensitivity to middle frequencies derives from the action of the pinna and ear canal. Figure 2.3, from Djupesland and Zwislocki (1972), shows the sound pressure transformation

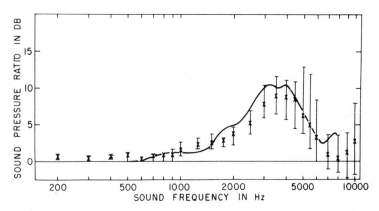

FIG. 2.3 The transformation in sound pressure between the eardrum and the entrance to the ear canal. Crosses indicate the means, vertical bars the interquartile ranges. The solid line reproduces earlier data of Wiener and Ross (1946). From Djupesland and Zwislocki (1972), by permission of the authors.

between the eardrum and a point 1 cm outside the tragus (the small projection at the entrance to the ear canal). The outer ear enhances the sound pressure at the eardrum for frequencies in the range 1–9 kHz, with a maximum enhancement at 3 kHz of about 15 dB. Another factor which contributes to the shape of the absolute threshold curve is the transmission characteristic of the middle ear. Transmission is most efficient for midrange frequencies and drops off markedly for very low and very high frequencies. This can account for the rapid rise in threshold at the low and high frequency ends of the audiogram.

The amplitudes of vibration corresponding to the SPLs at threshold are remarkably small. For example, the data of Dadson and King (1952) show that the root-mean-square pressure variation at threshold for a 3000 Hz tone is about $4 \times 10^{-3} \, \mu\text{N/cm}^2$. This corresponds to a displacement amplitude, at the entrance to the ear canal, of 6.25×10^{-10} cm, or 0.00625 nm. The action of the ear canal will increase the threshold displacement at the eardrum to about 0.03 or 0.04 nm, but this is still a very small value. Amplitudes of vibration on the basilar membrane may be even smaller; extrapolation from displacement amplitudes measured at high SPLs indicates threshold displacements of between 0.001 and 0.005 nm. It may be, however, that there is some nonlinearity in the behaviour of the basilar membrane, in which case such extrapolations are not justified (Rhode, 1971).

At low frequencies MAPs, measured under headphones, are greater than MAFs, by between 5 and 10 dB. A number of workers have shown that this is due to physiological noise of vascular origin, which is produced within the meatus when earphones are worn (Anderson and Whittle, 1971; Soderquist and Lindsey, 1972). The detectability of low frequency tones can be shown to vary according to their temporal position within the cardiac cycle (heartbeat). The level of this low frequency 'physiological noise' varies with the leakage of air around the headphone (this will depend in part on headband pressure), with the volume of the subject's meatus, and with the strength of his heartbeat. These sources of variance are lessened when circumaural headphones (which fit around the pinnae) rather than supra-aural headphones (which lie over and flatten the pinnae) are used. Thus circumaural earphones are preferable for use at low frequencies. However, at high frequencies these headphones are less reliable, and more difficult to calibrate than supra-aural headphones.

The highest audible frequency varies considerably with the age of the subject. Young children can often hear tones as high as 20 kHz, but for most adults threshold rises rapidly above about 15 kHz. The loss of sensitivity with increasing age (presbyacusis) is much greater at high frequencies than at low, and the variability between different observers is also greater at high frequencies. At the other end of the scale there seems to be no particular low frequency limit to our hearing. Whittle *et al.* (1972) measured thresholds for frequencies from 50 Hz down to 3.15 Hz, and showed that their results formed a continuum with the results at higher frequencies. However, for the 3.15 Hz tone the threshold level was about 120 dB SPL! It has been suggested (Johnson and von Gierke, 1974) that sounds below about 16 Hz are not heard in the normal sense, but are detected by virtue of the distortion products (harmonics) which they produce after being transduced through the middle ear. Thus the lower frequency limit for the 'true' hearing of pure tones probably lies about 16 Hz. This is close to the lowest frequency for which the attribute of pitch remains meaningful.

In many practical situations our ability to detect faint sounds is limited not by our absolute sensitivity to those sounds but by the level of ambient noise. In other words, detection will depend upon the masked threshold rather than the absolute threshold. In such cases the threshold as a function of frequency will depend upon the character of the ambient noise (e.g. frequency content, level, whether intermittent or continuous, etc). These problems are discussed more fully in Chapter 3.

Before finishing our discussion of absolute thresholds, we should mention that in clinical practice, and in audiology, thresholds are usually specified relative to the average threshold at each frequency for young, healthy listeners with 'normal' hearing. Thresholds specified in this way have units dB HL (hearing level). Thus, for example, a threshold of 40 dB HL at 1 kHz would mean that the patient had a threshold which was 40 dB higher than 'normal' at that frequency. Threshold in this case would correspond to about 46 dB SPL.

A plot of threshold as a function of frequency is called an *audiogram*. In psychoacoustic work audiograms are normally plotted with threshold increasing upwards, as in Fig. 2.1. However, in audiology threshold elevations are shown as hearing losses, plotted downwards. The average 'normal' threshold is represented as a horizontal line at the top of the plot, and the degree of hearing loss is indicated by how much the threshold falls below this line.

3   EQUAL-LOUDNESS CONTOURS

There are many occasions on which engineers and acousticians require some subjective scale corresponding to the loudness of a sound. Since complex sounds are often analysed in terms of their individual frequency components, a useful first step is to derive such a scale for pure tones. The most direct way of doing this is to use the technique of magnitude estimation, to determine the relationship between physical intensity and judged loudness. However, the validity of this technique has been questioned, and before discussing it (section 4) we will consider an alternative measure of loudness, which is not at first sight so straightforward, but which nevertheless has proved useful in practice, and which is not so controversial. The alternative is the loudness level, which tells us not how loud a tone is, but rather how intense a 1000 Hz tone must be in order to sound equally loud. The psycho-physical task required of the subject is a judgement of equal loudness with respect to two tones of different frequency. Results are usually presented in terms of equal-loudness contours. For example, the standard reference tone might be presented at 40 dB SPL. The subject is then presented with a tone of different frequency, say 500 Hz, and is asked to adjust its intensity until it sounds as loud as the 1000 Hz 40 dB tone. The loudness level of the 500 Hz tone is then defined to be 40 phons.

Thus the loudness level of any tone is the intensity level (in dB SPL) of the 1000 Hz tone to which it sounds equal in loudness. The unit of loudness level is the phon. Some typical results are shown in Fig. 2.4 (from Robinson and

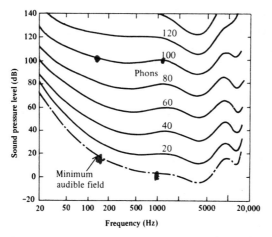

FIG. 2.4 Equal-loudness contours for various loudness levels. The absolute threshold curve is also indicated. Redrawn from Robinson and Dadson (1956), by permission of the authors and the Director of the National Physical Laboratory, UK.

Dadson, 1956). This figure shows equal-loudness contours for loudness levels from 20 phons to 120 phons, and it also includes the absolute threshold (MAF) curve. The equal-loudness contours are of similar shape to the threshold curve, but tend to become flatter at high loudness levels. This means that the rate of growth of loudness differs for tones of different frequency. For example, the absolute threshold for a 100 Hz tone is about 20 dB above that for a 1000 Hz tone (thresholds at 23 and 3 dB SPL). But for the 100 phon contour the intensities are nearly the same (102 and 100 dB SPL). For the same range of loudness, from threshold to 100 phons, the intensity of the 1000 Hz tone must be increased by 97 dB, while that of the 100 Hz tone must be increased by only 79 dB. Thus the rate of growth of loudness with increase in intensity is greater for low frequencies (and to some extent for very high frequencies) than for middle frequencies.

These findings have certain implications for the reproduction of sound; the relative loudness of the different frequency components in the sound will change as a function of the overall intensity, so that unless the sounds are reproduced at the same intensity as the original, the 'tonal balance' will be altered. This is one of the reasons why human voices often sound 'boomy' when reproduced at high levels via loudspeakers; the ear becomes relatively more sensitive to low frequencies at high intensities. Conversely, at low levels we are less sensitive to the very low and very high frequencies, so that many amplifiers incorporate a 'loudness' control which boosts the bass (and to some extent the treble) at low listening levels. Such controls are not usually effective, since they take no account of loudspeaker efficiency and size of room.

The explanation for the greater rate of growth of loudness at low frequencies may lie in the way the excitation patterns change as a function of intensity. For low frequencies the excitation patterns spread over a much larger area than for high frequencies (see Fig. 2.5). Thus an increase in

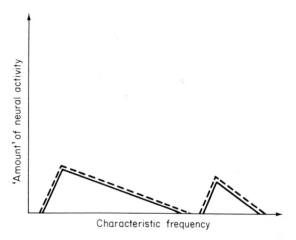

FIG. 2.5 Idealized 'excitation patterns' for a low frequency tone and a high frequency tone, both at moderate level. An increase in level, indicated by the dashed lines, produces a change in firing rate in a greater number of neurones for the low frequency tone than for the high frequency tone.

intensity will cause a change in the amount of excitation in a larger number of neurones at low frequencies. If a change in loudness is signalled as a change in the total number of neural firings, then this will lead to a more rapid growth of loudness at low frequencies.

The shapes of equal-loudness contours have been used in the design of sound level meters which attempt to give an approximate measure of the loudness of complex sounds. Such meters contain weighting networks, so that the meter does not simply sum the power at all different frequencies, but rather weights the power at each frequency according to the shape of the equal-loudness contours. At low sound levels low frequency components contribute little to the total loudness of a complex sound, so an 'A' weighting is used which reduces the contribution of low frequencies to the final meter reading. At high levels all frequencies contribute more or less equally to the loudness sensation (the equal-loudness contours being approximately flat), so that a more nearly linear weighting characteristic, the 'C' network, is used. The 'B' weighting is used for intermediate levels. Sound levels measured with these meters are usually specified in terms of the weighting used. Thus a given level might be specified as 35 dBA, meaning that the meter gave a reading of 35 dB when the 'A' weighting was used.

The sound level meters which we have described suffer from a number of problems. Firstly, they can only be reliably used with steady sounds of relatively long duration; the responses to transient sounds do not correspond to the subjective impressions of the loudness of such sounds. Secondly, they do not provide a satisfactory way of summing the loudness of components in widely separated frequency bands. As we shall see in Chapter 3, the loudness of a complex sound with a given amount of energy depends on whether that energy is contained within a narrow range of frequencies or is spread over a wide range of frequencies. Bauer *et al.* (1971) have described several stages in the development of a sound level meter which attempts to overcome these problems. These stages include:

1 The determination of equal-loudness contours for octave bands of pink noise. Such noise has constant energy in a given relative bandwidth (bandwidth divided by centre frequency), and is representative of many of the broadband sounds encountered in everyday life.
2 The determination of appropriate meter ballistics, so that the meter can cope with fluctuating and transient sounds.
3 The determination of a rule for adding loudness levels in different octave bands. The rule used actually involved the arithmetic addition of loudness levels in different bands.

A loudness level meter based on these principles was evaluated by asking subjects to make judgements of the relative loudness of a variety of complex sounds and comparing their judgements with the readings given by the meter. The results indicated a considerable superiority over the conventional loudness meter.

It should not be assumed that such meters give a 'true' estimate of the loudness of a given sound. The readings obtained are closely related to the decibel scale, which is a scale of physical magnitude rather than a scale of subjective sensation (see later). Thus it would be quite wrong to say that a sound giving a reading of 80 dB was twice as loud as a sound giving a reading of 40 dB. However, the meters do enable us roughly to compare the loudness of different complex sounds. We shall discuss below some of the models which attempt to provide more satisfactory estimates of the loudness of complex sounds.

4   THE SCALING OF LOUDNESS

We will not attempt here to discuss in detail the methods which have been used to construct scales of loudness, and the methods which have been used to validate them. The development of scales of loudness and of other sensory dimensions has been pioneered by S. S. Stevens, and the reader is referred to his work for further details (Stevens, 1957). Stevens proposed the sone as the unit of loudness, and we will discuss briefly how a sone scale of loudness could be constructed. One sone is defined arbitrarily as the loudness of a 1000 Hz tone at 40 dB SPL. The listener is asked to adjust the level of a 1000 Hz tone until it sounds half as loud as this standard of 40 dB. This loudness is labelled 0.5 sones. Similarly, a sound that is judged to be twice as loud will have a loudness of 2 sones. By continuing this process a wide range of intensities can be explored, and intermediate points can be obtained by a method of bisection, e.g. a tone whose loudness is judged to be halfway between that of a 2 sone tone and a 4 sone tone will have a loudness of 3 sones.

On the basis of his own observations on large numbers of subjects, and using the results of other workers, Stevens suggested that loudness, as defined by the sone scale, was a power function of physical intensity: $L = kI^{0.3}$ where k is a constant depending on the subject and the units used. In other words, the loudness of a given sound will be proportional to its intensity raised to the power 0.3. A simple approximation to this is that a two-fold change in loudness is produced by a 10 dB step in level.

The sone scale has been used by Zwicker and Scharf (1965), Zwicker (1958) and Stevens (1972) in models which allow the calculation of the loudness of complex sounds. We will not present these models in detail, since they are rather complicated. Although there are some differences in the models, in essence they involve the splitting of the complex stimulus into a number of frequency bands (usually third-octave bands), and the determination of the level in each one. The level in each band is then converted to a 'loudness' on the sone scale, using Steven's Power Law, and the loudness in each band is summed to give the total loudness.

There have been many criticisms of loudness scaling. The technique seems very susceptible to bias effects, so that results are affected by the range of stimuli presented, the first stimulus presented, the instructions to the subject, the range of permissible responses, symmetry of the response range (judgements tend to be biased towards the middle of the range available for responses), and various other factors related to experience, motivation, training, attention, etc. Very large individual differences are observed, and consistent results are only obtained by averaging many judgements of a large number of subjects. Warren (1970a) attempted to eliminate known bias effects by obtaining just a single judgement from each subject. Only those responses distributed symmetrically about the centre of the available range were considered as bias-free. He found that half-loudness corresponds to a 6 dB attenuation, rather than the 10 dB suggested by Stevens. However, considerable variability is also apparent in his data.

There are also theoretical objections to loudness scaling. One of these, pointed out by Treisman (1964), is that there are two stages involved in obtaining a loudness judgement, each of which may be governed by a different function. In the first stage the stimulus evokes a loudness sensation in the listener. It is the functional relationship between the stimulus magnitude and the sensation which we wish to determine. In the second stage the listener gives a number which is related *in some way* to the magnitude of the sensation. It is only if the relation between sensation and number is linear that the responses of the subject will directly indicate the relative magnitude of the sensation. If the listener is used to working with some other scale, such as a logarithmic scale, then the judgements will not give a direct indication of the loudness sensation. Unfortunately there is no easy way to determine what sort of number scale the listener is using.

A second theoretical objection is to the whole concept of asking a listener to judge the magnitude of a sensation. What we do in everyday life is to judge the 'loudness' of sound *sources*, so that our estimate is affected by the apparent distance of the sound source, the context in which it is heard, the nature of the sound, and so on. In other words, we are attempting to make some estimate of the properties of the source itself, and introspection as to the magnitude of the sensation evoked may be an unnatural and difficult process. This point of view has been well expressed by Helmholtz, who said that

> . . . we are exceedingly well trained in finding out by our sensations the objective nature of the objects around us, but that we are completely unskilled in observing these sensations *per se*; and that the practice of associating them with things outside of us actually prevents us from being distinctly conscious of the pure sensations
>
> (quoted in Warren, 1981).

It is not all clear that methods of calculating loudness using the 'psychological' sone scale give better agreement with loudness judgements than methods based on a physical analysis of the stimuli. Thus Corliss and Winzer (1964) say:

> The loudness of several complex sounds computed on the basis of Stevens' model did not agree with the results of Zwicker's model. The results were not related in any consistent way and both sets of computations were at variance with the subjects' response.

Similarly, Howes (1971) compared the loudness of broadband noise calculated by a method similar to Zwicker's, with the loudness calculated by summing weighted intensities of sub-bands of noise and obtaining the loudness of the sum. This 'power summation' method gave better agreement with actual loudness judgements than did Zwicker's method. Carter (1972) applied five different methods in the calculation of the loudness of repeated acoustic transients. A white noise was used as a comparison stimulus. The method predicting loudness most effectively in the face of variation in rise time and repetition rate of the transients was dBA, a measure obtained using a sound level meter with 'A' weighting (see section 3). This method was clearly superior to methods employing the sone scale.

At the present time there are a great many competing methods for calculating loudness, and no one method seems to be entirely successful in dealing with the great variety of sounds which are encountered in everyday life. There is certainly room for considerable scepticism when a statement such as 'Concorde is twice as loud as a Boeing 747' is made.

5   TEMPORAL INTEGRATION

It has been known for many years (Exner, 1876) that both absolute thresholds and the loudness of sounds depend upon duration. The studies of absolute threshold which were described earlier were all carried out with sounds, usually tone bursts, of relatively long duration, and it does appear to be the case that for durations exceeding about 500 ms threshold is independent of duration. However, for durations less than about 200 ms the sound intensity necessary for detection increases as duration decreases (remember that intensity is a measure of energy per unit time). A number of workers have investigated the relation between threshold and duration for tone pulses, over a wide range of frequencies and durations.

The early work of Hughes (1946) and Garner and Miller (1947) indicated that, over a reasonable range of durations, the ear appears to integrate the energy of the stimulus over time, in the detection of short-duration tone bursts. Ideally this would be expressed by the formula

$$I \times t = \text{constant} \qquad (1)$$

where I is the threshold intensity for a tone pulse of duration t. In other words, the threshold would depend only on the total amount of energy in the stimulus and not on how that energy was distributed over time. In practice the results are fitted better by the expression

$$(I - I_L) \times t = I_L \times \tau = \text{constant} \tag{2}$$

where I_L is the threshold intensity for a long-duration tone pulse and τ is a constant representing the 'integration time' of the auditory system. Notice that in this formula it is not the product of time and intensity which is constant, but the product of time and the amount by which the intensity exceeds the value I_L. Garner and Miller interpreted I_L as the minimum intensity which is an effective stimulus for the ear. They assumed that only intensities above this minimum value are integrated linearly by the ear.

Plomp and Bouman (1959) suggested an alternative way of accounting for the experimental results. They put forward the hypothesis that switching on a tone pulse of intensity I results in a sensory effect S that approaches its end value asymptotically according to an exponential function, this end value being proportional to I. Detection occurs when S exceeds a critical value S_0. According to this hypothesis the relation between S and I is given by

$$S = kI(1 - e^{-t/\tau}) \tag{3}$$

where t is the time after the start of the pulse, k is a constant and τ is a time constant which determines the rate of increase of S. Detection would occur when

$$kI(1 - e^{-t/\tau}) = S_0 \tag{4}$$

When t is much less than τ, equation (4) becomes identical with equation (2), but at longer durations there are differences. On the basis of a number of experiments, Plomp and Bouman concluded that their hypothesis gave a better description of the data than other hypotheses thus far used (including that of Miller and Garner). However, the data deviate from the predictions of their hypothesis at very short durations.

Plomp and Bouman found that the time constant of integration varies according to frequency, being around 375 ms at 250 Hz and 150 ms at 8000 Hz. Other workers have also found time constants which vary with frequency (e.g. Watson and Gengel, 1968), although the actual values of the time constants have not always been in agreement. On the other hand, Olsen and Carhart (1966) found for frequencies of 250, 1000 and 4000 Hz that changes in threshold with stimulus duration were similar for all stimuli, while Bilger and Feldman (1968) reported that results depend upon the particular method chosen to measure temporal integration.

The limits of complete energy integration have been studied using tone pulses of various durations but with equal energy (Green et al., 1957). In theory, complete integration would lead to constant detectability. Green and co-workers used as their measure of detectability the quantity d', which is derived from the theory of signal detection (see Chapter 3, section 9). They found that detectability was generally constant over the range of durations from 15 to 150 ms, but fell off for durations smaller or greater than this (see Fig. 2.6). A similar 'plateau' was found by Sheeley and Bilger

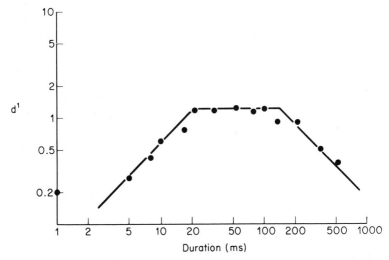

FIG. 2.6 The mean detectability (d') of equal energy tone bursts of frequency 1 kHz as a function of duration. Note the range of durations over which detectability is roughly constant. From Stephens (1973), by permission of the author.

(1964), although the plateau occurred at longer durations for low frequencies (250 Hz) and shorter durations at high frequencies (4000 Hz). The fall in detectability at longer durations is in line with previous studies, indicating that there is a limit to the time over which the ear can integrate energy (or a lower limit to the intensity which can be effectively integrated). The fall in detectability at very short durations may be connected with the inevitable spread of energy over frequency which occurs for signals of short duration (see Chapter 1, section 2). It may be that energy can only be integrated when it falls within a fairly narrow range of frequencies and that this range is exceeded for signals of very short duration. This idea is closely connected with the concept of the critical band, which is discussed in Chapter 3.

The effect of duration on loudness has also been measured extensively, but the results show considerable variability except for a general agreement that, at a given intensity, loudness increases with duration. Boone (1973) required subjects to match the loudness of tone bursts to that of a continuous reference tone. He found that for a frequency of 1 kHz the loudness was related to the total energy of the burst. He also found that the off-time between repeated bursts had an effect, and that this effect was frequency dependent. Stephens (1974) investigated the loudness of equal-energy tone bursts of various durations using two different techniques. In the first, subjects were required to give a numerical estimate of the loudness of tone bursts in relation to a standard which was presented initially and stated to have a loudness of 100. In the second, subjects were required to adjust the intensity of a fixed duration stimulus so that its loudness matched that of the tone burst being judged. Stephens also investigated the effect of different sets of instructions. He found that in most cases there was a plateau for a particular range of durations, indicating that equal energy means equal loudness, but that experimental paradigm and the exact wording of instructions did affect the results. One reason for this is that listeners find it difficult to separate the loudness and duration aspects of the stimuli in making their judgements. With both techniques the plateau tended to occur at shorter durations for higher frequencies. The influence of duration on loudness is discussed further in Chapter 3.

6   THE DETECTION OF INTENSITY CHANGES AND THE CODING OF LOUDNESS

The smallest detectable change in intensity has been measured for many different types of stimuli by a variety of methods. Harris (1963) called the two principal methods loudness modulation and loudness memory. Riesz (1928) used the former method, in which periodic smooth intensity changes are introduced into the signal (Riesz did this by mixing the outputs of two oscillators at slightly different frequencies) and the smallest detectable change in intensity is determined. The second technique involves the presentation of two stimuli, the observer being required to judge which is the more intense, i.e. the two-alternative forced-choice (2AFC) procedure is used. The intensity DL is usually defined as that intensity difference which produces 75% correct responses.

Harris (1963) has presented extensive data for both types of task. Since then many papers have appeared giving intensity DLs for a variety of stimuli. Although there are some minor discrepancies in the experimental results, the general trend is quite clear. For wideband noise, or for bands of noise of restricted frequency range, the smallest detectable intensity change is approximately a constant fraction of the intensity of the stimulus. If I is the intensity of a noise band, and ΔI is the smallest detectable change in intensity, then $\Delta I/I$ is roughly constant. In other words, Weber's Law holds. If we express the smallest detectable change in decibels, i.e. as $10 \log [(\Delta I + I)/I]$, then this, too, will be constant. Thus the just-detectable change in level, expressed in decibels, will be constant, regardless of the absolute intensity, and for wideband noise has a value of about 0.5–1 dB (Rodenburg, 1972). This holds from about 20 dB above threshold to 100 dB above threshold (Miller, 1947).

For pure tones the situation is somewhat different. Riesz's data for modulated tones, and data from a number of other workers using pulsed tones (2AFC task), show that Weber's Law does not hold (see, for example, Viemeister, 1972). Instead it is found that if ΔI (in dB) is plotted against I (also in dB), a straight line is obtained with a slope of about 0.9. Thus discrimination, as measured by the Weber fraction, improves at high levels. This has been termed the 'near miss' to Weber's Law. The data of Riesz for loudness modulation show a DL of 1.5 dB at 20 dB SL, 0.7 dB at 40 dB SL, and 0.3 dB at 80 dB SL (all at 1000 Hz).

Let us consider the implications of these findings in terms of the physiological coding of intensity in the auditory system. The two major factors which we have to explain are: (1) the auditory system is capable of detecting changes in intensity for a range of intensities of at least 100 dB; and (2) Weber's Law holds for the discrimination of bursts of noise but not for pure tones.

For many years it was thought that there were groups of auditory nerve fibres with widely differing thresholds (see, for example, Tasaki, 1954). Thus loudness could be coded simply in terms of which fibres were active. Then Kiang *et al.* (1965) and Kiang (1968) suggested that much of the range of thresholds in earlier studies resulted from pooling data across animals, poor stimulus control and poor physical condition of the animals. They reported that thresholds obtained within one animal, for nerve fibres with similar characteristic frequencies, fell within a much narrower range, typically about 20 dB. Further, the individual fibres reached saturation firing rate within 40 dB of threshold (see Fig. 1.15). If changes in intensity were signalled as changes in firing rates of neurones with similar CFs, then only a range of about 60 dB could be coded; for intensities greater than 60 dB above threshold all the neurones would be saturated (firing at their maximum rates).

Recently this position has been somewhat modified, since Liberman (1978) has reported that a small proportion of fibres in the auditory nerve have thresholds much higher than the majority. These 'high threshold' fibres have very low spontaneous firing rates, and thus are very easy to 'miss' using conventional methods of determining whether the electrode is in contact with a nerve fibre. Liberman used small electric shocks to search for the nerve fibres. A second modification to the position of Kiang (1968) comes from the discovery that not all auditory nerve fibres show saturation within 40 dB of threshold (Sachs and Abbas, 1974). Instead the function relating rate of firing to stimulus level shows a bend at 20–30 dB above threshold, with rate continuing to increase gradually over another 30–40 dB. This is called 'sloping saturation'. The functional significance of the high threshold fibres, and the fibres with sloping saturation, is not clear. It is possible that they are responsible for the coding of intensity and intensity changes at high sound levels. However, if this is the case it is surprising that intensity discrimination does not worsen at high sound levels.

As a result of a survey of a large number of nerve fibres, Palmer and Evans (1979) concluded that the proportion of nerve fibres with wide dynamic ranges (say 60 dB or more) is only about 10%. Further, at sound levels above about 60 dB SPL, of the small number of fibres which were not saturated all showed a substantial reduction in the slope of the rate versus intensity function. Thus changes in intensity resulted in only small changes in firing rate. These facts suggest that there may be some other mechanism for the coding of intensity changes at high intensities. One possibility lies in the way the excitation pattern of the stimulus would spread with increasing intensity (see Fig. 2.7). At high intensities the majority of neurones at the centre of the pattern would be saturated, but changes in intensity could still be signalled by changes in the firing rates of neurones at the edges of the pattern.

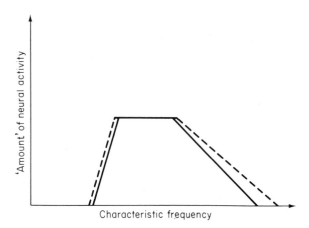

FIG. 2.7 Idealized, 'excitation pattern' for a tone at a high level. An increase in level, indicated by the dashed lines, produces no change in activity for the neurones in the centre of the pattern, since these are saturated. However, changes in neural activity do occur at the edge of the pattern. Note the greater growth of activity that occurs on the high frequency side.

It is not clear to what extent this argument could hold for the discrimination of wideband stimuli, such as white noise. In theory the excitation pattern for white noise has no edges, so that all fibres ought to be saturated by a noise of high intensity. However, we are not equally sensitive to all frequencies, as absolute threshold curves and equal-loudness contours indicate. Thus, although the nerve fibres with midrange characteristic frequencies would be saturated, this might not be the case for very low and very high frequencies. Furthermore, the stimuli have generally been presented via headphones which only pass a limited range of frequencies [in Miller's (1947) case the noise spectrum was only uniform ($\pm$ 5dB) between 150 and 7000 Hz]. Thus the acoustic stimuli would not have been truly wideband, even if the electrical signals were.

We see, then, that changes in firing rate for neurones at the edges of the excitation pattern evoked by the stimulus could provide an explanation for the wide dynamic range of the auditory system. Let us now consider the differences which have been observed in the discrimination data for pure tones and for bursts of noise. Several different models have been proposed to account for the 'near miss' to Weber's Law for pure tones. Zwicker (1956, 1970), who worked with amplitude modulated tones, suggested that a change in intensity can be detected whenever the excitation pattern evoked by the stimulus changes somewhere by (about) 1 dB or more. At high levels the high frequency side of the excitation pattern grows more rapidly with increasing intensity than the rest of the pattern. This is deduced from changes in the shapes of masking patterns for tones in noise as a function of intensity (see Chapter 3). This nonlinear growth in the excitation pattern means that a 1 dB change in excitation on the high frequency side will be produced by relatively smaller stimulus increments at high levels (see Fig. 2.7). In support of this idea, Zwicker reported that the addition of a high-pass noise, which masks the high-frequency side of the excitation pattern but does not actually mask the tone, causes the DL for amplitude modulation at high intensities to approach that found at low levels. (Masking is discussed in detail in Chapter 3.)

McGill and Goldberg (1968a, b) presented an account of intensity discrimination based on neural counting mechanisms. They suggested that stimulus energies are 'mapped' into neural impulses whose number fluctuates from trial to trial even for nonvarying stimuli. The number of neural impulses was assumed to follow a Poisson distribution. For this distribution the standard deviation equals the square root of the mean. If the mean number of neural impulses were proportional to stimulus energy (linear mapping), this would lead to a square root law for intensity discrimination ($\Delta I = k\sqrt{I}$, where k is a constant depending on the subject and the units used). However, if the mapping follows a power law, as suggested by Stevens, then depending on the value of the exponent ($0 < \alpha < 1$), a family of intensity discrimination functions is obtained which is bounded by Weber's Law on one side and the square root law on the other. An exponent of about 0.2 (so that the mean number of neural counts is proportional to $I^{0.2}$) produces a function which accords with the experimental data. Although this model is mathematically elegant, its assumptions about neural mapping are not well supported by physiological evidence. Further, the model does not take into account the spreading of the 'excitation pattern' which may be necessary to account for intensity discrimination at high levels.

A third explanation for the 'near miss' has been presented by Viemeister (1972), who suggested that the observers use information from aural harmonics. At high levels a single pure tone may produce in the ear of series of tones whose frequencies are multiples of the frequency of the tone which is physically presented. These tones, which are known as aural harmonics, behave like externally presented tones (e.g. they will 'beat' with a tone of slightly different frequency and they can be masked by bands of noise), and they probably arise as a result of some nonlinear process in the middle or inner ear. Aural harmonics are negligible at low levels, but grow rapidly with intensity at high levels, so that a given change in stimulus level (in dB) may produce a somewhat larger change in level (in dB) of one or more of the aural harmonics. Thus, if observers can detect changes in the levels of the aural harmonics, their performance will improve at high levels. To test this explanation, Viemeister investigated the intensity discrimination of pulsed sinusoids, with a frequency of 950 Hz, in the presence of various types of filtered noise. He found little effect with a low-pass noise, whose cutoff frequency was 800 Hz, but a bandpass noise centred at the second aural harmonic ($f = 1900$ Hz) or a high-pass noise with cutoff at 1900 Hz both degraded performance at high levels. With the latter stimulus Weber's Law was obtained.

Moore and Raab (1974) provided a further test of Viemeister's model by using stimuli specifically designed to eliminate information from aural harmonics, namely tonal maskers with frequencies corresponding to those of the aural harmonics. These stimuli did affect discrimination, but only when they were at levels in excess of those which would be required to mask the aural harmonics. Masking stimuli at levels which were lower, but which should have been sufficiently great to mask the aural harmonics (Clack *et al.*, 1972), had little effect on intensity discrimination, and did not eliminate the 'near miss'. Thus it seems likely that aural harmonics do not play an important role in intensity discrimination. This is confirmed by the results of Schacknow and Raab (1973) showing that the near miss is obtained for tone bursts of frequency 7000 Hz. It seems extremely unlikely that aural harmonics could provide usable cues at such a high frequency.

In a second experiment Moore and Raab investigated the intensity discrimination of tone bursts ($f = 1000$ Hz) in the presence of three types of noise: wideband, high-pass with cutoff frequency at 2000 Hz, and bandstop with cutoff frequencies at 500 Hz and 2000 Hz. Performance was unimpaired at low levels, but at high levels performance worsened, the greatest impairment being produced by the bandstop noise and the least by the wideband noise. This experiment confirms that information at frequencies other than the nominal frequency of the test tone is important, but it further indicates that information on both the high and low frequency sides of the test tone affects intensity discrimination at high levels; the bandstop noise, which disrupts both types of information, had a greater effect than the high-pass noise, which only disrupts information on the high frequency side.

It seems then that, at least for tones, information from the edges of the excitation pattern allows improved performance at high levels. Some problems still remain, however. Firstly, we have to explain why information from the edges of the pattern allows improved performance for tones, but not for bands of noise. Secondly, we have to explain why performance is not *worse* at high levels than at low levels when the edges of the excitation pattern are disrupted. For example, in the bandstop condition of Moore and Raab, the edges of the excitation pattern on both the low and high frequency sides were disrupted, so that at the high level, where most neurones at the centre of the pattern would have been saturated, performance should have been very poor. In fact, for this condition Weber's Law was found, so that performance was equally good at the high and low levels.

The answer to the first problem may be related to the stability of the edges of the excitation pattern; a narrow band of noise will produce a pattern with edges, but the edges will be unstable because of the fluctuating amplitude of the noise. It may be that improved performance at high levels only occurs with stimuli which produce excitation patterns with well-defined and stable edges. To answer the second problem it may be necessary to invoke some further mechanism for intensity discrimination. One possibility is that a regularity in the timing of neural impulses provides a cue as to the presence of a tone. When a tone is above threshold but is presented against a noise background, some neurones will be phase-locked to the tone, while neurones with characteristic frequencies far from that of the tone will show a quasi-random pattern of neural firing. When the tone is increased in intensity, more of the neurones will become phase-locked, and furthermore the degree of temporal regularity in the firing of neurones which are already phase-locked will increase, since the noise will now produce relatively less 'jitter'. Thus a change in temporal regularity of the patterns of neural firing will signal the intensity change of the tone. Such a mechanism would operate over a wide range of intensities, and would be little affected by saturation effects; temporal patterns of firing can alter even for neurones which are saturated. The mechanism would, however, be limited to frequencies below about 4–5 kHz.

It is possible that temporal patterns of neural firing contribute to the dynamic range of auditory neurones in another way. Hind (1972) has reported that "we have commonly observed phase-locking at intensities below that required to raise the discharge rate above the spontaneous level". Thus behavioural thresholds may be determined not by thresholds for increased

firing in primary auditory neurones, but by thresholds for the detection of
changes in temporal firing patterns. This would extend the effective dynamic
range of single neurones. Note that, even for noise stimuli, the temporal
patterns of firing are different from those for spontaneous activity (Ruggero,
1973). It is difficult to compare behavioural threshold with thresholds for
increased firing rates in auditory neurones, since the methods of specifying
stimulus level have not usually been comparable (cf. Elliot *et al.*, 1960;
Kiang, 1968). There is a slight tendency for behavioural thresholds to be
lower than 'neural' thresholds, but this discrepancy is also observed at high
frequencies, where cues to phase-locking would not be available. Thus the
role of temporal information in detection at low levels must remain in doubt.

In some situations the wide dynamic range of the auditory system can be
maintained even under conditions where cues related to phase-locking
would appear to be minimal. For example, Moore and Raab (1975) investigated the intensity discrimination of a band of noise which was presented in
the presence of a continuous bandstop background noise of sufficient intensity to disrupt information on both the high and low frequency sides of the
excitation pattern evoked by the noise band. Performance did worsen
slightly at high levels, but even at the highest levels used intensity discrimination was still quite good. Similar results have been reported by
Viemeister (1974). Thus, even for a stimulus with little temporal regularity,
such as a noise band, neural saturation appears to have little effect on
intensity discrimination. We should remember, however, that *any* change in
the spectral content of a sound will result in a change in the temporal
patterns of neural firing. When the level of a band of noise within a spectral
notch is incremented, more neurones will phase-lock to components within
the notch, and less to components in the passband of the bandstop background. Whenever components in a given frequency region are incremented
in level, there may be an increase in the degree of phase-locking to those
components. Thus even in the case of a noise in a bandstop background,
phase-locking may play a role in signalling intensity changes.

Evans and Palmer (1975) have reported measurements on single neurones
in the auditory nerve and cochlear nucleus of the cat, using stimulus
presentations similar to those of Moore and Raab (1974, 1975) and
Viemeister (1974). Firing rates of neurones were measured in response to
changes in intensity of stimuli presented in bandstop background noises. As
expected, the neurones in the auditory nerve did show saturation at high
levels, but in the cochlear nucleus some neurones responded to signal level
changes in the presence of bandstop noise over a very wide intensity range,
in many cases up to 100 dB above threshold. How the level signalling
information is carried to the cochlear nucleus, by primary neurones which
are presumably saturated, remains to be determined.

In summary, it seems likely that a number of different mechanisms play a role in intensity discrimination. For stimuli at low levels, intensity changes can be signalled both by changes in the firing rates of neurones at the centre of the excitation pattern, and by the spreading of the excitation pattern, so that more neurones are brought into operation. In addition, cues related to phase-locking may play a role in the detection of low-level tones. At high levels most of the neurones at the centre of the excitation pattern may be saturated but intensity changes can still be signalled by the spread of the pattern and by changes in firing rate at the edges of the pattern. For stimuli producing excitation patterns with stable edges, performance improves at high levels, and this may, in part, be related to a nonlinear growth of excitation on the high frequency side of the excitation pattern. For complex stimuli, the relative levels of different components may be signalled by the degree of phase-locking to the components. Thus an increase in the level of a tone in a noise background may be signalled by increased phase-locking to the tone, with a consequent increase in the temporal regularity of neural firings. Information related to phase-locking is available over a very wide dynamic range, but it is not available above about 5 kHz. An alternative possibility for the coding of intensity at high levels, is that information is carried by 'high threshold' neurones, and by neurones with sloping saturations.

7   LOUDNESS ADAPTATION, FATIGUE AND DAMAGE RISK

It is a property of all sensory systems that exposure to a stimulus of sufficient duration and intensity produces changes in the responsiveness of the system. Some changes occur during the presentation of the stimulus, so that its apparent magnitude decreases or it disappears completely (as sometimes happens for gustatory or olfactory stimuli). Other changes are apparent after the end of the stimulus; for example, shifts in threshold may occur. In general, such effects are much less marked in the auditory system than they are in, say, the visual system, although large threshold shifts are often observed after exposure to stimuli of very high intensity.

Hood (1950, 1972) has distinguished between auditory adaptation and auditory fatigue, and has emphasized that these are two quite distinct processes. The essential feature of fatigue is that it "results from the application of a stimulus which is usually considerably in excess of that required to sustain the normal physiological response of the receptor, and it is measured after the stimulus has been removed" (Hood, 1972). For example, a subject's threshold at a particular frequency might be measured, after which the subject would be exposed to a fatiguing tone of a particular frequency and intensity for a period of time. The threshold would then be measured again, and the shift in threshold would be taken as a measure of fatigue. Notice that this procedure is concerned with "the effect of an excessive stimulus upon a small and finite group of receptors, namely those which are normally brought into activity at near threshold intensities". Auditory fatigue defined in this way is more properly referred to as poststimulatory auditory fatigue, and the measure used is called temporary threshold shift (TTS).

Auditory adaptation has as its essential feature the process of 'equilibration'. The response of a receptor to a steady stimulus declines as a function of time until it reaches a steady level at which the energy expended by the receptor is just balanced by the metabolic energy which becomes available to sustain it. The psychological counterpart of this is a decline in the apparent magnitude of a stimulus (e.g. its loudness) during the first few minutes of presentation, followed by a period in which the apparent magnitude remains roughly constant. Auditory adaptation can be studied by means of loudness balance tests. For example, a tone of fixed intensity, say 80 dB SPL, is applied to the subject's left or test ear, and a loudness balance is made with a tone of the same frequency but variable level applied to the right or control ear. For a normal subject this balance will be obtained with an intensity of about 80 dB SPL. The tone in the right ear is now removed, but that in the left is continued for a further 3 min. Following this adaptation period, a loudness balance is established once again, and it is generally found that the tone in the right ear now produces a loudness match at a lower
● level, say 60 dB SPL. Thus the amount of adaptation corresponds to an intensity change of 20 dB. Notice that the measurement of the decrement of response takes place while the adapting stimulus is being applied.

There are several problems associated with this technique of simultaneous dichotic loudness balance (SDLB). Firstly, adaptation may occur in the control ear, either by means of central neural effects or by physical crossover of the sound, which occurs at 40–50 dB SL in the frequency range from 100 to 10 000 Hz (von Békésy and Rosenblith, 1951). Secondly, if the control tone is presented continuously during a loudness balance, this, too, may introduce adaptation in the control ear. Various other factors, such as the specific method of presentation, have also been shown to affect the results. Finally, it is not clear whether the balance is made on the basis of loudness *per se*, or on the basis of the position of the sound image within the head (see Chapter 5).

Recently a number of papers have appeared which indicate that if the test conditions are designed to eliminate binaural interaction between adapting and comparison tones, then suprathreshold loudness adaptation is essentially absent (e.g. Bray *et al.*, 1973). One technique makes use of a comparison tone whose frequency differs from that of the adapting tone. The adapting tone is presented continuously to one ear, while the comparison tone is presented intermittently to the other. This technique is called a simultaneous heterophonic loudness balance technique (the corresponding name for the case when adapting and comparison tones have the same frequency is homophonic). An alternative is to use a monaural heterophonic technique, where adapting and comparison tones are presented to the same ear, but are sufficiently different in frequency (say 500 Hz and 10 000 Hz) for adaptation to one to have little effect on the loudness of the other. A third technique requires the subject to adjust the intensity of a continuously presented sound so as to maintain it at constant loudness. If the subject increases the intensity of the sound with increasing duration of presentation, then this indicates that adaptation is occurring. Most of the workers using these techniques have reported that there is no significant loudness adaptation for adapting tones between 50 and 90 dB SPL. This has been taken to indicate that the effects which are observed for the homophonic SDLB test are mediated by central interactions, and should not be interpreted as indicating a genuine decrement in loudness for a continuously presented stimulus. On the other hand, there is at least one report (Weiler and Friedman, 1973) of significant (greater than 20 dB) adaptation obtained using a monaural heterophonic technique, so that not all adaptation phenomena can be attributed to binaural interactions.

In a recent review of loudness adaptation, Scharf (1981) has presented data obtained with a method of successive magnitude estimation. The listener is required to assign numbers to express the loudness of a sound at successive time intervals (see section 4 for a description of loudness scaling). The results indicate that adaptation occurs only for *low* level tones, below about 30 dB SL. This finding will be discussed in more detail in section 7.B. It is unfortunate that the different methods of measuring adaptation yield such different results, especially since there is no clear explanation of the differences. Clearly the results need to be treated with caution until such explanations are forthcoming.

Although there is a great deal of evidence that fatigue and adaptation are distinct phenomena, at both the physiological and psychological level, they are not always easy to distinguish. As Elliot and Fraser (1970) have pointed out,

> . . . the question continues to plague investigators as to whether, when the ear is stimulated, for example with a 60– or 80–dB tone, the changes observed during stimulation, or immediately after its cessation are primarily indicative of adaptation or of fatigue. Consequently, although the terms are well established, we are using them with the realization that they often do not refer to completely independent physiological processes.

We will not attempt here to give a detailed account of the physiological processes involved in fatigue and adaptation, or of the factors which affect these. For a review of these the reader is referred to Elliot and Fraser (1970). They conclude that ". . . stimulation results in reversible neural changes that indicate neural adaptation, reduction in hair-cell response, and in all probability, a variety of cochlear environmental changes that interfere with both hair-cell and nerve-cell functioning". In very general terms, the properties of adaptation (as defined by loudness balance tests) seem to parallel those of neural adaptation, while fatigue seems to be connected with hair cell changes.

A   Poststimulatory auditory fatigue

The most common index of auditory fatigue is the TTS, whose measurement was described briefly above. One problem with measuring the TTS is that the recovery process may be quite rapid, so that a threshold measurement has to be obtained as quickly as possible; but this in turn can lead to inaccuracies in the measurement. The most common method is to use a motor driven attenuator, which the subject controls so as to maintain the level of the tone as close as possible to threshold. Sometimes continuous tones are used, but since subjects often have difficulty in tracking these, pulsed tones are generally preferred.

There are five major factors which influence the size of the TTS: (1) the time between cessation of the fatiguing stimulus and the postexposure threshold determination—called the recovery interval (RI); (2) the intensity of the fatiguing stimulus (I); (3) the duration of the fatiguing stimulus (D); (4) the frequency of the fatiguing stimulus (F_c); and (5) the frequency of the test stimulus (F_t). We will briefly summarize the effects of each of these.

TTS generally becomes smaller the longer RI, although for many conditions the recovery curve is diphasic; recovery from the large TTS immediately following exposure is often followed by a 'bounce', particularly at high frequencies. Thus a valley at RI = 1 min is often followed by a bounce at RI = 2 min (see Fig. 2.8). Sometimes the initial recovery process may actually overshoot the original threshold level, so that a temporary sensitization occurs (Hughes and Rosenblith, 1957). The diphasic nature of the recovery curve has led to the suggestion that two processes are involved; a short lived recovery process which may correspond to neural activity, and a longer process which involves hair cell and metabolic changes. For RIs greater than 2 min, recovery is approximately linearly related to log RI, and this seems to hold for RIs from 2 min up to about 112 min (Ward, Glorig and Sklar, 1958). However, when the TTS at 2 min (denoted TTS_2) is greater than 40–50 dB, recovery may be much slower. Even when TTS_2 does not exceed 40 dB, recovery times may be as long as 16 h. Recovery over such long time intervals may indicate that tissue alterations, resulting from stimulation that exceeds the tissue's elastic limits, have occurred.

TTS generally increases with I, the intensity of the fatiguing stimulus, although there are some exceptions to this. At low intensities TTS changes

FIG. 2.8 Recovery curves illustrating the elevation in threshold produced by a fatiguing tone of 500 Hz at 120 dB SPL for 3 min. Test tones of 4 kHz (two subjects) and 1 kHz (one subject) were used, and each set of curves represents re-tests under identical conditions. Note the 'bounce' that occurs at 2 min for the 4 kHz test tones. From Hirsh and Ward (1952), by permission of the authors and *J. Acoust. Soc. Am.*

relatively little as a function of I, the TTS is symmetrically distributed about F_e, and is limited to its immediate neighbourhood. In other words, only test tones with frequencies F_t close to that of F_e show a TTS. As I increases, the TTS increases, the frequency range over which the effects occur increases, with the greatest increase above F_e, and the frequency of the maximum TTS shifts one half-octave or more above F_e. At high levels, and when F_t is above F_e, TTS grows very rapidly as a function of I. For fatiguing intensities above about 90–100 dB, TTS rises precipitously (see Fig. 2.9), and it has been suggested that this point of inflection indicates a division between fatigue which is physiological and transient in nature and fatigue which is more permanent and pathological in nature (Hood, 1950; Hirsh and Bilger, 1955). The upward frequency shift in F_t at which the maximum TTS occurs is not fully understood, but it may be related to the mechanical properties of the

FIG. 2.9 Increases in TTS with increases in the level of the 1 kHz fatiguing tone. Test tones of 1 kHz and 1.4 kHz were used. Note that for high exposure levels the function accelerates, and that the TTS is greater for a frequency above that of the fatiguing tone than for a tone at that frequency. From Hirsh and Bilger (1955), by permission of the authors and *J. Acoust. Soc. Am.*

basilar membrane. The nonlinearity observed by Rhode (1971) is consistent with shifts in the vibration envelope towards the basal (high frequency) end of the basilar membrane with increasing amplitude of a sinusoidal stimulus.

Fatigue generally increases with duration, and a number of workers have reported that TTS is linearly related to log D (Hood, 1950; Ward *et al.*, 1958). However, for low frequencies, particularly when the fatiguing stimulus is noise or a rapidly interrupted tone (Ward, 1963), the growth rate is reduced, probably because the aural reflex (a contraction of the middle ear muscles in response to intense sounds) reduces sound transmission. The log D function probably does not extend below a D of 5 min.

Fatigue effects are generally more marked at high frequencies, at least up to 4–6 kHz. Thus when the fatiguing stimulus is a broadband noise, maximum TTSs occur between 4 and 6 kHz. It is also the case that permanent hearing losses, resulting from exposure to intense sounds, or from old age, tend to be greatest in this region. Both of these may result from the greater stiffness of the high frequency portions of the basilar membrane, so that elastic limits are more easily exceeded.

Recently a number of studies have appeared reporting the effects of exposure to environmental noise of various kinds, including rock and roll music. Harris (1972) in a review of these concluded that

. . . the quieter bands may be harmless, but if the amplification/reverberation condition reaches 110 dBA, a sizeable fraction of persons would be adversely affected probably permanently; while a 120 dBA level, at which some music groups have registered, would create havoc with most audiograms.

B *Auditory adaptation*

We have already discussed some of the problems associated with the measurement of adaptation. One of the most reliable methods, and the one least beset by problems of interpretation, appears to be the method of successive magnitude estimation described by Scharf (1981), and we give initially his main conclusions:

A sound presented alone adapts only if it is below 30 dB SL. High-frequency pure tones adapt more than low-frequency tones or than noises, whether broad-band or narrow-band. Steady sounds adapt more than modulated sounds, and if the sound amplitude is modulated sufficiently adaptation may disappear altogether as when two tones beat together. People differ widely with respect to the degree of adaptation they experience. While most people hear the loudness of a high-frequency, low-level tone decline by at least half within one min, some others report no change in loudness and still others report that the tone disappears. No relation has been found, however, between the degree to which a person adapts and such individual characteristics as threshold, age, and sex, although there is some evidence that children under 16 years adapt less than adults. Free-field listening may produce less adaptation than earphone listening.

There have been comparatively few studies of the spread of adaptation to frequencies adjacent to that of the adapting tone, and most have used the SDLB technique, which we have seen suffers from difficulties of interpretation. Thwing (1955) used a 1000 Hz tone at 80 dB SPL as the adapting stimulus. For 15 seconds in every two minutes he presented a tone of a different frequency in the opposite ear, and at the same time adjusted the frequency in the test ear to match that of the comparison stimulus. The level of the comparison stimulus was adjusted to match the loudness in the test ear. Thwing found a maximum adaptation effect at the adapting tone frequency, with continuously decreasing effects on either side. He suggested that the adaptation is proportional to the extent to which the excitation patterns of the test and adapting stimulus overlap. More data are needed for the evaluation of this hypothesis.

8   LOUDNESS RECRUITMENT, ADAPTATION AND FATIGUE IN THE ASSESSMENT OF DEAFNESS

Hearing losses may be broadly categorized into two main types. The first type, conductive deafness, occurs when there is some defect, usually in the middle ear, which reduces the transmission of sound to the inner ear. For example, a growth may occur on the eardrum, or the bones in the middle ear may ossify or stick together. In general, this results in a more or less uniform hearing loss as a function of frequency, and the difficulty experienced by the sufferer can be well predicted from his threshold elevation. A simple hearing aid is usually quite effective in such cases, and surgery can also be effective.

The second type of hearing loss is called nerve deafness, or sensorineural hearing loss. Usually, the extent of the loss increases with frequency, but the difficulty experienced by the sufferer is not always well predicted from the audiogram. Sensorineural hearing loss may arise as a result of defects in many different parts of the auditory system, and the particular difficulties experienced by the sufferer, and the types of symptoms exhibited, depend on which part of the system is affected. Patients often have difficulty in understanding speech in noisy environments, and the condition is usually not completely alleviated by a hearing aid. Most sensorineural losses cannot be treated by surgery.

A   Recruitment

One phenomenon which often occurs when there are defects in the cochlea itself is loudness recruitment. This refers to an unusually rapid growth of loudness as the sensation level of a tone is increased, and it might be observed as follows. Suppose that a patient has a hearing loss at 4000 Hz of 60 dB in one ear only. If a 4000 Hz tone is introduced into his normal ear at 100 dB SPL (which would also be about 100 dB above threshold for that ear), then the tone which sounds equally loud in his poor ear will also be about 100 dB SPL. Thus a tone which is only 40 dB above threshold in his poor ear may sound as loud as a tone which is 100 dB above threshold in his good ear; the ear with recruitment seems to 'catch up' with the normal ear in loudness. Notice that although recruitment is normally regarded as pathological, a phenomenon very much like it occurs in normal listeners for tones of very high and very low frequency. The loudness of these tones grows more rapidly per decibel than does the loudness for tones of middle frequencies.

One method of detecting recruitment is based on the assumption that if loudness is increasing more rapidly than normal as the stimulus intensity is increased, then a smaller than normal intensity change will be required for a just-noticeable difference in loudness. Thus the difference limen for intensity (DL) should be abnormally small, particularly at low sensation levels, where the rate of growth of loudness is most rapid. This reasoning gives the basis for a number of clinical tests for recruitment, all of which assume that a smaller than normal DL will indicate the presence of recruitment. Unfortunately the reasoning is not sound. We know from the results with normal subjects that loudness grows more rapidly with sound intensity for low frequency tones than for middle frequency tones, but the DL for intensity is *not* smaller for low frequency tones. Similarly, in normal listeners the rate of growth of loudness with intensity is most rapid at low sound levels, but the intensity DL is *largest* at low sound levels. It appears that there is not necessarily a relationship between the rate of growth of loudness and the intensity DL. This makes sense if we assume that the size of the DL is determined by variability in the loudness sensation, as well as its rate of growth. At low sound levels, or in the impaired ear, the variability may well be increased.

In spite of the difficulties of interpretation, a small size of the DL *is* sometimes associated with recruitment. However this applies only to modulated tones, or tones where the increment to be detected is super-imposed on a steady background. Even in this case the test is not very reliable (Lamore and Rodenburg, 1980). Where the task is one of detecting a difference in intensity between two separate tone pulses, the intensity DL is generally somewhat *larger* than normal in cases of recruitment. In cases where the hearing disorder is in the auditory nerve rather than in the cochlea (and recruitment is generally not seen), the intensity DL may be considerably larger than normal (Fastl and Schorn, 1981).

A second technique for measuring recruitment is the alternate binaural loudness balance (ABLB) test, which can be applied when only one ear is affected. A tone of a given intensity at the good ear is alternated with a variable tone, of the same frequency, at the affected ear, and a loudness match is obtained. This is repeated at a number of different intensities, so that the rate of growth of loudness in the affected ear can be compared with that in the good ear. Hood (1972) has emphasized the importance of presenting the tones alternately at the two ears, rather than presenting sustained tones simultaneously at the two ears. The reason for this is that recruitment is essentially a function of the on-effect, the initial response to a stimulus; for sustained tones pathological adaptation (see below) may occur, so that the loudness decreases rapidly with increasing duration of the stimulus. Thus all tests designed to detect recruitment must involve either interrupted tones or abrupt changes in tonal intensity.

A third test for recruitment involves the measurement of loudness dis-comfort levels (LDLs). For most normal subjects a tone becomes un-comfortably loud when its level reaches 100–110 dB SPL. For a patient with a non-recruiting hearing loss the LDL may be much higher, whereas, if recruitment is present, the LDL will fall within the range for normal sub-jects. The phenomenon of recruitment probably accounts for a statement which is often heard from patients with this type of hearing loss: "Don't shout; you're talking loud enough, but I can't understand what you are saying!" The patient may not be able to hear very faint sounds, but sounds of high intensity are just as loud to him as to a normal listener. However, sounds which are easily audible may not be easily intelligible.

The physiological causes of recruitment are not entirely clear, but it occurs consistently in lesions of the cochlea, and is usually absent in conductive deafness and in retrocochlear deafness (deafness due to neural disturbances occurring at a higher point in the auditory pathway than the cochlea). It is probably connected with hair cell damage, and in particular with damage to the outer hair cells. If the responses of auditory nerve fibres to low level stimuli are determined primarily by input from the outer hair cells, then a loss of these hair cells would lead to an elevation in threshold. If, however, the response at high levels is determined primarily by input from the inner hair cells, and if these are normal, then response patterns at high levels will be normal. Thus the sensation of loudness at high levels will be normal, even though thresholds are elevated. Karlan, Tonndorf and Khanna (1972) have suggested that the inner and outer hair cells have different thresholds and different gains (rate of change of output as a function of the intensity of the stimulus), while Dallos *et al.* (1972) have suggested that potentials produced by inner hair cells are porportional to the velocity of the basilar membrane, and potentials generated by outer hair cells are proportional to the displacement of the basilar membrane. It is certainly the case that the outer hair cells are the most susceptible to damage (e.g. from intense auditory stimulation), and the anatomical evidence is consistent with the idea that it is the disproportion between the numbers of inner and outer hair cells that provides the basis for many types of loudness recruitment (Schuknecht, 1970). However, there have been reports (Dix and Hood, 1973) of recruitment caused by brain stem disorders.

Evans (1975) has suggested that recruitment may be associated with the abnormally broad tuning curves which are commonly found when the functioning of the cochlea is impaired (see Chapter 3, section 6). If tuning curves are abnormally broad, with shallow slopes, then the rate at which activity spreads across the nerve fibre array, with increasing intensity, will be greater than normal. This could be the basis of loudness recruitment. This explanation is not in conflict with explanations in terms of damage to the outer hair cells, since such damage does seem to be accompanied by broad tuning curves. The consequences of impairments in frequency selectivity will be discussed further in Chapter 3.

B   *Pathological adaptation*

Abnormal metabolic processes in the cochlea or auditory nerve sometimes result in a very rapid decrease in neural responses, although the on-effect may be normal or near-normal. The psychological correlate of this is adaptation, which is more extreme and more rapid than normal. It turns out to be the case that this effect is usually greater in defects of the nerve fibres than of the cochlea itself, and so pathological adaptation is useful in the differential diagnosis of cochlear and retrocochlear defects. There are several ways of studying this phenomenon, including the simultaneous dichotic loudness balance procedure which we described for normal adaptation. Since, however, pathological adaptation occurs at all intensity levels, it can be conveniently studied with tones close to threshold. One way of doing this is to measure the difference in threshold for continuous and interrupted tones. For patients with conductive deafness, or for normal subjects, there is little difference between the two types of threshold. For a patient with retrocochlear lesions the threshold for a continuous tone may be considerably higher than that for an interrupted tone. One very striking way of demonstrating this is first to determine the threshold for an interrupted tone. The intensity is then raised by 5 dB and the tone is presented continuously. After five or six seconds the sensation of tone will disappear completely, although for the normal listener the sensation would persist indefinitely. It is often necessary to raise the intensity of the tone by 20–30 dB before the sensation persists indefinitely for the subject with retrocochlear defects. It is easy to confirm that the effect is pathological adaptation rather than fatigue, by interrupting the tone at any time during the test; the original threshold is restored at once. These tests are known as tone decay tests.

It is clear that measures of recruitment and adaptation are of considerable use in the diagnosis of hearing disorders, and in the separation of different types of hearing loss. Such measures also give us a valuable insight into the relationship between normal and abnormal functioning of the auditory system, and thus provide pointers for the direction of research in these areas. Studies of what can go wrong with the auditory system help us to understand how it normally works, and conversely a more complete knowledge of how the normal system functions is essential if we are to be able to work out exactly what has gone wrong in cases of hearing loss. A knowledge of the underlying processes involved in adaptation and fatigue is important in the interpretation of clinical data, and also indicates the need, as Hood (1972) puts it ". . . for care in the design and execution of all audiological test procedures".

9   GENERAL CONCLUSIONS

In this chapter we have discussed a number of different aspects of the perception of loudness and the way it is coded in the auditory system. Absolute threshold curves show that we are most sensitive to middle frequencies, at least part of this sensitivity arising from the action of the outer and middle ear. Our absolute sensitivity is such that our ability to detect faint sounds would normally be limited by environmental noises, rather than by limits in the system itself. There is, however, considerable variability between different individuals, so that thresholds 20 dB on either side of the mean are still considered as 'normal'. Hearing losses with age are most marked at high frequencies, but unless some pathological condition occurs, the reception of frequencies important for speech perception deteriorates very little with age.

Equal-loudness contours allow us to compare the loudnesses of sounds of different frequencies. In general, the shapes of equal-loudness contours are similar to absolute threshold curves at low levels, but become flatter at high levels. Thus at high levels it is roughly true that tones of equal SPL sound equally loud regardless of frequency. The shapes of equal-loudness contours indicate that loudness grows more rapidly for low frequencies and for very high frequencies than for middle frequencies. This means that the tonal balance of recorded sounds, such as speech or music, may be affected by the level at which the sounds are reproduced. Equal-loudness contours are used in the design of sound level meters, so that the readings obtained give a better indication of the perceived loudness than would readings based simply on physical intensity.

The technique of magnitude estimation allows the construction of 'psychological' scales of loudness, the most common one being the sone scale suggested by S. S. Stevens. Such scales give a set of numbers which relate the perceived loudness of a given sound to its physical characteristics (such as intensity), and they have been utilized in models which allow the calculation of the loudness of any complex sound. The validity of such scales has been questioned, however, and at present there seems to be no well-established and generally accepted method for calculating loudness.

Absolute intensive thresholds and the loudness of sounds both depend upon duration. Over a certain range of durations (about 15–150 ms) the ear appears to integrate sound energy for the purpose of detection. Thus it is approximately true that threshold depends only on the total amount of energy in the stimulus, and not on how that energy is distributed over time. However, this does not hold at very long durations, probably because of the limited 'integration time' of the ear. At very short durations 'energy splatter' in the signal may also reduce its detectability. There is some evidence that the 'integration time' of the ear is shorter for high frequencies than for low. The loudness of short-duration sounds may also depend upon their total energy, but the results are much less clear-cut, and vary considerably according to the experimental technique used.

We are able to detect changes in intensity for a wide range of intensities and for many types of stimuli. In general, discrimination performance, as measured by the Weber fraction ($\Delta I/I$), is independent of level for bands of noise, but improves at high levels for pure tones. Various psychoacoustic experiments indicate that at high levels information in neurones with CFs above and (to a lesser extent) below the frequency of the test tone may be important in intensity discrimination. These results, together with neuro-physiological data, indicate that a number of different sources of information may be used in detecting intensity changes. These include the spreading of the excitation pattern with increasing level, the nonlinear growth of the excitation pattern on the high frequency side, and changes in the temporal patterns of neural firing.

Exposure to auditory stimulation produces two types of changes in the responsiveness of the auditory system: the apparent magnitude of the stimulus may decrease, a process known as adaptation, and the absolute threshold measured after exposure may increase, a process known as fatigue. There are many problems associated with the measurement of these processes, and they are not always clearly separable. However, the properties of adaptation seem to parallel those of neural adaptation, while fatigue seems to be connected with hair cell changes.

Fatigue, or temporary threshold shift (TTS), generally decreases with increasing recovery time, although a 'bounce' sometimes occurs about two minutes after cessation of the fatiguing stimulus. This may indicate that more than one process is involved in recovery. Recovery times vary considerably, but may be as long as 16 h, or more. TTS is generally small at low exposure intensities, but increases rapidly when the fatiguing stimulus is above about 90–100 dB SPL. This may indicate a division between fatigue which is physiological and transient in nature and fatigue which is more permanent and pathological in nature. Sound levels above 110–120 dB SPL may produce permanent hearing losses, particularly if the exposure is of long duration. Such sound levels are not uncommonly produced by rock and pop groups, and they may be easily obtained by many of the sets of headphones which are available on the domestic market.

Adaptation effects measured with the simultaneous dichotic loudness balance (SDLB) technique are generally quite rapid, the greatest adaptation occurring within one or two minutes of exposure. Adaptation measured in this way occurs at both high and low levels. In contrast, studies which avoid binaural interaction have shown that adaptation occurs only for low level tones (below 30 dB SL) and is strongest at high frequencies. The reasons for the discrepancies between the different methods remain to be explained.

In some cases of deafness, particularly when there is pathology of the cochlea itself, loudness recruitment may occur. Recruitment is an abnormally rapid growth of loudness with increase in intensity: the sufferer may have an elevated threshold, but intense sounds are as loud to him as to a normal listener. One method of detecting recruitment is based on the assumption that it will be associated with an abnormally small intensity DL, but this assumption does not appear to be well founded, and the method is not very reliable. When only one ear is affected recruitment can be detected by direct comparison with the good ear, using a loudness balancing technique. When both ears are affected recruitment may be revealed by a normal loudness discomfort level, but an elevated absolute threshold. Recruitment may be associated with hair cell damage, particularly to the outer hair cells. It is possible that it is produced by a loss of frequency selectivity; tuning curves appear to be broader in pathological cochleas.

Pathological adaptation may occur when there are abnormal metabolic processes in the cochlea or auditory nerve, although the effect is usually greater in the latter case. The adaptation is more rapid and more extreme than normal, and is most easily measured for tones close to threshold; a continuous tone just above threshold may fade after a time and eventually become completely inaudible. However, the tone may easily be made audible once again by interrupting it.

Recruitment and pathological adaptation are useful measures in the differential diagnosis of cochlear and retrocochlear lesions, and in addition they provide useful insights into the functioning of the auditory system. It is to be hoped that the future will see an increasing cooperation between clinical audiologists and otologists and the basic scientist. Theories about normal auditory functioning cannot be complete if they do not take into account the phenomena (such as recruitment) which are observed clinically, and clinical workers have much to gain from theories and data derived from studies of the normal human subject.

FURTHER READING

An extensive review of the perception of loudness may be found in:
Scharf, B. (1978). Loudness. In *Handbook of Perception*, Vol. 4 (eds E. C. Carterette and M. P. Friedman), Academic Press, New York.
A review and summary of the literature on loudness adaptation may be found in:
Scharf, B. (1981). Loudness adaptation. In *Hearing Research and Theory* (eds J. V. Tobias and E. D. Schubert), Academic Press, New York.

3 Frequency analysis, masking and the critical band

1   INTRODUCTION

It is a matter of everyday experience that one sound may be obscured, or rendered inaudible, in the presence of other sounds. Thus music from a car radio may mask the sound of the car's engine, provided that the music is somewhat more intense. Masking has been defined as:

(1) The *process* by which the threshold of audibility for one sound is raised by the presence of another (masking) sound. (2) The *amount* by which the threshold of audibility of a sound is raised by the presence of another (masking) sound. The unit customarily used is the decibel.

(American Standards Association, 1960.)

It is perhaps unfortunate that this definition includes the observed masking effect as well as the underlying masking processes. Further, the definition does not take into account the phenomenon of partial masking (Scharf, 1971), whereby the loudness of a sound may be decreased by another sound without actually becoming completely inaudible. For the moment, however, we will continue to use the ASA definition.

Hearing theorists have for many years been interested in the physical parameters which affect the masking of one sound by another. The experimental results can tell us a great deal about how the auditory system analyses and discriminates the various components in a mixture of sounds, and the limits of this analysing faculty may allow us to make certain inferences about the processes involved in masking. In addition, a knowledge of the rules governing the masking of one sound by another can be very useful in practical situations. For example, one might want to know the extent to which noise from new machinery in a factory will interfere with the ability of workers to hold conversations or to detect warning signals. One very general result which arose from the early experiments was that a signal will most easily be masked by a sound having frequency components close to, or the same as, those of the signal. This led to the idea that our ability to separate out the elements of a complex sound depends, at least in part, on the frequency resolving power of the basilar membrane. Fletcher, in 1940, formalized this idea with the concept of the critical band (see below). A different kind of masking, called central masking, has been described by Zwislocki (1971). In central masking the threshold of a signal presented to one ear is elevated by a masking sound presented to the other ear. The name 'central' is used because this masking cannot be ascribed to processes in the ear itself (i.e. peripheral processes) but must arise at or beyond the point in the auditory system where inputs from the two ears are combined (i.e. centrally). The threshold shift in central masking is generally small, and rarely exceeds 10 dB.

A second important physical parameter which affects masking is time. Most of this chapter will be devoted to simultaneous masking, in which the signal is presented at the same time as the masker. Later on we will discuss forward masking, in which a signal is masked by a preceding masker, and backward masking, in which the masker follows a signal.

2   THE CRITICAL BAND CONCEPT

Wegel and Lane (1924) published the first systematic investigation of the masking of one pure tone by another. They determined the threshold of audibility of a tone with adjustable frequency in the presence of a masker with fixed frequency and intensity. The graph plotting masked threshold as a function of the frequency of the adjustable tone is known as a masked audiogram. The results of Wegel and Lane were complicated by the occurrence of beats when the signal and masker were close together in frequency. Beats occur because of the changing phase relationship between the signal and masker, which causes the two sounds alternately to reinforce and cancel one another. The resulting amplitude fluctuations occur at a rate equal to the frequency difference between the two tones, and if this rate is not too rapid, audible loudness fluctuations occur. Beats can provide a cue to the presence of the signal even if the signal itself is not audible, and to avoid this problem later experiments (for example, Greenwood, 1961) have used a narrow band of noise as either the signal or masker. Such a noise has 'built in' amplitude fluctuations, and in addition does not produce regular beats when added to a tone.

The masked threshold curves obtained in these experiments show steep slopes on the low frequency side, of between 80 and 240 dB/octave for pure-tone masking, and 55–190 dB/octave for narrowband noise masking. The slopes on the high frequency side are less steep and depend to some extent on the level of the masker. A typical set of results is shown in Figure 3.1. Notice that on the high frequency side the slopes of the curves tend to become shallower at high levels. Thus if the level of a low frequency masker is increased by, say, 10 dB, the masked threshold of a high frequency signal may be elevated by more than 10 dB; the amount of masking grows non-

FIG. 3.1 Masked audiograms for a narrow band of noise centred at 410 Hz. Each curve shows the elevation in pure-tone threshold as a function of frequency for a particular level of the masking noise. From Egan and Hake (1950), by permission of the authors and *J. Acoust. Soc. Am.*

linearly on the high frequency side. This result has certain practical implications for the reproduction of sounds such as speech. Each frequency component in a speech sound will have a masking effect on adjacent frequency components. As the overall level is increased, the low frequencies become more and more effective in masking the higher ones, so that ultimately this 'upward spread of masking' results in a loss of audibility of the important information-carrying mid to high frequency components. The result is that reproduced speech is less intelligible at high overall listening levels. Overall these results confirm Mayer's (1894) observation that it is easier to mask a tone by a second tone of lower frequency than by one of higher frequency, and that frequencies near the signal are more effective than frequencies farther removed.

Fletcher (1940) attempted to account for many of the phenomena of masking with the concept of the auditory filter. He suggested that the peripheral auditory system behaves as if it contained a bank of bandpass filters, with continuously overlapping centre frequencies. When a listener is trying to detect a signal in a noise background, he will attend to the filter with a centre frequency close to that of the signal. Only the components in the noise which pass through the filter will have any effect in masking the signal. Thus the filter will pass the signal but remove a great deal of the noise, and threshold for the signal will be determined by the amount of noise passing through the auditory filter. Fletcher thought that the basilar membrane provided the basis for the filters. Each location on the basilar membrane will respond to a limited range of frequencies, so that each different point corresponds to a filter with a different centre frequency. This assumption is not necessary for the theory, and we should not rule out the possibility that other frequency selective mechanisms are involved (see section 6).

In order to account for the masking of tones by broadband noise Fletcher made a simplifying assumption. He approximated the shape of the auditory filter as a simple rectangle, with a flat top and vertical edges. For such a filter all components within the passband of the filter will be passed equally, and all components outside the passband will be removed. He called the width of the passband the *critical bandwidth*, but he also used the phrase 'critical band' as a convenient way of describing the concept of the auditory filter. Fletcher pointed out that the value of the critical bandwidth could be determined by measuring the threshold of a tone in broadband white noise, given the following hypotheses:

1 Only a narrow band of frequencies surrounding the tone—the critical band—contributes to the masking of the tone.
2 When the noise just masks the tone, the power of the noise inside the critical band is equal to the power of the tone.

Noise power is usually specified in terms of the power in a band of frequencies 1 Hz wide (say from 1000 Hz to 1001 Hz). This is called the noise power density, and is denoted by the symbol N_0. For a white noise N_0 is independent of frequency, so that the total noise power in a band of frequencies W Hz wide is $N_0 \times W$. According to Fletcher, when this width equals the critical bandwidth, the total power in the band will equal the power, P, of the tone at threshold. Thus W is equal to P/N_0, and by measuring P and N_0 we can evaluate W.

The first hypothesis has been confirmed by experiments in which the threshold of a tone is measured in noise of various bandwidths (Hamilton, 1957; Greenwood, 1961). Increases in noise bandwidth beyond a certain critical value have little effect on the threshold of a tone. However, the second hypothesis has turned out not to be strictly accurate (Scharf, 1970); at most frequencies this hypothesis leads to estimates of the critical bandwidth which are about 2.5 times smaller than estimates obtained by more direct methods (see later). For this reason the values obtained by Fletcher's method (see, for example, Hawkins and Stevens, 1950) are called critical ratios, and the term 'critical bandwidth' is reserved for more direct measurements of the bandwidth of complex stimuli or of maskers at which the pattern of responses obtained in various psychoacoustical tasks changes. The difference between the critical ratio function and the generally accepted critical band function is illustrated in Fig. 3.2.

Although Fletcher approximated the auditory filter as a simple rectangle,

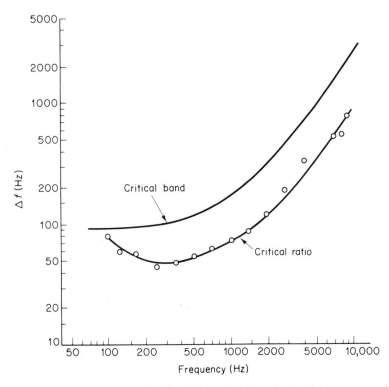

FIG. 3.2 A comparison of the width, Δf, of the critical band as determined by direct measures and as determined from the critical ratio. From Zwicker *et al.* (1957), by permission of the authors and *J. Acoust. Soc. Am.*

he was well aware that the filter was not perfectly rectangular. Indeed the masked audiograms shown in Fig. 3.1 are clearly incompatible with such a shape; a tone or narrow band of noise may mask another tone for frequency separations considerably exceeding the critical bandwidth. We are led to consider the critical band as resembling a filter with sloping edges; the critical bandwidth then becomes some measure of the 'effective' bandwidth of this filter. We will now describe some attempts to measure the characteristics of the auditory filter, in other words, to derive the shape of the auditory filter.

Although the masked audiograms shown in Fig. 3.1 can give us some clue as to the shape of the auditory filter, there is a serious problem in their interpretation. It seems almost certain that the width and shape of the auditory filter change with centre frequency. When the signal frequency is altered, the auditory filter to which the listener attends will alter correspondingly; the listener will attend to the filter which gives the best signal-to-masker ratio. Thus a different auditory filter will be used for each signal frequency, and the shape of the masked audiogram will reflect this. Indeed one way of interpreting the masked audiogram is as a crude indication of the excitation pattern of the masker: the signal will be detected when the excitation it produces is some constant proportion of the excitation produced by the masker in the frequency region of the signal. Thus the threshold of the signal as a function of frequency will be proportional to the masker excitation. The masked audiogram will be parallel to the excitation pattern of the masker, but shifted vertically by a small amount.

In order to determine the shape of the auditory filter at a given centre frequency, it is necessary to keep the frequency of the *signal* fixed. One method of doing this involves a procedure which is analogous in many ways to the determination of a neural tuning curve, and the resulting function is often called a psychophysical tuning curve (PTC). To determine a PTC the signal is fixed in level, usually at a very low level, say, 10 dB SL. The masker can be either a sinusoid or a narrow band of noise, but noise is generally preferred to avoid the complication of beats when the masker frequency is close to that of the signal. For each of several masker frequencies, the level of the masker needed just to mask the signal is determined. Because the signal is at a low level it is assumed that it will produce activity primarily in one auditory filter. It is assumed further that at threshold the masker produces a constant output from that filter, in order to mask the fixed signal. Thus the PTC will tell us the masker level required to produce a fixed output from the auditory filter as a function of frequency. Normally we determine a filter characteristic by plotting the output from the filter for an input varying in frequency and fixed in level (see Chapter 1, section 4 and Fig. 1.4). However, if the filter is linear the two methods will give the same result. Thus, if we assume linearity, the shape of the auditory filter can be obtained simply by inverting the PTC. Examples of some PTCs are given in Fig. 3.3.

The PTCs in Fig. 3.3 are very similar in general form to the neurophysiological tuning curves in Fig. 1.13. Remember that the neural tuning curves are obtained by determining the level of a tone required to produce a fixed output from a single neurone, as a function of the tone's frequency. The similarities in the procedures and the results encourage us to believe that the basic frequency selectivity of the auditory system is established at the level of the auditory nerve, and that the shape of the human auditory filter (or PTC) corresponds to the shape of the neural tuning curve. However, there is a need for caution in reaching this conclusion. In the determination of the neural tuning curve only one tone is present at a time, whereas for the PTC the masker and signal are presented simultaneously. This turns out to be an important point, and we will return to it in section 5. A second problem is that the neural tuning curve is derived from a single neurone, whereas the PTC inevitably involves activity over a group of neurones with slightly different characteristic frequencies. Returning to the

FIG. 3.3 Psychophysical tuning curves (PTCs) determined in simultaneous masking, using sinusoidal signals at 10 dB SL. For each curve the solid diamond below it indicates the frequency and level of the signal. The masker was a sinusoid which had a fixed starting phase relationship to the brief, 50 ms, signal. The masker level required for threshold is plotted as a function of masker frequency (logarithmic scale). The dashed line shows the absolute threshold for the signal. From Vogten (1974), by permission of the author.

filter analogy, we have assumed in our analysis that only one auditory filter is involved, but it might be the case that the listener does not attend to just one filter. When the masker frequency is above the signal frequency the listener might do better to attend to a filter centred just below the signal frequency. If the filter has a relatively flat top, and sloping edges, this will considerably attenuate the masker at the filter output, while loosing very little of the signal. By 'shifting' the filter the listener can achieve a better performance. This strategy is known as 'off-frequency listening', and there is now good evidence that humans do indeed listen 'off-frequency' when it is advantageous to do so. The result of off-frequency listening is that the PTC has a sharper tip than would be obtained if only one auditory filter were involved (Johnson-Davies and Patterson, 1979; O'Loughlin and Moore, 1981).

Patterson (1976) has described an ingenious method of determining auditory filter shape which prevents off-frequency listening. The method is illustrated in Fig. 3.4. The signal is fixed in frequency, and the masker is a noise with a bandstop or notch centred at the signal frequency. The deviation of each edge of the noise from the centre frequency is denoted by Δf. The width of the notch is varied, and the threshold of the signal is determined as a function of notch width. Since the notch is symmetrically placed around the signal frequency, the method cannot reveal asymmetries in the

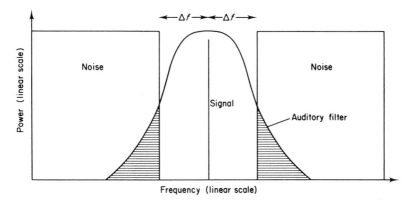

FIG. 3.4 Schematic illustration of the technique used by Patterson (1976) to determine auditory filter shape. The threshold of the sinusoid signal is measured as a function of the width of a spectral notch in the noise masker. The amount of noise passing through the auditory filter centred at the signal frequency is proportional to the shaded areas.

auditory filter, and the analysis assumes that the filter is symmetric on a linear frequency scale. This assumption appears not unreasonable, at least for the top part of the filter and at moderate sound levels; PTCs are quite symmetric around the tips. For a signal symmetrically placed in a band-stop noise, the optimum signal-to-masker ratio at the output of the auditory filter will be achieved with a filter centred at the signal frequency, as illustrated in Fig. 3.4. Shifting the filter, say, upwards will reduce the amount of noise passing through the filter from the lower band, but this will be more than offset by the increase in noise from the upper band.

As the width of the spectral notch is increased, less and less noise will pass through the auditory filter. Thus the threshold of the signal will drop. The amount of noise passing through the auditory filter will be proportional to the area under the filter in the frequency range covered by the noise. This is shown as the shaded areas in Fig. 3.4. If we assume that threshold corresponds to a constant signal-to-masker ratio at the output of the filter, then the change in signal threshold with notch width will tell us how the area under the filter varies with Δf. The area under a function between certain limits is obtained by integrating the value of the function over those limits. Hence by differentiating the function relating threshold to Δf, the height of the filter is obtained. In other words, the height of the filter for a given deviation, Δf, from the centre frequency is equal to the slope of the function relating signal threshold to notch width, at that value of Δf.

A typical auditory filter derived using this method is shown in Fig. 3.5. It has a rounded top and quite steep skirts. Unlike the simple rectangular filter, a filter with this shape cannot be completely specified with a single number, the critical bandwidth. However, some sort of summary statistic is

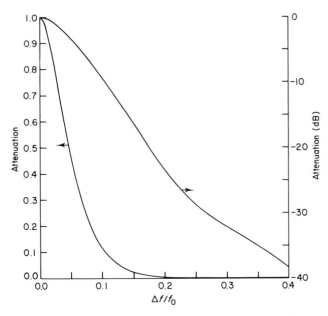

FIG. 3.5 A typical auditory filter shape derived using Patterson's (1976) method. Only half of the filter is shown, since it is assumed to be symmetrical. The abscissa is the deviation from the centre frequency divided by the centre frequency. The left ordinate shows the attenuation in linear power, using the centre of the filter as a reference level. The right ordinate shows attenuation in dB (cf. Fig. 1.4). The arrows indicate the axis to which each curve is to be referred.

useful, and one common measure is the width of the filter at which the response has fallen by a factor of two in power, i.e. by 3 dB (see Chapter 1, section 4). The 3-dB bandwidths of the auditory filters derived using Patterson's method are typically between 10% and 15% of the centre frequency. An alternative measure is the equivalent rectangular bandwidth (ERB). The ERB of a given filter is equal to the bandwidth of a perfect rectangular filter which has a transmission in its passband equal to the maximum transmission of the specified filter and transmits the same power of white noise as the specified filter. In other words, if we take a rectangular filter and scale it to have the same maximum height and area as our filter, then the bandwidth of the rectangular filter is the ERB of our filter. The equalization of height and area is done with the filter characteristic plotted in linear power co-ordinates. The ERBs of the auditory filters derived using Patterson's method are typically between 11% and 17% of the centre frequency. These values are quite close to the estimates of the critical bandwidth obtained in other ways, as will be described in the following sections.

One question we may ask is whether the listener can only attend to one critical band at a time. The answer to this is obviously no, since many of the complex signals which we can perceive and recognize occupy more than one critical band; speech is a prime example of this. Indeed we shall see later that the perception of timbre seems to depend, at least in part, on the distribution of activity across different critical bands. However, in order to predict whether a complex sound will be detected in a given background noise, it is usually sufficient to calculate the detectability of the most prominent frequency components. If we know the shape of the auditory filter centred at each component, then we can calculate the amount of noise passing through the filter, and the signal-to-noise ratio at the output of the filter. If this ratio exceeds some criterion amount in any filter, then the signal will be detected. The criterion amount corresponds to a signal-to-noise ratio of about 1:2.5 or −4 dB; the signal will be detected if its level is not more than 4 dB below that of the noise at the output of the filter.

This model has practical applications, since it allows the prediction of appropriate levels for warning signals in factories and aircraft. In the past, when no theoretical model was available, the signals were often set at excessively high levels, to err on the side of 'safety'. The result was that when a signal 'went off' it was extremely aversive, and disrupted speech communication. The application of the auditory filter model has shown that sometimes signal levels can be reduced by 20 dB (a factor of 100 in power) and remain clearly audible (Patterson and Milroy, 1980).

Another question which arises is whether there is only a discrete number of critical bands, each one adjacent to its neighbours, or whether there is a continuous series of overlapping critical bands. For convenience, data relating to critical bands have often been presented as though the former were the case. For example, Scharf (1970) presented a table showing critical bandwidths for 24 successive critical bands, the upper cutoff frequency for each band being the same as the lower cutoff for the next highest band. While this method of presentation is convenient, it seems clear that critical bands are continuous rather than discrete; there has been no experimental evidence for any discontinuity or break between different critical bands. Thus we may talk about the critical band around any frequency in the audible range which we care to choose.

Since Fletcher first described the critical band concept, a large number of different types of experiment have shown that listeners' responses to complex sounds differ according to whether the stimuli are wider or narrower than the critical band. Further, these different experiments give remarkably similar estimates both of the absolute width of the critical band and of the way the critical band varies as a function of frequency. Thus the critical band phenomenon pervades and summarizes a great variety of data, and provides a valuable guide in the planning of experiments and the analysis of data. For example, it may be used as an indication of the spectral resolution of the auditory system at different centre frequencies. Some of the types of experiment in which critical band phenomena have been observed are described below.

A   *The loudness of complex sounds*

Consider a complex sound of fixed energy (or intensity) having a bandwidth (the range of frequencies over which the energy is spread) of W. If W is less than the critical bandwidth, then the loudness of the sound is more or less independent of W; the sound is judged to be about as loud as a pure tone of equal intensity lying at the centre frequency of the band. However, if W is increased beyond the critical bandwidth, the loudness of the complex begins to *increase*. This has been found to be the case for bands of noise (Zwicker *et al.*, 1957) and for complexes consisting of pure tones whose frequency separation is varied (Sharf, 1961, 1970) (see Fig. 3.6). Thus, for a given

FIG. 3.6 The loudness level in phons of a band of noise centred at 1 kHz, measured as a function of the width of the band. For each of the curves the overall SPL is constant and is indicated in the figure. The dashed line shows that the bandwidth at which loudness begins to increase is the same at all levels tested (except that no increase occurs at the lowest level). From Feldtkeller and Zwicker (1956), by permission of the authors and publisher.

amount of energy, a complex sound will be louder if the energy is spread over a number of critical bands, than if it is all contained within one critical band. This finding has been incorporated in the models described in Chapter 2, which allow the calculation of the loudness of almost any complex sound (see, for example, Zwicker and Scharf, 1965).

The increase in loudness with increasing bandwidth can be understood if we assume that when the bandwidth of a sound is sufficient to occupy more than one critical band, the loudness in adjacent, but nonoverlapping, bands is summed to give the total loudness. Consider the effect of taking two tones very close together in frequency, so as to occupy one critical band, and increasing their frequency separation so that two critical bands are occupied. The intensity in each band will now be half of what it was, since only one tone is present in each band. According to Steven's Power Law, $L = kI^{0.3}$ (see Chapter 2, section 4). Thus halving intensity is equivalent to a reduction in loudness to 0.81 of its original value. The total loudness in the two bands will be $2 \times 0.81 = 1.62$ times the original value. Thus increasing bandwidth beyond the critical band results in an increase in loudness.

A corresponding explanation can be offered in terms of the neurophysiological data. When the two tones are very close in frequency they will, to a large extent, excite the same set of neurones. If the two tones are separated in frequency, they will excite essentially independent sets of neurones. Now at moderate and high intensities the firing rates of individual neurones change relatively slowly as a function of intensity. Thus the decrease in neural firings as a result of halving the effective intensity exciting each set, will be more than offset by the doubling of the number of neurones involved. If, then, loudness is at least related to the total number of neural impulses evoked by the stimulus, it is clear that the loudness of the complex will be greater when the components are widely separated. The argument can easily be extended to cover multicomponent complex tones and bands of noise.

At low sensation levels (around 10–20 dB SL) the loudness of a complex sound is roughly independent of bandwidth. This also is easy to explain. At these low levels firing rates change relatively rapidly with intensity, and so does loudness. The loudness of a single critical band changes almost in direct proportion to intensity, so that increasing the spread of energy from one to two critical bands, for example, produces two component bands each half as loud as the original sound (Scharf, 1970). The total loudness will thus equal that of the original single band, so that loudness is independent of bandwidth. At very low sensation levels (below 10 dB), if we distribute the energy of a complex sound over a wide range of frequencies, then at no frequency will the individual components be audible, nor will there be enough systematic effect on the nervous system for the widely separate components to interact to make the whole audible. Accordingly, near threshold, loudness must decrease as the bandwidth of a complex sound is increased from a subcritical value. As a consequence, if the intensity of a complex sound is increased slowly from a subthreshold value, the rate of growth of loudness will be greater for a wide-band sound than for a narrow-band sound.

B   *The threshold of complex sounds*

When two tones with a small frequency separation are presented together, a sound may be heard even when either tone by itself is below threshold.

Gässler (1954) measured the threshold of multitone complexes consisting of evenly spaced sinusoids. As the number of tones in a complex was increased, the threshold, specified in terms of total energy, remained constant, until the overall spacing of the tones reached the critical bandwidth. Thereafter the threshold increased. Similar results are found when bands of noise are substituted for the multitone complexes. These results indicate that the energies of the individual components in a complex sound will summate, in the detection of that sound, provided that the components lie within a critical band. However, components lying outside the critical band contribute little to the detectability of the sound.

C   *Two-tone masking*

Zwicker (1954) measured the threshold for a narrow band of noise, of centre frequency f, in the presence of two tones, with frequencies on either side of f. He increased the frequency separation of the two tones, starting with a small separation, and found that threshold for the noise signal remained constant until the separation reached a critical value, after which it fell sharply. He took this critical value to be an estimate of the critical bandwidth. Unfortunately the interpretation of this experiment is complicated. One problem is that the lower of the two tones may interact with the noise band to produce a distortion product, or combination tone (combination tones are discussed more fully in Chapter 4, section 3). The listener may detect this distortion product even though the signal itself is inaudible. When precautions are taken to mask the distortion product, then the threshold for the signal does not show an abrupt decrease, but decreases smoothly with increasing frequency separation between the two tones (Patterson and Henning, 1977).

In principle the measurement of threshold with a two-tone masker can be used to derive an estimate of the auditory filter shape in an even simpler way than using a bandstop noise. The value of the threshold for a given separation of the tones from the noise signal should give a direct indication of the height of the filter at that distance from the centre frequency. Again, however, it is necessary to make some assumptions about filter symmetry. Patterson and Henning assumed that the filter was symmetric on a linear frequency scale, and used tones whose arithmetic mean frequency equalled the signal frequency. Others, including Zwicker (1954), assumed that the filter was approximately symmetric on a logarithmic frequency scale, and hence used tones with a geometric mean frequency equal to that of the signal. Although there are differences between the results of these different workers, estimates of the critical bandwidth obtained using two-tone maskers are broadly in line with those obtained using other methods. For an extensive review of results obtained using two-tone maskers, the reader is referred to Rabinowitz *et al.* (1980).

D   *Sensitivity to phase*

The sounds which we encounter in everday life often change in frequency and amplitude from moment to moment. In the laboratory the perception of such sounds is often studied using either frequency-modulated or amplitude-modulated sine waves. Such waves consist of a carrier frequency (a sine wave) upon which some other signal is impressed. In amplitude modulation (AM) the carrier's amplitude is varied so as to follow the magnitude of a modulating sine wave, while the carrier frequency remains unchanged. In frequency modulation (FM) the carrier's instantaneous frequency is varied in proportion to the modulating signal's magnitude, but the amplitude remains constant. The two types of waveform are illustrated in Fig. 3.7.

Although these waveforms are quite complex, they are periodic, and so they can be analysed into a series of sinusoidal components. For an AM wave the results of the analysis are very simple: the spectrum contains just three frequency components. If the carrier frequency is f_c and the modulating frequency is g, then the three components are $f_c - g$, f_c and $f_c + g$ (all in Hz). For an FM wave the spectrum is somewhat more complex, but if the depth of modulation (which is related to the size of the frequency swing) is small, then the FM wave can also be considered as consisting of three components: $f_c - g$, f_c and $f_c + g$. Under some conditions an AM wave and an FM wave may have identical frequency components, the only difference between them being in the relative phase of the components. If, then, the two types of wave are perceived differently, the difference is likely to arise from a sensitivity to the relative phase of the components.

Zwicker (1952) measured one aspect of the perception of such stimuli, namely the just detectable amounts of amplitude or frequency modulation, for various rates of modulation. He found that for high rates of modulation, where the frequency components are widely spaced, the detectability of FM and AM was equal when the components in each type of wave were of equal amplitude. However, when all three components fell within a critical band, AM was more easily detectable than FM. Thus it appears that we are only sensitive to the relative phase of the components, in the detection of modulation, when those components lie within a critical band.

It is not at present clear whether this finding can be generalized to the perception of suprathreshold levels of modulation, or to other aspects of our sensitivity to phase. Indeed there is some evidence to the contrary. For example, it has been shown that subjects can respond to cues associated with phase changes between octave complexes (e.g. 500 Hz and 1000 Hz), in which the components are separated by more than a critical band (Raiford and Schubert, 1971; Lamore, 1975). Further work is needed to clarify the nature of these discrepancies, and to determine the applicability of the critical band concept to the phase sensitivity of the ear.

FIG. 3.7 Waveform of an amplitude-modulated wave (upper) and a frequency-modulated wave (lower).

E   *The discrimination of partials in complex tones*

According to Ohm's (1843) Acoustical Law, the ear is able to separate out the individual sinusoidal components in a complex periodic sound. This ability is called 'frequency analysis', although that term is also used to describe a more general and basic process entering any psychoacoustic task involving frequency resolution. Plomp (1964) used a complex tone with 12 sinusoidal components to investigate the frequency analysing power of the auditory system. The listener was presented with two comparison tones, one of which was of the same frequency as a partial in the complex; the other lay halfway between that frequency and the frequency of the adjacent higher or lower partial. The listener had to judge which of these two tones was a component of the complex. Plomp used two types of complex: a harmonic complex containing harmonics 1 to 12, where the frequencies of the components were integral multiples of that of the fundamental; and a non-harmonic complex, where the frequencies of the components were mistuned from simple frequency ratios. He found that for both kinds of complex only the first five to eight components were discriminable. If it is assumed that a partial will only be distinguished when it is separated from its neighbour by at least one critical band, then the results can be used to estimate the critical band. Above 1000 Hz the estimates obtained in this way coincide with other critical band measures. Below 1000 Hz the estimates are about two-thirds as large. When Plomp repeated the experiment using a two-tone complex, he found that the partials could be distinguished at smaller frequency separations than were found for multitone complexes.

Thus, while the results are roughly in line with other measures of critical bandwidth, there are discrepancies, especially at low frequencies. It is possible that the analysis of partials from a complex sound depends in part on factors other than pure frequency resolution. Some indication of this is given by the work of Soderquist (1970). He compared musicians and non-musicians in a task very similar to that of Plomp, and found that the musicians were markedly superior. This result could mean that musicians have narrower critical bands, but this is unlikely if the critical band reflects a basic physiological process, as is generally assumed (Scharf, 1970). It seems more plausible that some other mechanism is involved in this task and that musicians, because of their greater experience, are able to make more efficient use of this mechanism. Haggard (1974) also reports comparisons of different measures of the critical bandwidth, and suggests that discrepancies at low frequencies may be explained by the intervention of non-critical band mechanisms. This problem is discussed more fully in the following section.

3   THE NATURE OF THE CRITICAL BAND AND MECHANISMS OF MASKING

Figure 3.8 shows the value of the critical bandwidth as a function of centre frequency. It may be seen that data from a large number of experiments produce quite similar estimates of the critical bandwidth. It seems that

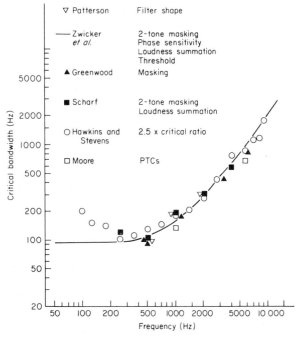

FIG. 3.8 The value of the critical bandwidth as a function of frequency. The results of several different sets of measurements are shown. Adapted from Scharf (1970), by permission of the author.

sound energy within a critical band is treated differently from energy outside the band, and that subcritical stimuli are treated similarly with respect to masking, loudness and threshold. The mechanism is analogous in many ways to a system of bandpass filters; stimuli within the same filter are not treated separately, whereas stimuli falling in different filters are. We should remember, however, that the critical band is *not* a rectangular filter, and that the value of the critical bandwidth is only an estimate of one aspect of the filter characteristic. Thus is some cases there are perceptual interactions between stimuli which are separated by much more than one critical band. Examples may be found in the masked audiograms of narrowband maskers and in our sensitivity to changes in relative phase. Sometimes, also, our analysing abilities appear to be greater than would be predicted from the critical bandwidth. For example, at low frequencies partials can be heard out from complex tones when they are separated by somewhat less than a critical band.

A   The origin of the auditory filter

The locus of the critical band mechanism is still uncertain, although the frequency-resolving power of the basilar membrane is almost certainly its initial basis. However, the patterns of vibration observed on the basilar membrane are quite broad in comparison with critical band estimates (von Békésy, 1960), which suggests that some sharpening mechanism must be involved. Single neurones in the auditory nerve appear to be more sharply tuned (see Chapter 1), and this has led to the suggestion that there is a 'second filter' located between the basilar membrane and the neurones. One possible way in which a sharpening of frequency selectivity might be achieved is by a process of lateral inhibition or lateral suppression. In such a process weak inputs to one group of receptors (hair cells or neurones) are suppressed by strong inputs to adjacent receptors. Von Békésy (1960) suggested that lateral inhibition caused the broad patterns of excitation on the basilar membrane to be transformed into sharply circumscribed areas of excitation surrounded by areas of inhibition. He called the combined area of excitation and inhibition the neural inhibitory unit, and Zwislocki (1965) calculated the size of this unit to correspond to the critical bandwidth.

Carterette *et al.* (1969) attempted to provide psychoacoustic evidence for such lateral inhibition in an experiment using bands of noise with very sharp spectral edges. They reasoned by analogy with the visual situation in which a bright band of light is viewed against a dark background. The edges of such a band look brighter than the centre of the band, while the area of the background adjacent to the band looks darker than the rest of the background. This phenomenon is generally ascribed to lateral inhibition; receptors responding to the edge of the band will be inhibited less than receptors responding to the centre of the band, owing to the adjacent dark area, thus producing a 'bright' band. The 'dark' band in the background can be explained similarly by assuming a spread of inhibition from receptors responding to the edge of the light band. The situation is illustrated schematically in Fig. 3.9. The 'bright' and 'dark' bands are known as Mach bands.

Carterette and co-workers argued that neural responses to the noise bands should be enhanced in those neurones responding to the edges of the noise band, by analogy with the 'bright' bands in the visual situation. They suggested that this enhanced neural response to the noise should be revealed by an elevated masked threshold for tones whose frequencies coincided with the edges of the band, and they claimed to find exactly this effect. However, similar work by Rainbolt and Small (1972) failed to show any edge effects, and the consensus of opinion is that such experiments do not provide clear evidence for lateral inhibition. Nevertheless, effects of the type predicted by Carterette and co-workers do occur with masking which is not simultaneous (see section 4).

If the critical band mechanism does depend on some neural inhibitory process, then it is reasonable to expect that the process would take several

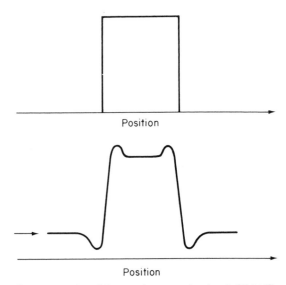

Position

Position

FIG. 3.9 Schematic representation of the neural response to a band of light. The upper part of the figure is the luminance profile of the stimulus and the lower part is the neural response, which is influenced by lateral inhibition. Notice the elevation of neural activity at the edge of the band and the reduction below the spontaneous level (indicated by the arrow) just outside it.

milliseconds to become effective; work on lateral inhibition in other sensory systems has indicated a time constant of about 30 ms. Some critical band experiments have indicated that the time required for the critical band to be effective is considerably less than this. For example, Port (1963) found that measures of loudness summation for short-duration stimuli (as short as 1 ms) gave the same value for the critical band as was found at long durations. Other experimental results, involving thresholds (e.g. Zwicker, 1965a, b; Srinivasan, 1971) have been taken to indicate a wider critical band at short durations. At the present time the reasons for the discrepancies are not entirely clear. Zwicker and Fastl (1972) in a review of this area concluded that the results which have been taken to indicate a wider critical band at short durations can, in fact, be explained in other ways, so that it is not necessary to assume a development of the critical band with time. Rather, the critical band mechanism may be viewed as a system of filters which are permanently and instantaneously present. This makes it unlikely that any neural inhibitory process is involved in the formation of the critical band. It is possible, however, that some form of lateral suppression might operate at a very early stage in the processing of the auditory stimulus, for example at the level of the hair cell (Sellick and Russell, 1979). Such a process could operate very fast. We will return to the question of lateral suppression and the 'second filter' in section 5.

B   *The mechanism of masking—swamping or*
     suppression?

It is clear that Fletcher's original conception of the critical band as a system of filters, each responding to a limited range of frequencies, has not been modified in any fundamental way by more recent work. However, Fletcher's ideas about the mechanisms involved in masking have not stood up so well. He suggested that masking involved the saturation of certain channels (i.e. critical bands) by the masking stimulus. Once a channel was saturated, the response of that channel would not change when a signal was presented, so that the signal would be masked. Thus for Fletcher masking involved a 'pre-emption' of certain channels by the masking stimulus. This concept of masking does not fit in very well with the known properties of the auditory nervous system. For example, even a tone at a very low level (say 20 dB SL) can have a masking effect on tones of adjacent frequencies, while at the same time it is unlikely that such a tone would produce any neural saturation.

There are now two common conceptions of the mechanism by which masking occurs. The first, which is most common among psychologists, is that masking involves the *swamping* of the activity evoked by the signal. If the masker produces a significant amount of activity in the channels (auditory filters or critical bands) which would normally respond to the signal, then the activity added by the signal may be undetectable. Consider, for example, the case of a tone together with a wideband white noise. When the tone is at its masked threshold, the level of the tone is about 4 dB *less* than the level of the noise in the critical band around the tone. This is the average discrepancy between critical bands and critical ratios; 4 dB corresponds to a power ratio of about 2.5:1. The combined excitation produced by the tone plus noise will be about 1.5 dB higher in level than that produced by the noise alone. Thus one might argue that 1.5 dB represent the minimum increment in excitation necessary for detection of the tone. If the tone is much lower in level than the noise passing through the critical band, then it will produce a negligible increment in excitation. For example, if the difference in levels is 20 dB, the increment in level will be less than 0.05 dB. Thus the excitation produced by the tone will be 'swamped' by that produced by the masker. We should note that the task required of the subject may differ somewhat according to the manner of stimulus presentation. For a steady tone presented in a continuous background noise, the subject would have to detect that the excitation at some location (in one critical band) exceeded that at surrounding locations. Thus the subject would have to detect that there was a peak in the pattern of excitation (see, for example, Greenwood, 1961; Schubert, 1969). If, on the other hand, the tone was interrupted, or presented intermittently, the subject could compare the level in the same critical band on successive occasions. This might make the task somewhat easier. Whichever of these two is appropriate, masking will only take place if the masker produces excitation in the channels (critical bands) which would otherwise respond to the signal.

An alternative view of masking, which is quite popular among neuro-physiologists, is that the masker *suppresses* the activity which the signal would evoke if presented alone. This is most easily explained by analogy with the 'two-tone suppression' observed in single neurones of the auditory nerve, which was described in Chapter 1, section 6. The neural response to a tone at the characteristic frequency (CF) of a neurone may be suppressed by a tone which does not itself produce excitatory activity in that neurone. The suppression may be sufficient to drive the firing rate of the neurone down to its spontaneous rate, and we might argue that this corresponds to the masking of the tone at CF. In the more general case, the second 'masking' tone might fall within the excitatory area of the neurone, and produce an increase in net firing rate. We could not then determine from the firing *rate* whether suppression was occurring, but we could determine this by looking at the proportion of the activity of the neurone which is phase locked to the original tone. Using this measure, it is clear that suppression can occur for suppressing tones which are well inside the excitatory area of the neurone. Masking in this case might correspond both to swamping and suppression.

At the moment there seems to be no clear way of distinguishing between these two mechanisms of masking. However, there is general agreement that the threshold of a signal in simultaneous masking is quite well predicted by modelling the auditory system as a system of *linear* filters. Suppression is a markedly nonlinear process; the response to two simultaneous inputs is not the linear sum of the responses to each input separately. The fact that the linear model works so well encourages the belief that swamping is the major mechanism of simultaneous masking. This is in accord with the conclusion of the previous section, that effects of suppression are not revealed in simul-taneous masking. A possible reason for this will be presented in section 5. We should, however, not rule out the possibility that suppression plays some role in simultaneous masking, and that it influences the results of other measures of the critical band. For example, suppression may well affect the loudness of complex sounds, and the way loudness changes with bandwidth.

C   *The neural code used for signal detection*

So far we have discussed the basis of the auditory filter, and the mechanism by which the neural activity evoked by the signal might be 'masked'. We turn now to a consideration of what aspect of the neural activity evoked by the signal might be used for detection. The most common assumption is that the *amount* of activity is critical, and that neural firing *rates* are the important variable. However, an alternative possibility is that information in the temporal patterns of neural firing is used. The theoretical issues involved are in many ways similar to those which we discussed in relation to the intensity discrimination of signals in noise. Indeed, many researchers would consider that the detection of a signal in a masker is equivalent to the detection of an increment in intensity.

One major problem in explaining masking in terms of the distribution of the amount of activity across neurones with different CFs comes from a consideration of neural saturation. As was discussed in Chapter 2, section 6, the majority of neurones at a given CF will be saturated for a stimulus more than 60 dB above threshold. Thus if we add a tone to a high-level white noise, the majority of neurones with CFs close to that of the tone will be saturated by the noise, and little or no change in amount of activity will be observed. We would expect on the basis of this that the signal-to-noise ratio required at threshold would increase markedly at high sound levels. In fact, however, the signal-to-noise ratio at threshold is remarkably constant over a wide range of levels (Hawkins and Stevens, 1950), except perhaps for high frequencies (Moore, 1975). This leads us to suspect that some other form of information must be available to signal the presence of the tone at high levels.

One source of information which is available over a very wide range of intensities is contained in the temporal patterns of neural firing. In response to a single pure tone, neural firings tend to occur at a particular phase of the stimulating waveform, so that intervals between successive nerve firings are multiples of the period of that tone. This phase-locking occurs for stimulating frequencies up to about 5 kHz. In response to a complex stimulus, the pattern of phase-locking observed in a given neurone will depend upon which components in the stimulus are most effective in driving that neurone. For example, in response to two tones which are nonharmonically related, discharges may be phase-locked to one tone, or the other, or both tones simultaneously. Which of these occurs is determined by the relative intensities of the two tones and their frequencies in relation to the response area of the neurone. When phase-locking occurs to only one tone of a pair, each of which is effective when presented alone, the temporal structure of the response may be indistinguishable from that which occurs when that tone is presented alone. Thus the dominant tone appears to 'capture' the response of the neurone. This effect appears to be partly mediated by suppression of the nondominant tone, although in general it will arise from a mixture of swamping and suppression.

It is possible that the 'capture' effect underlies the masking of one tone by another. Clearly, the results we have described apply only to the responses of single auditory nerve fibres, and their application to the responses over an ensemble of nerve fibres is not entirely clear. However, recent recordings of the responses of many different nerve fibres within the same animal, indicate that information about the relative levels of components in complex sounds *is* contained in the time patterns of neural impulses, even at sound levels sufficient to produce saturation in the majority of neurones (Kim and Molnar, 1979; Sachs and Young, 1980). In general the temporal patterns of response will be dominated by the most prominent frequency components in the complex stimulus, with the result that there may be little or no phase-locking to weak components which are close in frequency to stronger ones. Thus it seems reasonable to suggest that a tone (with a frequency below about 5 kHz) will be masked when its presence produces no detectable effect on the time pattern of nerve impluses evoked by the stimulus as a whole. This argument can easily be applied to the masking of a tone by wideband noise. A tone will evoke neural firings with a well-defined temporal pattern; the time intervals between successive nerve firings will be integral multiples of the period of the tone. A noise will evoke, in the same neurones, a much less regular pattern of neural firings. Thus we might argue that a tone will be detected when the nerve fibres responding to it show a certain degree of temporal regularity in their patterns of firing. If the temporal regularity is less than this amount the tone will be masked. Notice that the neurones involved in the detection of the tone will be those with CFs close to that of the tone. The action of the auditory filter will be important in reducing the contribution of the noise to the neural responses, and the neurones with CFs close to the tone frequency will be the ones showing the greatest degree of temporal regularity.

The idea that we use the temporal patterns of neural firing to analyse complex stimuli can provide an explanation for the discrepancies observed by Plomp (1964) in human subjects' abilities to analyse partials from two-tone complexes and multitone complexes. As was mentioned earlier, Plomp found that a partial could only be 'heard out' from a multitone complex if that partial were separated from neighbouring partials by about one critical bandwidth. However, for a two-tone complex the partials could be identified for separations less than this. Figure 3.10 shows some idealized excitation patterns for a two-tone complex and a multitone complex. For a multitone complex the excitation at CFs corresponding to the higher partials arises from the interaction of several partials of comparable effectiveness. Thus there is no CF where the temporal pattern of response will be determined primarily by one partial. However, for a two-tone complex there will be certain CFs (indicated by arrows) where the temporal pattern of response will be dominated by one or the other of the component tones; this would correspond to the capture effect which we described earlier. Thus the temporal patterns of firing in these neurones could signal the individual pitches of the component tones. This could explain why partials are more easily heard out from a two-tone complex than a multitone complex.

It should be emphasized that the extent to which the auditory system is

and the course of masking as a function of time is determined; and (3) forward masking, in which the probe follows the masker (also known as post-stimulatory masking). Foward masking is just one of three conceptually distinct processes which may affect the threshold of a probe presented after another sound; the other two are adaptation and fatigue, which were discussed in Chapter 2. Forward masking is distinguished from adaptation and fatigue primarily by the range of time intervals involved, although the separation is rarely clear-cut. Forward masking is generally considered to be limited to a time of a few hundred milliseconds after the cessation of the masker.

We summarize below the main features of nonsimultaneous masking, based on the work of Elliot (1971) and others.

1   The nearer in time to the masker that the signal occurs, the more is its threshold elevated. This always occurs when the masker level is above 40 dB SL. Sometimes the curve relating threshold to the time delay between masker and signal is U shaped, showing 'sensitization', or a lowering of threshold, when the signal occurs soon after a 'not too intense' stimulus of similar frequency characteristics (Moore and Welsh, 1970).

2   More backward than forward masking occurs for very short time intervals between the signal and the masker (we will denote such a silent interval by the symbol Δt). Also, in simultaneous masking the threshold is more elevated for a signal occurring soon after the onset of the masker than for a signal occurring later.

3   Most backward or forward masking occurs within about $\pm$ 100 ms of the masker onset or termination.

4   Masking is more pronounced when signal and masker are presented to the same ear, although dichotic listening also produces backward masking and small amounts of forward masking.

5   The amount of masking increases with increasing masker duration for Δt between 1 and 20 ms, but is approximately independent of masker duration outside this range.

6   Both backward and forward masking are influenced by the relation between the frequencies of the signal and the masker (just as in the case of simultaneous masking). Frequency selective backward masking may occur over time intervals up to 100 ms. In forward masking the threshold may be elevated for frequencies outside a narrow masker band, when the masker is of short duration (25 ms). This is another example of threshold experiments indicating a wider critical band at short durations (see section 3).

7   Increments in masker intensity do not produce corresponding increments in amount of forward and backward masking. For example, if the

masker level is increased by 10 dB, the masked threshold may only increase by 3 dB. This contrasts with simultaneous masking, where, at least for wideband maskers, threshold usually corresponds to a constant signal-to-masker ratio.

8 The masking of a probe signal in a short temporal gap between two maskers is greater than would be predicted from a simple summing of the amounts of backward and forward masking, i.e. the two types of masking interact.

The basis of forward and backward masking is still not clear. Forward masking could be explained in terms of a reduction in sensitivity of recently stimulated cells, or in terms of a persistence in the pattern of neural activity evoked by the masker. Backward masking is more difficult to explain, since it is the interference of a later masker with a signal which is physically completed, although clearly the processing of that signal cannot be complete. Further, backward masking occurs over time intervals which are longer than those required for the development and decay of the travelling wave pattern along the basilar membrane. Thus physiological processing of the stimulus is also implicated; the excitation pattern from one signal, or the central activity involved in its processing, must persist for some time after the cessation of that signal if the later activity produced by a more intense signal can overtake and obscure that from the earlier signal.

Elliot (1967) has suggested that a number of distinct but interacting phenomena are required to explain the data summarized in points 1–8. One such phenomenon is the time-dependent organization of *frequency contours*, for stimuli containing narrow band(s) of frequencies. According to Elliot, frequency contours are representations, at one or more levels in the auditory system, of the edges of a band or bands. Elliot suggested that a time-dependent organization of the frequency contours would explain the finding that in forward masking by brief narrowband maskers threshold may be elevated for frequencies outside the narrow masker band; the narrowband masker would initially produce a wideband representation within the auditory system, and the narrowband characteristics would only develop after a certain processing time had elapsed. It is not clear whether this explanation is appropriate. The problem is analogous in many ways to that of the time course of the development of the critical band, and some experiments indicate that the critical band is present even for stimuli of short duration (see above).

Duifhuis (1973) has suggested that at short Δt values (less than about 20 ms) the dominant component in both forward and backward masking results from a temporal overlap of cochlear responses. That is to say, the vibrations evoked by the first stimulus on the basilar membrane will not have completely died away before the second stimulus arrives. If this is the case, then backward and forward masking effects at short Δt values should be more pronounced for low frequencies than for high (de Boer, 1969a, b). A comparison of the results of different workers (Elliot, 1962; Gruber and Boerger, 1971; Patterson, 1971) reveals that this is indeed the case. Further, Duifhuis (1971) has demonstrated that for short Δt's the masked threshold is affected by the relative phase of the masker and the signal, as would be expected if there were a temporal overlap of the patterns of vibration on the basilar membrane (although the phase effect could occur at higher levels in the auditory system if phase is preserved).

While at least part of the observed masking at short Δt's might be explained in terms of peripheral mechanisms, such as fatigue and temporal overlap of vibration patterns, is is clear that, for backward masking, higher neural levels must be involved. This is suggested not only by the length of time over which the effects last, but also by the fact that backward masking effects are observed in dichotic listening. Further, these effects occur both for simple stimuli, such as tones and bands of noise (Deatherage and Evans, 1969), and for complex stimuli, such as speech sounds (Darwin, 1971). Darwin's results show that the extraction of complex auditory features from a target can be disrupted by the subsequent dichotic presentation of a sound sharing certain features with the target.

The data summarized above indicate that there is a lack of symmetry between forward and backward masking effects. For example, more backward than forward masking occurs at very short Δt's, for both monaural and dichotic presentations of the masker and the probe. This lack of symmetry, and the fact that effects greater than would be predicted from a simple summation are observed in situations involving both forward and backward masking, indicate that different underlying processes may be involved in these two types of masking. Again, effects exceeding simple summation have been found both for tone stimuli (Elliot, 1969; Patterson, 1971) and for speech stimuli (Dirks and Bower, 1970).

In summary, the empirical phenomena of forward and backward masking are now fairly well known, although the exact masking functions obtained depend to some extent on the specific experimental situation used. The nature of the underlying processes is less well understood. Contributions from a number of different sources may be important, these contributions being related to different neural levels in the auditory system. At the pheripheral level temporal overlap of patterns of vibration may be important at short Δt values. Also at this level some sort of temporary fatigue effect may play a role in forward masking. At higher neural levels a persistence of the excitation pattern evoked by the stimulus seems to be required. The nature of the interactions between the excitation patterns of the signal and masker remains uncertain.

5   EVIDENCE FOR LATERAL SUPPRESSION FROM NON-
      SIMULTANEOUS MASKING

We described earlier Rainbolt and Small's (1972) replication of the work of
Carterette *et al.* (1969), measuring the thresholds of sinusoids in bands of
noise with sharp spectral edges. Rainbolt and Small concluded that there
were no edge effects indicative of any form of lateral suppression. Houtgast
(1972) has argued that simultaneous masking is not an appropriate tool for
detecting the effects of lateral suppression. Its use is based upon the assumption that when the nervous activity corresponding to some frequency region
is influenced by lateral suppression (e.g. at the edges of a bandpass noise
with a sharp cutoff in frequency), the masked threshold for a test tone would
also be affected near that frequency. Houtgast argued that, in simultaneous
masking, the masking stimulus and the test tone are processed
simultaneously in the same channel. Thus any suppression in that channel
will affect the nervous activity caused by both the test tone and the masking
noise. In other words, the signal-to-noise ratio in a given frequency region
will be unaffected by lateral suppression, and thus the threshold of the test
tone will remain unaltered.

Houtgast suggested that this difficulty could be overcome by presenting
the masker and the test tone successively (i.e. by using a forward masking
technique). If lateral suppression does occur, then its effects will be seen in
the forward masking threshold curve provided that: (1) in the chain of levels
of neural processing the level at which the lateral suppression occurs is not
later than the level at which most of the forward masking effect arises; (2)
the suppression built up by the masker has decayed by the time that the test
tone is presented (otherwise the problems described for simultaneous masking will be encountered).

Houtgast used a repeated-gap masking technique, in which the masker
was presented with a continuous rhythm of 150 ms on, 50 ms off. Probe
tones, with a duration of 20 ms, were presented in the gaps. He used as
maskers high- and low-pass noises with sharp spectral cut-offs (96 dB/octave),
and also a sound with a spectral peak (tone plus noise). The masking curves
obtained showed edge effects, similar to Mach bands in vision; both 'bright'
band and 'dark' band effects could be discerned. No such effects were
observed in the case of simultaneous masking. Thus forward masking does
reveal the type of effects which a suppression process would produce.

Houtgast also noted a very remarkable feature of the repeated-gap technique; when the bursts of probe tone are just above the threshold, they
sound like a continuous tone. Only at higher levels of the probe tone is the
perception in accord with the physical time pattern, namely a series of tone
bursts. Houtgast called the level of the probe tone, at which its character

changed from pulsating to continuous, the pulsation threshold. He showed that the existence of such a pulsation threshold is a very general feature of alternating stimuli, and is not restricted to the alternation of two stimuli with a frequency component in common. However, the phenomenon does not occur when the masker contains no frequency component in the neighbourhood of the probe tone. He suggested the following interpretation of the phenomenon: "When a tone and a stimulus S are alternated (alternation cycle about 4 Hz), the tone is perceived as being continuous when the transition from S to tone causes no (perceptible) increase of nervous activity in any frequency region." In terms of patterns of excitation this suggests that "the peak of the nervous activity pattern of the tone at pulsation threshold level just reaches the nervous activity pattern of S". Given this hypothesis, the pulsation threshold for a test tone as a function of frequency can be considered to map out the apparent spectrum of the stimulus S (i.e. its excitation pattern) on the nervous activity level. The pulsation threshold curve will thus reflect both the frequency-analysing properties of the cochlea and the effects of lateral suppression.

Following the pioneering work of Houtgast, many workers have reported that there are systematic differences between the results obtained using simultaneous and nonsimultaneous masking techniques. One major difference is that nonsimultaneous masking reveals effects which can be directly attributed to suppression. A good demonstration of this involves a psychophysical analogue of neural two-tone suppression. Houtgast (1973, 1974) measured the pulsation threshold for a 1 kHz 'signal' alternating with a 1 kHz 'masker'. He then added a second tone to the 'masker' and measured the pulsation threshold again. He found that sometimes the addition of this second tone produced a *reduction* in the pulsation threshold, and he attributed this to a suppression of the 1 kHz component in the 'masker' by the second component. If the 1 kHz component is suppressed, then there will be less activity in the frequency region around 1 kHz, producing a drop in the pulsation threshold. The second tone was most effective as a 'suppressor' when it was somewhat more intense than the 1 kHz component, and above it in frequency. A 'suppression' of about 20 dB could be produced by a 'suppressor' at 1.2 kHz. Houtgast mapped out the combinations of frequency and intensity over which the 'suppressor' produced a 'suppression' exceeding 3 dB. He found two regions, one above 1 kHz and one below, and the regions were similar to the suppression areas which can be observed in single neurones of the auditory nerve (see Fig. 1.18). Similar results have been found using a forward masking technique (Shannon, 1976).

A second major difference between the two types of masking is that the frequency selectivity revealed in nonsimultaneous masking is greater than that revealed in simultaneous masking. A well-studied example of this is the psychophysical tuning curve (PTC), which was discussed in section 2. PTCs are obtained by determining the level of a masker required to mask a fixed signal as a function of masker frequency. We pointed out earlier the general resemblance in shape of the PTC and the neural tuning curve. PTCs determined in forward masking, or using the pulsation threshold method, are typically sharper than those obtained in simultaneous masking. An example is given in Fig. 3.11. The difference is particularly marked on the high

FIG. 3.11 Comparison of psychophysical tuning curves (PTCs) determined in simultaneous masking (squares) and forward masking (circles). The signal was a brief 1 kHz sinusoid with a level of 10 dB SL. The masker level required for threshold is plotted as a function of masker frequency. From Moore (1978).

frequency side of the tuning curve. According to Houtgast (1974) this difference arises because the internal representation of the masker (its excitation pattern), is sharpened by a suppression process, with the greatest sharpening occurring on the low frequency side. In simultaneous masking, the effects of suppression will not be seen, since any reduction of the masker activity in the frequency region of the signal will be accompanied by a similar reduction in signal evoked activity. In other words, the signal-to-masker ratio in the frequency region of the signal will be unaffected by the suppression. In forward masking, on the other hand, the suppression will not affect the signal. For maskers with frequencies above that of the signal, the effect of suppression will be to increase the masker level required to mask the signal. Thus the suppression will be revealed as an increase in the high frequency slope of the PTC. According to this explanation, the PTC in simultaneous masking does not indicate the level of the masker required to produce a fixed *amount* of activity in the signal channel (critical band). Rather, it indicates the masker level required to produce a constant *signal-*

to-masker ratio within that channel. The PTC determined in nonsimultaneous masking would, however, indicate the masker level required to produce a fixed amount of activity in the signal channel. Thus the nonsimultaneous PTC would provide a better analogue of the neural tuning curve.

Although this explanation is appealing, it is not the only way of accounting for the sharper PTC obtained in nonsimultaneous masking. An alternative explanation is that, in simultaneous masking, the low level signal may be suppressed by the masker, so that it falls below absolute threshold. The neural data indicate that tones falling outside of the region bounded by the neural tuning curve can produce suppression. Thus the PTC in simultaneous masking might map out the boundaries of the more broadly tuned suppression region. The signal in nonsimultaneous masking could not be suppressed in this way, so that, as for the other explanation, the nonsimultaneous PTC provides a better analogue of the tuning curve. A major difference between these two explanations is that the first assumes that suppression will sharpen the excitation pattern of a single sinusoidal component, whereas the second assumes only that one component may suppress another; suppression will not necessarily affect the internal representation of a single component. At the present time there is no clear consensus as to which of these two views is correct. We should also remember that the shape of the PTC is likely to be influenced by off-frequency listening (see section 2), so that even in nonsimultaneous masking it will not correspond accurately to the neural tuning curve (O'Loughlin and Moore, 1981).

Several other methods of estimating frequency selectivity have indicated sharper tuning in nonsimultaneous masking. For example, auditory filter shapes estimated in forward masking using a notch noise masker (as described in section 2), have 3-dB bandwidths abut 17% less and slopes about 50% greater than those estimated in simultaneous masking (Moore and Glasberg, 1981). This encourages us to believe that a general consequence of suppression is an enhancement of frequency selectivity.

We may conclude that results from nonsimultaneous masking do show clearly the types of effects which would be expected if a suppression mechanism were operating. The level at which the effects occur is uncertain, but the commonest assumption has been that they arise at a very early stage in auditory processing, possibly at or close to the point of transduction of mechanical movements to neural impulses. Houtgast has pointed out that the high frequency sides of PTCs in simultaneous masking and of tuning curves on the basilar membrane have similar slopes (about 100 dB/octave), whereas the slopes obtained in nonsimultaneous masking resemble those found for the tuning curves of primary auditory neurones (200–500 dB/oct). Thus it is possible that the sharp tuning seen in auditory nerve fibres includes the effects of suppression. However, it also seems clear that suppression on its own is not sufficient to account for the differences between basilar membrane and neural tuning. The biggest differences occur on the *low-frequency* sides of tuning curves; the basilar membrane behaves almost as a low-pass filter whereas neural tuning curves have a distinct bandpass characteristic. Suppression as measured psychophysically appears to have little, if any, effect on the low frequency side of the tuning curve (or the high frequency side of the excitation pattern). Furthermore, psychophysical estimates of frequency selectivity obtained in simultaneous masking, which presumably *do not* include the effects of suppression, still indicate a well-tuned bandpass characteristic. It appears, then, that we cannot identify suppression with the 'second filter'; some other frequency selective mechanism must be involved in producing the bandpass character of neural and psychophysical tuning. Suppression might be a part of the action of the 'second filter', or it might act as an independent 'third filter', albeit a nonlinear filter, whose action is not revealed in simultaneous masking.

6   THE 'SECOND FILTER'

In recent years the 'second filter' has been the subject of intensive research. Some workers have argued that there is no need to postulate a second filter; rather we should assume that the amplitude or velocity of vibration at a given point on the basilar membrane does not represent the effective input to the hair cells (see, for example, Tonndorf, 1970). Other variables, such as the shearing motion between the basilar membrane and the tectorial membrane, might be more sharply tuned. However the case for a 'second filter' has been strengthened by the observation of Robertson and Manley (1974) that the normal sharp tuning seen in auditory neurones can be altered by reducing the oxygen supply to the animal. Slowing the rate of ventilation makes the tuning curves less sharp, and at the same time decreases the sensitivity around the tip. These changes are reversible. Similar effects have been reported by Evans (1975), who also found that a reversible degradation in tuning could be produced by the ototoxic agents cyanide and frusemide. It appears that the normal sharp tuning of auditory nerve fibres depends upon a mechanism which is physiologically vulnerable, and that the loss of the sharp tuning is accompanied by an elevation in threshold. Evans and Harrison (1975) used the drug kanamycin to produce selective damage to the outer hair cells of the cochlea. They found that the threshold and tuning properties of auditory nerve fibres are dependent on the integrity of the outer hair cells, even though the great majority of fibres innervate only inner hair cells.

   Evans (1975) has pointed out that in fibres affected by anoxia or ototoxic drugs the tuning properties approximate those of the basilar membrane. Thus, in the absence of the physiologically vulnerable 'second filter', the tuning properties of the auditory nerve can be accounted for in terms of basilar membrane mechanics. Evans has suggested that damage of a similar nature may occur in human deafness of cochlear origin, with a consequent widening of the critical band. The evidence for this, and the perceptual consequences of it, will be discussed in the following section.

Robertson (1976) has reported that conditions which lead to a loss of sharp tuning in primary auditory neurones also result in the disappearance of two-tone suppression. This suggests that suppression is linked in some way to the 'second filter'. However, Evans (1980) has challenged this view, pointing out that if the tuning curve is broadened, then the excitatory area may cover the normal suppression regions, making it difficult to measure suppression. He has shown that it is possible to show weak two-tone suppression even when the tuning curve is markedly broadened. Thus the connection between suppression and the 'second filter' remains a matter of speculation.

7   FREQUENCY SELECTIVITY IN THE HEARING IMPAIRED

There is now a good deal of evidence that hearing impairments produced by a disorder of the cochlea are commonly associated with a loss of frequency selectivity. Zwicker and Schorn (1978) measured psychophysical tuning curves (PTCs) in six different groups of subjects: normal hearing, conductive hearing loss, degenerative hearing loss (produced by ageing or progressive hereditary loss), noise-induced hearing loss, otosclerosis and Menière's disease. They found that the PTCs of the last four groups, where the hearing loss is assumed to involve a defect in the cochlea, were considerably flatter than those in the first two groups, where no defect of the cochlea is involved. This indicates a loss of frequency selectivity. Florentine *et al.* (1980) used several of the tasks which have been used to measure critical bands in normally hearing subjects (section 2), and found that in patients with cochlear impairments all of the measures indicated a broadening of the critical band. In our own laboratory we have found that auditory filter shapes estimated using a bandstop noise masker are much broader than normal in cases of cochlear impairment. Pick *et al.* (1977) estimated auditory filter shapes in a different way, but came to essentially the same conclusion. They also found that there was a correlation between threshold elevation and filter bandwidth; higher absolute thresholds tended to be associated with broader filters.

It is worth considering the perceptual consequences of a loss in frequency selectivity. The first major consequence will be a greater susceptibility to masking by interfering sounds. When we are trying to detect a signal in a noisy background we will 'listen' to the auditory filter(s) giving the best signal-to-noise ratio. In the normal ear, where the auditory filter is relatively narrow, all of the background noise except a narrow band around the signal frequency will be attenuated at the filter output. In the impaired ear, where the filter is broader, much more of the noise will get through the filter, so that the detectability of the signal will be reduced. Thus background noises will severely disrupt the detection and discrimination of sounds, including speech. This may partly account for the great difficulties experienced by those with cochlear impairments, in following speech in noisy situations such as in pubs or at parties.

A second, but related, difficulty is that of perceptually separating two or more simultaneously presented sounds. Our ability to do this depends on more than just frequency selectivity (see Chapter 6, section 3), but the critical band mechanism undoubtedly plays a role. Thus, when the auditory filter is broader than normal, it will be much more difficult to hear out one voice from a mixture of voices. Holding a conversation when two people are talking at once can be very difficult for the hearing impaired person.

A third difficulty arises in the perceptual analysis of complex sounds, such as speech or music. We will see in Chapter 6 that the perception of timbre seems to depend upon the critical band mechanism. When the ear's frequency selectivity is impaired, the ability to detect differences in the spectral composition of sounds, and hence in timbre, will be reduced. Thus it may be more difficult for the impaired listener to tell the difference between different vowel sounds, or to distinguish different musical instruments.

We should note that the provision of a hearing aid which simply amplifies sound will not help in the least to overcome any of the difficulties described in this section. The aid may help to make sounds audible, but it does not correct the impaired frequency selectivity.

8   GENERAL CONCLUSIONS

A great many of the phenomena discussed in this chapter can be understood by considering the peripheral auditory system as containing a band of bandpass filters with continuously overlapping centre frequencies. The basilar membrane appears to provide the initial basis of the filtering process, but some other frequency selective mechanism, the 'second filter', may also be involved. The general properties of the frequency analysis carried out by the auditory system are summarized in the critical band concept; listeners' responses to complex stimuli will differ depending on whether the components of the stimuli fall within one critical band or are spread over a number of critical bands. The critical band is revealed in experiments on masking, loudness summation and threshold. We should remember, however, that the auditory filter is not a simple rectangle; rather it has a rounded top and sloping sides. The value of the critical bandwidth should not be regarded as a complete specification of the filter, but merely as a rough indication of filter bandwidth. The processes underlying masking are not well understood. Masking may correspond to a 'swamping' of the neural activity of the signal, a suppression of that activity by the masker, or a mixture of the two. The neural code carrying information about the signal is also uncertain. A common assumption is that the *amount* of neural activity in neurones with different characteristic frequencies is important. However, this form of information would not be very effective at high intensities, where the majority of neurones may be saturated. An alternative is that the *time pattern* of neural activity may carry information, but this will only apply for stimulating frequencies below 4–5 kHz.

The processes underlying the phenomena of forward and backward masking are also poorly understood. A number of stages can be distinguished in these processes, which may be related to different levels of neural activity. It is likely that forward masking takes place at a fairly peripheral level in the auditory system, whereas backward masking may involve higher levels, occurring at least partly after the point of binaural interaction. Houtgast and others have shown that nonsimultaneous masking reveals suppression effects similar to the suppression observed in primary auditory neurones. This suppression is not revealed in simultaneous masking, possibly because suppression in a given frequency region does not affect the signal-to-masker ratio in that region. One result of suppression is an enhancement in frequency selectivity, mainly on the high frequency side of the tuning curve (the low frequency side of the excitation pattern).

Although suppression may make a contribution to frequency selectivity, it is not to be identified with the 'second filter'. Some other mechanism is probably involved. There is now a good deal of evidence that part of the ear's frequency selectivity is physiologically vulnerable. This has been shown both in neurophysiological studies in animals, and in psychophysical studies in patients with hearing impairments of cochlear origin. The reduction in frequency selectivity produced by damage to the cochlea may correspond to a loss of the 'second filter'. The broadening of the auditory filter in hearing-impaired people can produce several perceptual deficits which are not corrected by a conventional hearing aid.

9   APPENDIX: SIGNAL DETECTION THEORY

A   *Introduction*

A great deal of Chapters 2 and 3 has been concerned with the measurement of thresholds. Classically, a threshold has been considered as that intensity of a stimulus above which it will be detected and below which it will not. It has been known for many years that this viewpoint is unsatisfactory; if the intensity of a stimulus is slowly increased from a very low value, there is no well-defined point at which it suddenly becomes detectable. Rather there is a range of intensities over which the subject will sometimes report a signal and sometimes will not. Thus a plot of percentage correct detections against the intensity of the stimulus (such a plot is called a psychometric function) typically has the form shown in Fig. 3.12. A further problem is that a

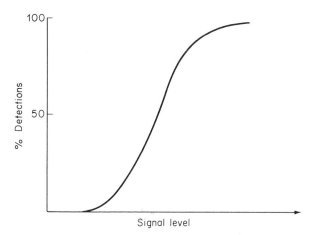

FIG. 3.12 A typical psychometric function showing how the percentage of detection of a signal varies with signal level.

subject's performance may be altered by changing the instructions, while at the same time the stimulus itself has remained unaltered. Thus it seems that factors not directly associated with the discriminability of the signal may influence the subject's performance. Signal detection theory provides a means of separating factors relating to criterion, motivation and bias from factors relating to purely sensory capabilities. It also enables us to account for the fact that responses may vary from trial to trial even when an identical stimulus is presented on each trial.

B   *The basic idea of signal detection theory*

The theory assumes that decisions are based upon the value of some internal variable x. The nature of x is not precisely specified. One might consider it to correspond to the 'sensory impression' evoked by the stimulus, or one might think of it in more physiological terms; x might correspond to the number of neural firings occurring in some particular channel during the presentation time of the stimulus. The important point is that such a variable exists, and that its average value is monotonically related to the intensity of the stimulus, i.e. increases in the intensity of the stimulus will, on average, increase the value of x. The second important assumption of the theory is that the value of x will fluctuate from trial to trial, even though the same signal is presented. This variability may arise from two sources. The signal may actually be presented against a variable background, such as a noise, so that fluctuations in physical intensity occur. Alternatively, or in addition, the source of the variability may be neural; most neurones exhibit a pattern of random firings in the absence of external stimulation, so that the presence of a stimulus will be signalled as an increase in firing rate superimposed upon this pattern of random activity. Even in neurones with low spontaneous activity the response to a fixed stimulus may vary from trial to trial.

We see then that although the average value of x will depend on whether a signal is present or absent, on any given trial the observer will never be absolutely sure that a signal has occurred, because of the inherent variability of x. Of course, if we make the signal sufficiently intense, the increase in x will be large compared with this variability, and thus the uncertainty becomes vanishingly small. But for faint signals the best that the observer can do is to make a guess on the basis of the value of x which occurred on that particular trial.

To proceed further, we have to make certain assumptions about the distribution of x. Since x is a random variable, we cannot predict its exact value on any trial, but we can specify the probability that x will fall within a specified range of values. One way of doing this is to plot a probability density function, $f(x)$. The expression $f(x)$ simply implies that f is a function of x. A probability density function, $f(x)$, is defined in such a way that the probability of x lying between x and $x + \mathrm{d}x$ (where $\mathrm{d}x$ represents a small change in the value of x) is equal to $f(x)$ multiplied by $\mathrm{d}x$. A probability density function is illustrated in Fig. 3.13. The probability that x lies between

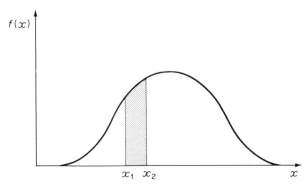

FIG. 3.13 A probability density function. The probability of x lying between the two values x_1 and x_2 is given by the shaded area under the curve. The total area under the curve is 1.

two values, x_1 and x_2, is given by the area under the curve between these two points. Since, on any given trial, some value of x must occur, the total area under the curve is equal to 1.

Consider the situation where an observer is given a series of trials, on some of which a signal is present and on some of which it is absent. To describe this situation we need to specify two probability density functions; one describes the distribution of values of x when no signal is present (this is often denoted by $f(x)_N$, the suffix N referring to the 'noise', either external or neural, which gives rise to this distribution), and the other describes the distribution of values of x where a signal does occur (often denoted $f(x)_{SN}$). It is usually assumed that these two distributions are normal, or Gaussian, and that they have equal variances. There are some theoretical reasons for making this assumption, but normal distributions are also chosen because results are easier to handle in terms of the mathematics involved. The distributions are usually plotted with standard deviation units along the abscissa; in other words, they are scaled so as to have a standard deviation of unity. They will appear as in Fig. 3.14. For each of these two distributions

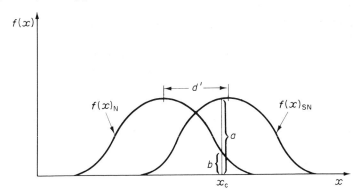

FIG. 3.14 The two distributions (probability density functions) which occur in response to 'noise' alone [$f(x)_N$], and 'noise' plus signal [$f(x)_{SN}$]. The separation between the means of the two curves, denoted by d', gives a measure of the discriminability of the signal. The criterion value is labelled x_c, and the ratio of the heights of the curves at x_c, namely a/b, gives the likelihood ratio, β.

the mean value of x corresponds to the peak in the distribution, and the separation between the two peaks, denoted by d', gives a measure of the separation of the two distributions, and thus of the discriminability of the signal.

The theory assumes that the subject establishes a cutoff point corresponding to a particular value of x, which we may denote x_c. If, on any given trial, the value of x which actually occurs is greater than x_c, the subject will report that a signal was present; otherwise he will report no signal. Just what value of x_c is chosen will depend upon the instructions to the subject, the probability of a signal, the system of rewards of punishments, previous experience and motivation. Since the exact nature of x is not specified, we cannot assign a number to x_c. To overcome this problem a new quantity is introduced—the likelihood ratio, β. This is defined as the ratio of the heights of the two distributions at x_c, i.e. as $f(x_c)_{SN}/f(x_c)_N$. In other words, the quantity β is equal to the likelihood ratio that a central effect of magnitude x_c arose from the presentation of a signal plus noise as opposed to noise alone. In Fig. 3.14 β would be equal to a/b. In contrast to d' which gives us a pure measure of the discriminability of the signal, β is related to the criterion of the subject and gives us a measure of his degree of caution independent of any changes in sensory capability.

In a given experiment we can measure the proportion of times the subject responds yes when a signal was present, $P(H)$ (this is called the probability of a hit), and the proportion of times he responds yes when a signal is absent, $P(F)$ (this is called the probability of a false alarm). From these proportions, and given our assumption that the distributions are normal and of equal variance, it is easy to calculate the values of d' and β. A simple example of how this is done is given in Welford (1968: p. 33). In practice the situation is even easier than this, since tables exist giving the values of d' and β for any given values of $P(H)$ and $P(F)$.

The major advantage of signal detection theory, then, is that it enables us to separate changes in performance related to purely sensory factors from changes related to motivational or criterion factors. Notice that this can only be done by measuring the proportion of false alarms as well as the proportion of hits. Classical methods of determining thresholds, ignoring as they did the former measure, were not able to achieve this separation. We should note further that according to this theory there is no such thing as a sensory threshold; any given intensity of a signal presented to an observer will have associated with it a certain value of d', but there will be no particular value of the intensity which corresponds to threshold.

In practice, if we are interested in comparing the discriminability of different types of signals, we can measure the intensity of the signal needed to produce a particular value of d'. Alternatively, we can use a task which attempts to eliminate the effects of bias or criterion, so that threshold can be arbitrarily defined as corresponding to a particular percentage correct. One type of task which has proved useful in this respect is the two-alternative forced-choice (2AFC) task, in which there are two observation intervals, only one of which contains the signal. The theory assumes that for each observation interval a particular value of x occurs, and that the subject simply chooses the interval in which the largest value of x occurs. It turns out to be the case that results in a 2AFC task can be simply related to those in a 'single interval' task; 76% correct in 2AFC corresponds to a d' of 1.

C   *Application of signal detection theory to theories of masking*

Although we do not need to specify the nature of x in order to apply this theory, many workers have considered what x might be. The question is equivalent to enquiring about the nature of the processes involved in masking—what features of a signal, or of its representation at a neural level, enable us to distinguish it from a masking stimulus. Some workers have considered that the masking of a tone by a noise can be explained purely in terms of the statistics of the stimuli; in other words, the variability of x arises primarily from the inherent variability of the stimuli rather than from any 'internal variability'. An example of this type of approach is given by the work of Jeffress (1964). He assumed that all stimuli are filtered, so that only a narrow band of frequencies in the noise contributes to the masking of the tone, i.e. he assumed a critical band mechanism. After this is an envelope detector, and following this a criterion device. Jeffress showed that this model gave a good fit to much of the data obtained in detection experiments. Other workers (e.g. Swets *et al.*, 1962) have assumed that stimulus energy rather than the stimulus envelope is the feature on which decisions are based. Again, however, it is necessary to assume a critical band mechanism.

This class of models, in which variability in the signals rather than variability in the observer limits performance, may be considered as describing different types of 'ideal observer'. These models have never been intended as complete descriptions of the human observer, since it is clear that internal variability does play a significant role; human observers rarely if ever achieve the performance levels which would be predicted as 'ideal'. This does not mean, however, that they are of no value. Rather, they provide "a class of normative models with which the observer's performance can be compared" (Tanner and Sorkin, 1972).

FURTHER READING

Many of the phenomena associated with the critical band are reviewed in:
Scharf, B. (1970). Critical bands. In *Foundations of Modern Auditory Theory*, Vol. 1 (ed. J. V. Tobias), Academic Press, London and New York.
The following monograph has as its central theme the action of the ear as a frequency analyser. It is clearly written, and contains a discussion of several aspects of frequency selectivity which are beyond the scope of this book:
Plomp, R. (1976). *Aspects of Tone Sensation*. Academic Press, London and New York.

Signal detection theory and its applications are covered in detail in:
Green, D. M. and Swets, J. A. (1974). *Signal Detection Theory and Psychophysics*. Kreiger, New York.

4 Pitch perception

1   INTRODUCTION

In this chapter we will consider the perception of the pitch of both pure and complex tones. Pitch may be defined as "that attribute of auditory sensation in terms of which sounds may be ordered on a musical scale" (American Standards Association, 1960). In other words, pitch is that attribute in which variations constitute melody. Pitch is related to the repetition rate of the waveform of a sound; for a pure tone this corresponds to the frequency and for a periodic complex tone to the fundamental frequency. There are, however, exceptions to this simple rule, as we shall see later. Since pitch is a subjective quality, it cannot be measured directly. Assigning a pitch value to a sound is generally understood to mean specifying the frequency of a pure tone having the same subjective pitch as the sound.

2   THEORIES OF PITCH PERCEPTION

The classical place theory of hearing has two distinct postulates. The first is that the stimulus undergoes some sort of spectral analysis in the inner ear, so that different frequencies (or frequency components in a complex stimulus) excite different places along the basilar membrane, and hence neurones with different characteristic frequencies. The second is that the pitch of a stimulus is related to the pattern of excitation produced by that stimulus; for a pure tone the pitch is generally assumed to correspond to the position of maximum excitation. The first of these two postulates is now almost universally accepted, and has been confirmed in a number of independent ways, including direct observation of the movement of the basilar membrane (see Chapter 1). The second is still a matter of dispute. An alternative to the place theory, which will be called the temporal theory, suggests that the pitch of a stimulus is related to the time pattern of the neural impulses evoked by that stimulus. Nerve firings tend to occur at a particular phase of the stimulating waveform, and thus the intervals between successive neural impulses will approximate integral multiples of the period of the stimulating waveform. The reader will recall that in Chapter 3 the possible role of this temporal information in masking was discussed.

Neither of these theories can account for our perception of pitch over the whole of the audible range; von Békésy (1960) has shown that the patterns of vibration on the basilar membrane do not shift as a function of frequency for frequencies below 50 Hz. On the other hand, the synchrony of nerve impulses to stimulus cycles has not been observed for frequencies above 5 kHz (Rose *et al.*, 1968). Thus there is a large range of frequencies over which either or both of these mechanisms could be operating. A difficulty for the place theory arises when we consider complex tones. These produce patterns of excitation along the basilar membrane which do not show a single well-defined maximum; rather there is a distribution of excitation, whose maximum, or maxima, may not correspond to the fundamental component. However, the perceived pitch, in general, still corresponds to this component. We shall discuss later how the place theory may be modified to account for this.

A   *The perception of pure tones*

In this section we shall discuss theories which attempt to explain how we perceive and discriminate pure tones. However, the ultimate aim is to produce a theory which is consistent with the data for both pure and complex tones. We shall see later on that there are close relationships between these two types of data, and that these relationships point to a unified framework in which to order the data. The main topics which we shall discuss in relation to pure tones are the size of the frequency difference limen (the smallest detectable change in frequency, abbreviated DL), and changes in the size of the DL and other aspects of our perception of pure tones which occur as a function of frequency. We shall see that these changes can provide important insights into the ways in which complex tones are perceived.

A basic problem for any theory of hearing is to account for the remarkably small size of the frequency DL; for a frequency of 1 kHz and at a moderate intensity a change of about 3 Hz can be detected, and with practice some observers achieve even smaller DLs. This is a particular problem for the place theory, since the patterns of vibration which have been observed on the basilar membrane seem much too broad to account for this acuity.

We have to remember that the basilar membrane may not be the only frequency selective mechanism in the cochlea. We discussed in Chapter 3, section 6, the possibility that there was a 'second filter' following the basilar membrane. It is also possible that the effective stimulus for the hair cells is not indicated correctly by the amplitude or velocity of vibration of the basilar membrane. For the purposes of this chapter we will continue the discussion as if the basilar membrane were the basic frequency-analysing mechanism. However, where the phrase 'basilar membrane' is used, for the rest of this chapter it should be taken to mean 'basilar membrane plus any other peripheral filtering mechanism'.

To determine whether 'place' information is sufficient to account for frequency discrimination it is perhaps more appropriate to use neural measures of frequency selectivity such as the tuning curve. This is attractive since, contrary to what is often supposed (and written), there is little evidence for progressive sharpening at higher levels in the auditory system (Møller, 1972). However, comparisons of human psychophysical data with animal neural data are difficult, particularly since the most commonly studied animals hear over a different range of frequencies from man. At any given CF, human neural tuning curves probably differ in bandwidth and slope from those in the cat or monkey. For this reason it is desirable to use psychophysical measures of frequency selectivity to determine whether 'place' information is sufficient to account for the frequency discrimination of pure tones.

Zwicker (1970) has attempted to account for the size of the DL in terms of changes in the 'excitation pattern' evoked by the stimulus when the frequency is altered. Zwicker inferred the shapes of the 'excitation patterns' from masked audiograms such as those shown in Fig. 3.1. The threshold of a sinusoidal signal is measured as a function of frequency in the presence of a fixed narrowband noise masker. It is assumed that the threshold of the signal is proportional to the amount of excitation produced by the masker in the frequency region of the signal. Thus the shape of the excitation pattern evoked by the masker will be the same as the shape of the masked audiogram. Provided the noise masker has a very narrow bandwidth, its excitation pattern will resemble that produced by a pure tone. The excitation patterns at different centre frequencies have similar shapes if they are plotted with critical bandwidth units along the abscissa rather than frequency (above 500 Hz, this corresponds roughly to plotting on a logarithmic frequency scale). According to Zwicker's model, a change in frequency will be detected whenever the excitation on the steeply sloping low frequency side of the excitation pattern changes by 1 dB or more (see Fig. 4.1). Maiwald (1967) has shown that the steepness of this slope is almost independent of the level and the frequency of the exciting tone, and has a value of 27 dB/bark (a bark is a unit of one critical bandwidth). Thus Zwicker's model would predict that the frequency DL at any given frequency should be a constant fraction (1/27) of the critical bandwidth at that frequency.

The frequency DLs obtained by the modulation method (e.g. Shower and Biddulph, 1931) do conform fairly well to these predictions. This method involves shifting the frequency of the test tone up and down about four times per second and determining the minimum detectable frequency shift. However, Henning (1966) has shown that the method is unreliable, especially at

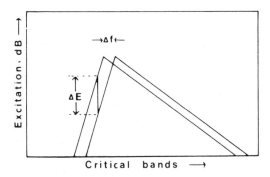

FIG. 4.1 Schematic representation of the patterns of excitation evoked by two tones of slightly different frequency. According to Zwicker, the patterns will have a similar shape, regardless of frequency, when they are plotted in terms of critical bands rather than frequency. The greatest difference in excitation for the two patterns occurs on the steeply sloping low frequency side. A change in excitation, ΔE, of 1 dB or more is assumed to be detectable.

high frequencies, since here frequency changes may be accompanied by correlated loudness fluctuations; the response of headphones on real ears is generally very irregular at high frequencies, and there is also a loss of absolute sensitivity of the observer at high frequencies (see the right-hand half of Fig. 2.1). These loudness fluctuations may provide observers with usable cues in the detection of frequency modulation. A generally better method is the two-interval forced choice (2IFC) task, in which a subject is presented on each trial with a pair of successive tone pulses and is asked to judge whether the first or the second had the higher pitch. This is varied randomly from trial to trial, and the frequency DL is usually taken as that frequency separation between the pulses for which the subject achieves 75% correct responses.

Some results using this method are given in Table II (data from Moore, 1974). The table also shows the critical band values given by Scharf (1970)

Table II. The second and third columns show the frequency DLs (mean of three subjects) and the values of the critical bandwidth for each of the frequencies shown in the first column. The fourth column shows the value of the ratio (critical band)/(frequency DL) for each frequency

Frequency	Frequency DL, Δf (Hz)	Critical band (CB) (Hz)	CB/Δf
250 Hz	0.70	100	143
500 Hz	0.83	114	137
1 kHz	1.80	160	89
2 kHz	3.8	300	79
4 kHz	12.9	660	51
6 kHz	38	1130	30
8 kHz	96	1650	17

and the ratio of the critical band to the frequency difference limen, which according to Zwicker's model should be approximately constant. It may be seen that the ratio varies by a factor of over 8 to 1 in the range considered. Further, at low frequencies the subjects are doing considerably better than would be predicted on the basis of this model.

One of the key assumptions of Zwicker's model is that the masked audiograms, such as those shown in Fig. 3.1, give a correct indication of the shapes of excitation patterns. There are, however, two reasons why this might not be the case. The first is that the steepness of the low frequency edge of the pattern may be increased by suppression, but the effects of suppression are not seen in simultaneous masking (see Chapter 3, section 5). The second is that the signal threshold may not be directly proportional to the excitation produced by the masker in the frequency region of the signal; the observer may listen 'off-frequency' to improve his performance. The first of these two problems can be overcome by using a nonsimultaneous method, such as the pulsation threshold method (see Chapter 3, section 5). However, off-frequency listening is more difficult to deal with, and the calculation of its effects can be rather complex (Verschuure, 1978).

An alternative way of testing Zwicker's model is to use a stimulus which has energy distributed over a range of frequencies. The slope of the physical spectrum of the stimulus will then place an upper limit on the slope of the excitation pattern. This approach was adopted by Moore (1972, 1973a). He measured the frequency DL for tone pulses of various durations. For a short-duration tone pulse the frequency spectrum contains energy at frequencies other than the nominal frequency, f, of the tone pulse. This effect is quite a general one; whenever a stimulus is altered from its steady state (e.g. by switching on or off), energy is spread or 'splattered' into adjacent frequency regions (see Chapter 1, section 2). The shorter the tone pulse is made, the wider the range of frequencies over which the energy is spread (see Fig. 4.2). Below some critical duration the slope of the spectral envelope will be less than the slope of the excitation pattern evoked by a long-duration pure tone. Thus, if Zwicker's model is correct, this physical slope will limit performance at short durations. Given these assumptions, and assuming that a 1 dB change is detectable, it may be shown that

$$\Delta f \times d > 0.24$$

where Δf is the frequency DL for a tone pulse of duration d. (See Moore, 1973a, for details of the calculations involved.) The results showed that at short durations observers did better than predicted for all frequencies up to 5 kHz. At about this frequency the DLs showed a sharp increase in value (see Fig. 4.3). This is in accord with previous findings (Henning, 1966). Further, when the results are plotted in terms of the relative increase in DL for each frequency (Fig. 4.4), a clear kink is observed between 4 and 6 kHz.

FIG. 4.2 The spectrum of a short tone pulse of frequency 1 kHz, with a rectangular envelope and a duration of 10 ms. With shortening duration the energy spreads over a wider range of frequencies, and the slope of the envelope of the spectrum becomes less steep.

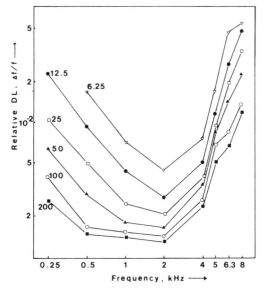

FIG. 4.3 Relative frequency DLs, $\Delta f/f$, as a function of frequency. The parameter is duration of the tone pulses in msec. Both scales are logarithmic. Notice the sharp increase in the size of the DLs which occurs around 5 kHz.

These results are consistent with a change in mechanism at about 5 kHz. It seems that a model based on shifts in excitation patterns is inadequate to explain the results for frequencies below this. The inadequacy of this type of model has been confirmed by other experimental results (Feth, 1972; Moore, 1972, 1973a–c). Other types of place model have been suggested (e.g. Corliss, 1967, Henning, 1967; Siebert, 1968, 1970), but none of these is completely satisfactory in explaining either the DL size at short durations or

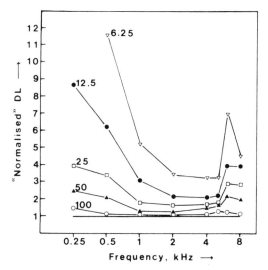

FIG. 4.4 This figure shows the same data as Figure 4.3, plotted in terms of 'normalized' DLs. For each frequency the 'normalized' DL is obtained by dividing the DL for a given duration by the DL for duration 200 ms. Plotting the results in this way enables us to see more clearly the effect of shortening duration. Notice the 'kink' in the curves at about 5 kHz.

the changes which occur at about 5 kHz. It seems that we must seek some alternative mechanism, the obvious candidate being the temporal theory. The loss of neural synchrony at about 5 kHz would explain the changes which occur at this frequency, and would also explain certain other changes in the way that pure tones are perceived. One such change is a loss of 'musical pitch' for pure tones above 5 kHz; a sequence of such tones does not produce a sense of melody. This has been confirmed by experiments involving octave matches (these become erratic when the higher tone lies above 5 kHz) and by experiments involving musical transposition. For example, Attneave and Olson (1971) asked subjects to reproduce sequences of tones (e.g. the NBC chimes) at different points along the frequency scale. Their results showed an abrupt breakpoint at about 5 kHz, above which transposition behaviour was erratic.

It seems quite clear that some sort of change occurs at around 5 kHz, and the fact that this change occurs at the same frequency at which the phase-locking of neural impulses ceases to exist is highly suggestive. However, there are still considerable difficulties involved with a temporal model. One of these is that so far there has been no evidence of a physiological mechanism which would carry out the time measurements involved with sufficient accuracy. The DL size at 1 kHz requires that a time interval of 1 ms be measured with an accuracy of about 3 μs. When we consider that there is a certain 'jitter' in the initiation of nerve impulses, which, according to de Boer (1969a), has a standard deviation of about 100 μs for a 1 kHz tone, the problem becomes even more acute; the mechanism must also be required to 'average' over time and over different auditory nerve fibres.

Recently Goldstein and Srulovicz (1977) have shown that it is possible to predict the dependence of the frequency DL on frequency and duration by assuming that the auditory system processes the time intervals between successive nerve impulses, ignoring higher order temporal dependencies. Thus the absence of physiological or anatomical evidence for an appropriate time measuring mechanism should not be discouraging, particularly since similar problems exist in explaining our ability to resolve interaural time differences of a few microseconds in localization judgements (see Chapter 5), yet clearly we do have this ability (Tobias, 1972).

Von Békésy (1963) suggested a further problem associated with a temporal theory, that "an increase in firing rate should produce not only an increase in loudness, but, if pitch is assumed to be connected with firing rate, a rise in pitch as well". Thus it should be difficult for the auditory system to separate out pitch and loudness. This problem disappears if we assume that pitch is not connected with firing rate *per se* but with the time intervals between nerve firings, or bursts of nerve firings. Consider, for example, a neurone which is firing, on average, on every fourth cycle of the stimulus. If the intensity of the stimulus is now increased, the firing rate may increase, so that the neurone fires on every third cycle, but the firings remain locked to a particular phase of the stimulating waveform, and the intervals between firings remain integral multiples of the period of that waveform. In fact nerve firings tend not to occur as regularly as this (Rose *et al.*, 1968), but the physiological evidence indicates that phase-locking is maintained over a wide range of intensities, so that the timing information in a single fibre, or over a group of fibres, will convey the same pitch regardless of changes in the overall rate of firing.

The two mechanisms we have been discussing are not, of course, mutually exclusive; it is likely that place information is available over almost all of the auditory range but that temporal mechanisms allow greater efficiency in certain types of tasks for frequencies up to 5 kHz. If this interpretation is correct, we see that a true sense of musical pitch is only obtained for frequencies where a temporal mechanism is operating, and it is interesting to note that the highest orchestral notes have frequencies lying just below 5 kHz.

B   *The pitch of complex tones*

As was stated earlier in this chapter, the classical place theory has difficulty in accounting for the way in which we perceive complex tones. For such tones the pitch does not, in general, correspond to the position of maximum excitation on the basilar membrane. A striking example of this is provided by the 'phenomenon of the missing fundamental'. Consider, as an example, a sound consisting of short impulses (clicks) occurring 200 times per second. This sound has a low pitch, which is very close to the pitch of a 200 Hz pure tone, and a sharp timbre. It may be shown to contain harmonics with frequencies 200, 400, 600, 800 . . . etc. Hz. However, it is possible to remove (electronically) the 200 Hz component, and it is found that the pitch does not alter; the only result is a slight change in the timbre of the note. Indeed, we can eliminate all except a small group of high harmonics, say 1800, 2000 and 2200 Hz, and the low pitch still remains, although the timbre will now be markedly different.

Schouten (1940) called this low pitch associated with a group of high harmonics the residue. He pointed out that the residue is distinguishable, subjectively, from a fundamental component which is physically presented or from a fundamental which may be introduced (at high sound pressure levels) by nonlinear distortion in the ear. Thus it seems that the perception of a residue pitch does not require activity at the point on the basilar membrane which would respond maximally to a pure tone of similar pitch. This is confirmed by a demonstration of Licklider (1956) which showed that the low pitch of the residue persists even when the low frequency channels are masked with low frequency random noise. Thus it seems that low pitches may be perceived via those neural channels that normally respond to the high or middle frequency components of a signal.

Several models have been proposed to account for the residue effect and for certain other phenomena associated with the perception of complex tones (see later). These models may be divided into two broad classes. The first class (which we will call 'pattern recognition' models) assumes that the pitch of a complex tone is derived from neural signals corresponding to more primary sensations, such as the pitches of the individual partials. The second class of model involves the assumption that pitch is based on time interval measurement. In particular, it has been suggested that the pitch of a complex tone is related to the time interval between peaks in the fine-structure of the signal close to adjacent envelope maxima (Schouten, Ritsma and Cardozo, 1962). If nerve firings tend to occur at these peaks, then this time interval will be present in the time pattern of neural impulses. Let us examine each class of model in more detail.

C   *Pattern recognition models*

Thurlow (1963) suggested that pitch arises on the basis of place information (i.e. according to the spatial pattern of activity on the basilar membrane), but the response is mediated by vocal activity. This vocal activity may be overt or subliminal, or involve only auditory imagery. Thurlow's mediation hypothesis suggests that the subject produces either overtly or covertly a comparison signal whose fundamental frequency is adjusted so that its harmonics coincide with those of the complex tone presented. The perceived pitch will correspond to that fundamental frequency. A similar type of theory, but one not requiring an active matching process, has been suggested by Whitfield (1967, 1970). He suggests that a complex tone gives rise to a series of active groups of nerve fibres in the central auditory pathway, separated by groups of inactive fibres. Although each of these groups corresponds to one of the partials of the complex, we do not normally hear these as such. Rather, we hear a unitary experience of a complex sound to which we ascribe a pitch. The total pattern in the auditory pathway corresponds to this pitch. Clearly, there is a whole group of patterns to which the same pitch is attributed by the system. Whitfield suggests that these patterns are learned as a result of our exposure to harmonic complex sounds (which in nature usually include the fundamental) from the moment the auditory system commences to function. The absence or distortion of a part of the pattern (e.g. by removing the fundamental) will not entirely destroy the normal sensation. The mechanism will try for the best fit among known patterns; the interpretation put on the available data is that which is 'most likely'.

   Both of these theories are inadequate in the sense that they do not state exactly what components of a complex stimulus are important in determining the pitch of the complex as a whole. For example, Whitfield (1970) says that "pitch is related to some weighted average of all the components", and that "the way in which this average is taken is complex". To see why this point is important let us consider the experiments of Schouten *et al.* (1962). They investigated the pitch of amplitude modulated sine waves, which may be shown to contain just three sinusoidal components. Thus a 2000 Hz sine wave (the 'carrier' frequency) modulated 200 times per second contains components at 1800, 2000 and 2200 Hz, and has a pitch which is similar to that of a 200 Hz sine wave. This would be predicted by either of the theories discussed above. Consider now the effect of shifting the 'carrier' frequency to, say, 2040 Hz. The complex now contains components at 1840, 2040 and 2240 Hz. This stimulus would be very unlikely to occur naturally; how will the subject choose the appropriate matching pattern? One possibility is that he makes his judgement on the basis of the spacing between adjacent partials, in which case the pitch would be unaltered. On the other hand, the partials correspond to the 46th, 51st and 56th harmonics of a 40 Hz fundamental, and so an appropriate matching stimulus would have the same pitch as a 40 Hz sinusoid. In fact, the perceived pitch, in this particular case, corresponds roughly to that of a 204 Hz sinusoid. In addition, there is an ambiguity of pitch, so that matches around 185 Hz and 227 Hz are also found.

While it is possible to explain these results in terms of *post hoc* arguments about the weighting of the various components, it seems that Whitfield's model is not sufficiently precise to allow us to predict the pitch of any given complex tone. A model which does not suffer from this defect has been proposed by Walliser (1968, 1969a–c). His model does not specify the mechanisms by which the pitch of a complex tone will be perceived, but provides a rule for determining the 'periodicity pitch', or residue pitch, of complex tones. There are two parts to the rule: (1) The pitch corresponding to the frequency difference between neighbouring partials (i.e. the envelope repetition rate) is approximately determined. This may be inferred from the pitch differences between adjacent partials (for high repetition rates where partials are well separated), or it may be determined from 'the roughness sensation' (for low repetition rates where the partials are closely spaced). The 'roughness sensation' seems to be related to fluctuations in the envelope of the stimulus. (2) A subjective subharmonic of the lowest present partial is found, such that the pitch of this sub-harmonic lies as close as possible to the pitch determined in (1).

To illustrate the working of the rule consider again the example discussed above, of a complex tone with components at 1840, 2040 and 2240 Hz. The envelope repetition rate, which is the same as the spacing between adjacent partials, is 200 Hz. The lowest partial is 1840 Hz, and the subharmonic of this which lies closest to 200 Hz is 204.4 Hz (1840 divided by 9). This corresponds closely to the perceived pitch.

Terhardt (1972a, b) has modified and elaborated this model, suggesting that a residue pitch will always be a subharmonic of a dominant partial rather than simply the lowest partial. By dominant he means 'partials which are resolvable', i.e. which can be heard out from the complex as a whole. Terhardt suggests that these dominant partials lie in the frequency region between 500 and 1500 Hz. According to this model, then, a residue pitch will only be heard when at least one partial can be analysed from the complex. When the partials are too close together in frequency, they will no longer be resolvable, and no residue pitch will be heard.

Terhardt (1974) has extended this model still further to include a learning phase. Since speech frequently contains harmonic complex tones (see Chapter 7), we are repeatedly exposed to such tones from the earliest moments in life. Terhardt suggested that as a result of this exposure we learn to associate a given frequency component with the subharmonics of that component; these will occur together in harmonic complex sounds. After the learning phase is completed, stimulation by a single pure tone will produce pitch cues corresponding to subharmonics of that tone. When a harmonic complex tone is presented, the pitch cues corresponding to these subharmonics will coincide at certain values. The largest number of co-incidences will occur at the fundamental, and this will determine the overall pitch of the sound. This is illustrated below, for a complex tone consisting of three components: 800, 1000 and 1200 Hz.

	Frequency of component, Hz		
	800	1000	1200
Frequencies of subharmonics	400	500	600
	266.7	333.3	400
	200	250	300
	160	*200*	240
	133.3	166.7	*200*

It may be seen that the greatest number of coincidences in the subharmonics occurs at 200 Hz, which corresponds to the perceived pitch. For non-harmonic complex tones, such as those used by Schouten *et al.* (1962), there will be no exact coincidences, but the frequency at which there are several near coincidences predicts the perceived pitch quite well. Notice that this model requires that more than one partial can be analysed from the complex tone in order for a residue pitch to be perceived.

An alternative model, although one still dependent on the resolution of individual frequency components in a complex tone, has been presented by Goldstein (1973). In this model the pitch of a complex tone is derived by a central processor which receives information only on the frequency, and not on the amplitude or phase, of individual components. The processor presumes that all stimuli are periodic and that the spectra comprise successive harmonics (which is the usual situation for naturally occurring sounds). The processor finds the harmonic series which provides the 'best fit' to the series of components actually presented. For example, if we present components at 1840, 2040 and 2240 Hz (as in the experiment by Schouten and co-workers described above), then a harmonic complex tone with a fundamental of 204 Hz would provide a good 'match'; this would have components at 1836, 2040 and 2244 Hz. The perceived pitch is in fact close to that of a 204 Hz sinusoid. According to this model, errors in estimating the fundamental occur mainly through errors in estimating the appropriate harmonic number. In the above example the presented components were assumed by the processor to be the 9th, 10th and 11th harmonics of a 204 Hz fundamental. However, a reasonable fit could also be found by assuming the components to be the 8th, 9th and 10th harmonics of a 226.7 Hz fundamental, or the 10th, 11th and 12th hamonics of a 185.5 Hz fundamental. Thus the model predicts the multimodal pitch matches which are actually observed for this stimulus. The extent to which such multimodal pitch matches occur will depend upon the accuracy with which the frequencies in the stimulus are represented at the input to the central processor.

All of the models which we have described in this section depend on the spectral resolution of individual components in the stimulus. It is predicted that no 'residue' pitch will be heard if no frequency components can be analysed or 'heard out' from the complex. We will discuss the experimental evidence relating to this in section 3.A. The mechanism by which individual partials would be analysed from a complex tone has not generally been specified, although Terhardt (1972a, b) has suggested that this could operate via an extended place principle, and that the basic determinant of the pitch of a complex sound is the spatial pattern of activity on the basilar membrane. This is not a necessary assumption for these models. Indeed Goldstein (1973) was careful to state that

> . . . the concept that the optimum processor operates on signals representing the constituent frequencies of complex-tone stimuli does not necessarily imply the use of tonotopic or place information *per se* as the measure of frequency. For example, temporal periods of pure tones are not ruled out as the measure of frequency.

As we saw in the section on pure tones, there is quite good evidence that temporal mechanisms play a part in our perception of pure tones, at least for frequencies up to 5 kHz. Thus it is likely that the analysis of partials from a complex tone, and the determination of their pitches, relies at least in part on temporal mechanisms. Given this assumption, these models could still hold, but the basic data on which they operated would be the temporal patterns of firing in different groups of auditory neurones.

We shall discuss later some of the experimental evidence which is relevant to these models. Let us now turn to the second main type of model—the 'temporal' model.

D   Temporal models

Consider again the example of a pulse train of repetition rate 200/s, containing harmonics at 200, 400, 600 . . . Hz. The lower harmonics in this sound will be analysed into effectively separate locations on the basilar membrane, and the timing of the neural firings derived from these locations will relate to the frequencies of those harmonics rather than to the repetition rate of the complex as a whole. However, the patterns of vibration on the basilar membrane corresponding to the higher harmonics will overlap to some extent, so that the waveform on the basilar membrane will result from the interference of a number of harmonics, and will show a periodicity the same as that of the input waveform. The timing of neural impulses derived from such a region would then relate to the repetition rate of the original input waveform. This is illustrated in Fig. 4.5 (see also Figs 1.5, 1.10, 1.11 and 1.19).

These considerations lead to a theory whose development is mainly due to Schouten (1940, 1970). We summarize below the major points of his theory.

Hz

6300

5000

4000

3150

2500

2000

1600

1250

1000

800

630

500

400

315

250

200

160

periodic pulse

TIME →

1 The ear analyses a complex sound into a number of components each of which is separately perceptible.

2 Some of these components correspond with individual partials present in the input waveform. These components have a pure tone quality.

3 One or more components may be perceived which do not correspond with any individual sinusoidal oscillation, but which are a collective manifestation of some of those oscillations which are not or are scarcely individually perceptible. These components (residues) have an impure, sharp tone quality.

4 The ear ascribes a pitch to a residue by virtue of the periodicity of the total waveform of the harmonics which are responsible for this residue.

5 The pitch ascribed to a complex sound is the pitch of that component to which the attention, by virtue either of its loudness or of its contrast with former sounds, is most strongly drawn.

In general, the residue is the most prominent component in a complex sound, and thus the pitch of the whole sound will be given by the pitch of the residue. We see, then, how a low pitch may be signalled through those neural channels which normally respond to the high or middle frequency components of a complex sound.

Notice a major difference between this model and the pattern recognition models, such as Walliser's model. The pattern recognition models require that at least one partial in the complex sound should be analysable from the complex in order for a low residue pitch to be heard, whereas Schouten's model requires that at least two harmonics are interacting in order for the residue to be heard. And according to Schouten's model, a residue pitch may still be heard when none of the individual components is separately perceptible.

Let us consider how Schouten's model deals with the complex tone which we discussed earlier in relation to the pattern recognition models; this contained components of 1840, 2040 and 2240 Hz. If we compare the waveform of this signal and the waveform of a signal containing components at 1800, 2000 and 2200 Hz, we see that, while the envelope repetition rates are the same, the time interval between corresponding peaks in the fine structure of the waveform is slightly different (see Fig. 4.6). Since these signals contain only a narrow range of frequency components, the waveforms on the basilar membrane will not be greatly different from those of the physically presented signals; the basilar membrane will not separate the

---

FIG. 4.5 A simulation of the responses on the basilar membrane to periodic impulses of rate 200 pulses per second. Each number on the left represents the frequency which would maximally excite a given point on the basilar membrane. The waveform which would be observed at that point, as a function of time, is plotted opposite that number. This figure can be compared with Fig. 1.9, which represents the envelope of responses to the same stimulus. From Plomp (1968), by permission of the author.

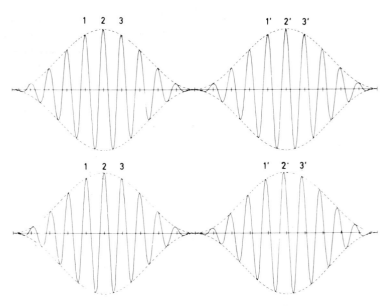

FIG. 4.6 Waveforms for two amplitude modulated sine waves. In the upper waveform the carrier frequency (2000 Hz) is an exact multiple of the modulation frequency (200 Hz). Thus the time intervals between corresponding peaks in the fine-structure, 1-1', 2-2', 3-3', will be 5 ms, the period of the modulation frequency. In the lower waveform the carrier frequency is shifted slightly upwards. Thus 10 complete cycles of the carrier occur in slightly less than 5 ms, and the time intervals between corresponding points on the waveform, 1-1', 2-2', 3-3', will be slightly shorter than 5 ms. The lower waveform has a slightly higher pitch than that of the upper. From Plomp (1968), by permission of the author.

individual components to any great extent. Thus, if nerve firings tend to occur at peaks in the fine structure of the waveform close to envelope maxima, the timing of the nerve impulses will convey slightly different pitches for the two stimuli. These differences in the time pattern of neural impulses have been observed by Javel (1980). Notice that for the signal containing components at 1840, 2040 and 2240 Hz the time intervals between nerve firings will fall into two groups, one slightly longer than 5 ms (the period of a 200 Hz tone) and one slightly shorter than 5 ms. The shorter of these two time intervals would correspond to a pitch of about 204 Hz, which is what is normally reported, but Schouten *et al.* (1962) did also report an ambiguity of pitch, so that sometimes the perceived pitch corresponded to the longer of these two time intervals.

We see that it is necessary to refine Schouten's original theory, particularly with respect to point 4. The pitch of the residue will be determined by the time interval between peaks in the fine structure of the waveform (on the basilar membrane) close to adjacent envelope maxima. If more than one possible time interval is present, the pitch will correspond, in general, to the shortest, although sometimes ambiguity of pitch may occur. If we consider the representation of the signal on a neural level, in terms of the time pattern of nerve firings, then, just as was the case for pure tones, the time intervals between nerve firings rather than the overall rate of firing will be important. If the system were simply counting, say, the number of impulses per second, then the pitch shifts observed by Schouten and co-workers would not have occurred.

3   EXPERIMENTAL EVIDENCE RELEVANT TO THE PATTERN RECOGNITION AND TEMPORAL MODELS

Both the 'pattern recognition' models and Schouten's model give a fair description of what Schouten *et al.* (1962) called the 'first effect of pitch shift'; for an amplitude modulated sine wave there is a slight upward shift in pitch when the carrier frequency is increased from a value which is an exact multiple of the modulation rate. This pitch shift would be predicted from the shifts which occur in the time intervals between peaks in the fine-structure of the waveform close to adjacent envelope maxima (as in Fig. 4.6). However, the experimental data reveal that the pitch shifts actually observed are consistently slightly larger than predicted, particularly for high harmonic numbers (when the carrier frequency is high relative to the modulation rate). The extra pitch shift, over and above the predicted 'first effect of pitch shift', was called the 'second effect of pitch shift' by Schouten and co-workers.

This 'second effect' is explained in various ways by the different models. Recall that Walliser's model required the determination of a subjective subharmonic of a dominant partial. Ward (1954) showed that subjective octave intervals between pure tones correspond to frequency ratios slightly greater than 2. Walliser (1968) confirmed these results and derived a scale of subjective harmonics as a function of objective harmonics. From this scale one predicts that a pitch determined as a subjective subharmonic will be slightly different from that calculated as an objective (i.e. mathematically perfect) subharmonic, and thus the 'second effect' is explained. The same reasoning can explain the finding that a periodic sound of repetition rate g periods/s is sometimes reported to have a pitch slightly different from that of a pure tone of frequency g Hz (Walliser, 1968; Terhardt, 1971).

Terhardt (1972a, b) has suggested a way in which the 'octave enlargement' phenomenon could arise. He says "our sense of musical intervals, and thereby of the octave interval, is acquired; we acquire the knowledge of harmonic relations in earliest life, when we learn to recognize and to understand speech sounds" (Terhardt, 1972c). He presents evidence showing that for a complex tone containing a fundamental and a number of harmonics, the pitch of the fundamental component is shifted slightly downwards, whereas the pitches of the 2nd and higher harmonics are shifted upwards. Thus the pitch intervals between the 1st and 2nd harmonics will be enlarged compared with the corresponding intervals for successive pure tones. By exposure to these sounds we 'learn' an octave interval which is slightly enlarged. Lindqvist and Sundberg (1971) consider this explanation unlikely, since the perceptual size of the octave, if picked out from harmonic sounds, would vary substantially, especially in vowel sounds, owing to the frequent variations of the relative levels of the two lowest partials.

An alternative explanation of the 'second effect of pitch shift' is suggested by the work of Smoorenburg (1970). He investigated the pitch perception of stimuli containing only two frequency components. Sometimes these are perceived as having a single pitch corresponding to that of the (absent) fundamental, although the pitch is generally rather weak (see later for further data on this type of stimulus). Smoorenburg found that a shift of the frequencies away from a harmonic situation resulted in a pitch shift. For high harmonic numbers the shift was larger than could be accounted for either by a temporal model or by a pattern recognition model, such as Walliser's. The large pitch shift, which is analogous to the second effect of pitch shift observed by Schouten and co-workers, can be explained by taking into account certain types of combination tones—in particular, those with pitches corresponding to frequencies $f_1 - K(f_2 - f_1)$, where f_1 and f_2 are the frequencies of the tones which are physically presented and K is an integer. A combination tone may be defined as a perceived tone not present in the sensations produced by the constituent components of the stimulus when they are presented singly. Combination tones of this type, and particularly those with a pitch corresponding to frequency $2f_1 - f_2$, have been shown to be audible even at moderate intensities (Plomp, 1965; Goldstein, 1967). Smoorenburg suggested that these combination tones, rather than the physically presented partials, are dominant in determing the pitch of the complex in cases where a large pitch shift occurs. He showed that when the combination tones are masked by bands of noise, the large pitch shift is diminished, although at the same time the clarity of the pitch sensation is diminished.

Notice that this type of combination tone corresponds to a lower partial of the complex which is physically presented. For example, if two tones with frequencies 1800 Hz and 2000 Hz are presented, the combination tone will have a frequency of 1600 Hz ($[2 \times 1800] - 2000$). In the case of tones which are harmonically related, the combination tone will have a frequency corresponding to a lower harmonic of the same fundamental frequency. For primary tones of, say, 1840 Hz and 2040 Hz, the combination tone will have a frequency of 1640 Hz.

Combination tones can explain the second effect of pitch shift in terms of both Schouten's and the 'pattern recognition' models. For the former we must assume that the waveform on the basilar membrane results from the interference of physically presented partials and combination tones. For the latter we must assume that the pitch of a complex tone is determined from information relating to individual partials, combination tones included.

A   *The existence region of the tonal residue*

Ritsma (1962) investigated the audibility of residue pitches, for amplitude modulated sinusoids containing three components, as a function of the modulation rate and the harmonic number (carrier frequency divided by modulation rate). Later (Ritsma, 1963) he extended the results to complexes with a greater number of components. He found that the tonal character of the residue pitch existed only within a limited frequency region. When the harmonic number was too high (above about 20), only a kind of high buzz of undefinable pitch was heard. He found, further, that some harmonics below 5 kHz had to be present for a residue pitch to be heard, and that the modulation rate had to be below about 800 Hz. Other workers (Plomp, 1967; Moore, 1973c) have found, using complex tones with a greater number of components, that residue pitches can be perceived for repetition rates up to about 1400 Hz.

Let us consider the implications of these results for the models we have been discussing. According to the pattern recognition models, a residue pitch will only be heard when at least one partial is analysable from the complex. In Chapter 3 we discussed Plomp's (1964) experiments which showed that for a partial within a multitone complex only the first 5–8 harmonics are separately perceptible, although the limit was somewhat higher for two-tone complexes. Since Ritsma (1962) found a tonal residue for complexes which only contained harmonics around the 20th, it would seem that under some conditions we can hear a residue pitch when none of the individual components is separately perceptible. We can describe these results in terms of the critical band concept; roughly speaking, components separated by a critical band or more will not interact, and will be separately perceptible, whereas components within a critical band will interact and will not produce separate pitches. Thus Ritsma's results would indicate that a low residue pitch can be heard when the components do not fall in separate critical bands and so should not be separately perceptible. On the other hand, Terhardt (1970) investigated another aspect of the critical band phenomenon—the frequency difference between two simultaneously presented pure tones which is necessary to give a perception of two separate pitches; he found that the curve of 'pitch separation' was almost identical with the lower boundary of the 'existence region of the tonal residue'.

There are a number of difficulties in making these comparisons. Firstly, individual differences can be very great (see, for example, Moore, 1973c).

Thus comparing the results of different individuals in different experiments is a dubious procedure, especially when few subjects have been used. Secondly, in this particular comparison, it is not clear whether the results for two-tone complexes, or those for multitone complexes, are the more appropriate ones for comparison. Finally, it is likely that Ritsma's results were influenced by the presence of combination tones, as has since been pointed out by Ritsma himself (1970).

Moore (1973c) carried out a series of experiments in an attempt to resolve these difficulties. He first determined that the lowest partial in a multitone complex was more easily audible than any of the other partials. In fact, it was about as easily audible as a partial in a two-tone complex. He then determined the audibility of the lowest partial in a multitone complex as a function of the frequency separation of the partials. A condition was included where a band of noise was present in the frequency region below the lowest partial. The functions relating audibility to separation were then compared with the frequency separation of the harmonics for which a complex tone produced a well-defined pitch, using the same set of subjects. Again a 'noise' condition was included, so that combination tones in the frequency region below the lowest presented partial could not influence the results. Moore found that for high harmonic numbers there was a range of conditions over which a residue pitch could be heard when none of the individual partials would have been separately perceptible.

More recently Moore and Rosen (1979) investigated subjects' abilities to identify simple melodies which were 'played' by varying the repetition rate of pulse trains. The pulse trains were filtered so as to contain only high, unresolvable harmonics, and a low frequency noise was present to mask combinations tones. In order to determine whether these stimuli evoked a sense of musical interval, performance was compared with that obtained when the tunes were played as a pattern of sinusoidal frequencies in which the pitch changes were clearly audible, but the musical intervals had been distorted; the musical scale was either 'compressed' or 'expanded'. This preserves the pitch contour but makes the musical intervals sound 'wrong'. Moore and Rosen found that performance was superior for the high-pass filtered pulse trains, and concluded that simuli containing only high, unresolvable harmonics can evoke a sense of musical interval, and hence of pitch. The pattern recognition models cannot account for this. We should note, however, that the pitch of high-pass filtered pulse trains is much less clear than that heard when lower harmonics are present.

B   *The principle of dominance*

Ritsma (1967a) carried out an experiment to determine which components in a complex sound are most important in determining its pitch. He presented complex tones in which the frequencies of a small group of harmonics were multiples of a fundamental which was slightly higher or lower than the fundamental of the remainder. The subject's pitch judgements were used to determine whether the pitch of the complex as a whole was affected by the shift in the group of harmonics. Ritsma found that

> for fundamental frequencies in the range 100 Hz to 400 Hz, and for sensation levels up to at least 50 dB above threshold of the entire signal, the frequency band consisting of the third, fourth and fifth harmonics tends to dominate the pitch sensation as long as its amplitude exceeds a minimum absolute level of about 10 dB above threshold.

This finding has since been confirmed in other ways (Ritsma, 1967b; Bilsen and Ritsma, 1967).

Thus Ritsma introduced the concept of dominance:

> . . . if pitch information is available along a large part of the basilar membrane the ear uses only the information from a narrow band. This band is positioned at 3–5 times the pitch value. Its precise position depends somewhat on the subject.
>
> (Ritsma, 1970)

This concept has a number of implications. Firstly, it explains why the second effect of pitch shift becomes more marked as the harmonic number is increased. For low harmonic numbers the partials contributing most to the pitch sensation are those which are physically present in the stimulus. For higher harmonic numbers the combination tones lie in the dominant region, and thus their contribution is more marked. Secondly, the concept of dominance may help us decide whether the components involved are interacting or are being separately analysed in the auditory system. It seems, however, that there is no clear-cut answer to this question. For the normal range of fundamentals that are used in these experiments (up to 1000 Hz), the 3rd, 4th and 5th harmonics do lie in a region where individual partials are well analysed, but the overlap of vibration patterns on the basilar membrane would also be sufficient to provide temporal information about the periodicity of the input waveform. Thus, in the dominant region, both spectral and temporal analyses would appear to be possible.

C   *Evidence for the role of central mechanisms in the perception of complex tones*

Houtsma and Goldstein (1972) conducted perhaps the first experiment which clearly demonstrates that a 'residue'-type pitch may be heard when there is no possibility of an interaction of components in the cochlea. They investigated the perception of stimuli which comprised just two successive harmonics. Subjects were required to recognize melodies corresponding to the (missing) fundamentals. Harmonic numbers were randomized from note to note, so that the subjects could not use cues associated with the pitches of individual harmonics in order to recover the melody. They found that performance was good for low harmonic numbers, but fell to chance level for harmonic numbers above about 10–12. They found further that subjects were able to identify melodies when the stimuli were presented *dichotically* (one harmonic to each ear). At high intensities monotic performance was superior to dichotic, whereas at low levels (20 dB SL) there was no difference between the two conditions. Houtsma and Goldstein suggested that the differences at high intensities resulted from the influence of combination tones, which would lower the effective harmonic number. They considered that if an allowance were made for the effect of combination tones, then there would be essentially no difference between the monotic and dichotic conditions.

These results cannot be explained in terms of Schouten's model, or indeed in terms of any model which requires an interaction of components on the basilar membrane (e.g. von Békésy, 1961). They imply that "the pitch of these complex tones is mediated by a central processor operating on neural signals derived from those effective stimulus harmonics which are tonotopically resolved". In other words, these experiments clearly indicate that the pitch of a complex tone can be mediated by some sort of pattern recognition process. However, it is not yet entirely clear that the findings apply to the pitches of complex tones in general. The pitch of a two-tone complex is not very clear; indeed, many observers do not hear a single low pitch, but rather perceive the component tones individually (Smoorenburg, 1970). Residue pitches are generally much more distinct when greater numbers of harmonics are present, and while Goldstein (1972) has reported similar results for complex tones with up to six components, no full report of this work has yet appeared. It does seem to be the case that two-tone complexes only produce a residue pitch for harmonic numbers below about 10, whereas the limit is somewhat higher for multitone complexes (Ritsma, 1962; Moore, 1973c). Thus some factor other than our ability to analyse individual components from complex tones affects the upper limit of the 'existence region'.

Houtgast (1976) has reported an even more extreme example of hearing a 'residue' pitch in the absence of interaction of components. He showed that, provided a context was provided to focus the attention of the subject on pitches in a particular range, a single harmonic was capable of evoking the perception of a low 'residue' pitch. He set up his experiment as follows. Subjects were presented with two successive harmonic complex signals which differed in fundamental frequency by 3%. On each trial the subject had to say whether the pitch of the second was higher or lower than that of the first. The signals did not have any harmonics in common, so that subjects could not simply listen to the pitches of the individual harmonics in order to perform the task. The first signal always contained six harmonics and had a clear unambiguous pitch. The second signal initially had three harmonics, but after a certain number of trials this number was reduced to two, and finally to one. In the absence of any background noise performance was very poor, and was at chance level (50%) for the one-component signal. Thus a single sinusoidal component in quiet does not allow the subject to infer the 'fundamental'. However, when the experiment was conducted with a background noise, performance *improved* considerably; a score of 80% was obtained for the one-component signal. It appears that a single sinusoidal component has the potential to evoke subharmonic pitches. When the sensory information is made ambiguous, by the presence of a background noise, these potential pitches are more likely to be perceived. If the subject's attention is focussed in a particular pitch range, then the subharmonic pitch in this range may be the dominant percept.

Yet another demonstration that interaction of components is not essential for the perception of a 'residue' pitch is provided by an experiment of Hall and Peters (1981). They investigated the pitch associated with stimuli consisting of three harmonics which were presented successively rather than simultaneously. Each sinusoidal component lasted 40 ms, and there was a 10 ms pause between components. They found that, in the absence of a background noise, only pitches corresponding to the individual components were heard. However, when a background noise was present, pitches corresponding to the missing fundamental were heard. This result resembles that of Houtgast (1976), except that it was not necessary to provide a prior context to direct the subject's attention. It appears that noise enhances a synthetic mode of pitch perception, in which information is combined over different frequency regions and over time to produce a 'residue' pitch. In quiet, an analytic mode of perception is more likely, so that the individual components are heard separately.

We may conclude, then, that the pitch of a complex tone can be derived from neural signals corresponding to individual partials in the complex, at least for stimuli with low harmonics and containing only a small number of harmonics. It is still not established whether the information about these partials is coded in terms of place or in terms of the temporal patterns of nerve firing. Houtsma and Goldstein (1972) concluded that "all the constraints could conceivably be met by mechanisms based on either time or place information". But it is noteworthy that residue pitches are only observed when harmonics (or combination tones) are present with frequencies below 5 kHz (Ritsma, 1962, 1963; Moore, 1973c). We saw earlier in this chapter that it is likely that temporal mechanisms are important in the perception of pure tones for frequencies up to about 5 kHz, but that above this only place mechanisms could operate. Thus residue pitches are only heard when harmonics are present in the frequency region where temporal information is available.

D   *Pitches based upon purely timing
     information*

To avoid some of the difficulties associated with harmonic stimuli, a number
of workers have investigated pitches evoked by stimuli which contain no
spectral peaks, and which therefore would not produce a well-defined
maximum on the basilar membrane. Such pitches presumably cannot arise
on the basis of place information, and so provide evidence for the operation
of temporal mechanisms.

Miller and Taylor (1948) presented random noise which was turned on
and off abruptly, and periodically, at various rates, by an electronic switch.
Provided that care is taken to eliminate switching transients (clicks), the
interrupted noise will have a uniform spectrum. They reported that the noise
had a pitchlike quality for interruption rates between 100 and 250 Hz. More
recently Pollack (1969) has shown that some subjects are able to adjust
sinusoids to have the same pitch as the interrupted noise for interruption
rates of the noise up to 2000 Hz. They adjust the frequency of the sinusoid to
be roughly equal to the interruption rate of the noise. These experiments
support the idea of a temporal analysis in the auditory system, but the pitch
sensation for this type of stimulus is not very clear. This could be because the
exact waveform of the noise in successive samples is different. Many subjects do not report a pitch sensation at all, although most can hear that
something pitchlike changes when the interruption rate is changed. This
phenomenon, that a pitch is heard more clearly if it is varied, seems to be
quite a general one, and is often marked for residue pitches.

A number of experiments have been reported showing pitch sensations as
a result of the binaural interaction of noise stimuli. Huggins and Cramer
(1958) fed white noise from the same noise generator to both ears, via
headphones. The noise to one ear went through an all-pass filter, which
passed all audible frequency components without change of amplitude, but
produced a phase change in a small frequency region. A faint pitch was
heard corresponding to the frequency region of the phase transition, although
the stimulus presented to each ear alone was white noise, and produced no
pitch sensation. The effect was limited to frequencies below about 1 kHz. A
phase shift of a narrow band of the noise would tend to be handled as a
difference in localization by the auditory system (see Chapter 5), so that this
band would be separated in subjective space from the rest of the noise. This
spatial separation presumably produces the pitchlike character associated
with that narrow band.

Fourcin (1970) used two noise sources, which we shall denote n_1 and n_2. n_1
was led via headphones to the two ears, producing a sound image localized in
the middle of the head. n_2 was also fed to both ears, but the input to one ear

was delayed by a certain time, τ, producing a second sound image localized to one side. Sometimes the observer simply heard two separate sound images, neither of which had a pitch. At other times, however, a faint pitch was heard, whose position was not well defined, but which was generally centrally located. When the observed pitches were matched to pure tones (of frequency f), the matches lay along the line $1/\tau = 4f/3$.

Bilsen and Goldstein (1974) reported that a pitch may be perceived when just one noise source is used, presented binaurally, but with a delay at one ear. For delays shorter than about 2 ms a single noise image is reported, whose perceived position depends on the delay. For longer time delays the image remains at the side of the head and becomes more diffuse, and, in addition, "a faint but distinct pitch image corresponding to $1/\tau$ appears in the middle of the head". As for the pitches reported by Fourcin, the effect is an essentially low frequency one; the highest pitch matches reported by Bilsen correspond to frequencies of about 500 Hz.

The exact mechanism which gives rise to these pitches remains to be elucidated. Since in all three of the experiments producing pitches by binaural interaction the stimuli presented to each ear separately conveyed no spectral information, timing information must be used in the creation of a central pattern of neural activity from which the pitch is extracted. In other words, information about the relative phases of components in the two ears must be preserved up to the point in the auditory system where binaural interaction occurs. We shall see in Chapter 5 that we are only able to use phase differences between the two ears in the localization of sounds for frequencies up to about 1500 Hz, and it seems that pitches perceived by binaural interaction are limited to this region. The necessity for binaural interaction means that there is no particular obligation to regard 1500 Hz as a limit for temporal coding in general. A feature of all these pitches is that they are very faint, and indeed many observers do not hear them at all. They may arise from the operation of a mechanism which is not normally involved in pitch extraction, but is primarily concerned with the localization of sound, and the extraction of signals from noise. Indeed, one of the models put forward to explain the pitches of these stimuli, and to account for the factor of 4/3 which was found in Fourcin's experiments (Bilsen and Goldstein, 1974), is based on Durlach's equalization and cancellation model, which is a model designed to account for the detection of signals in noise under binaural listening conditions (see Chapter 5). Nordmark (1970) has pointed out there are many similarities in the systems involved in pitch and localization, especially when periodic stimuli are used. The relationship of the faint pitches heard with noise stimuli to the much clearer pitches observed in situations where spectral information is available is not, at the moment, clear.

4   A CRUDE MODEL FOR THE PITCH PERCEPTION OF COMPLEX TONES

It is now quite clear that the perception of a particular pitch does not depend on a high level of activity at a particular place on the basilar membrane, or in a particular group of peripheral neurones. The pitch of complex tones will, in general, be mediated by harmonics higher than the fundamental, so that similar pitches may arise from quite different distributions of neural activity. For stimuli containing a wide range of harmonics, the harmonics in a region around the 3rd, 4th and 5th will tend to dominate the pitch percept. These harmonics lie in the range where it is possible to resolve and hear them out as separate entities. This supports the 'pattern recognition' models of pitch perception. However, it is possible to hear a 'residue' pitch when the harmonics are too high to be resolved. This cannot be explained by the 'pattern recognition' models, but can be explained by the temporal model. The temporal model, on the other hand, cannot account for the fact that it is possible to hear a 'residue' pitch when there is no possibility of the components of the complex tone interacting in the peripheral auditory system.

It seems that none of the theories presented so far can account for all of the experimental data. We next present a crude schematic model which incorporates features of both the temporal model and the 'pattern recognition' models, and which can account, in a qualitative way, for all of the data. The model is illustrated in Fig. 4.7. The first stage in the model is a bank of bandpass filters with continuously overlapping centre frequencies. These are the auditory filters or critical bands. The outputs of the filters in response to a complex tone will have the form shown in Fig. 4.5. The filters responding to low harmonics will have outputs which are approximately sinusoidal in form; the individual harmonics will be resolved. The filters responding to higher harmonics will have outputs corresponding to the interaction of several harmonics. The waveform will be complex, but will have a repetition rate corresponding to that of the input.

The next stage in the model is the transduction of the filter outputs to neural impulses. The temporal pattern of firing in a given neurone will reflect the temporal structure of the waveform driving that neurone. Say, for example, that the input has a fundamental frequency of 200 Hz. The fourth harmonic, at 800 Hz, will be well resolved in the filter bank, and hence the neurones with CFs close to 800 Hz will respond as if the input were an 800 Hz sinusoid. The time intervals between successive nerve impulses will be multiples of the period of that tone, i.e. 1.25, 2.5, 3.75, 5.0 . . . ms (cf. Fig. 1.17). Neurones with higher CFs, say around 2000 Hz, will be driven by a more complex waveform. The temporal structure of the response will be correspondingly complex. Each peak in the fine structure of the waveform is capable of evoking a spike, so that many different time intervals will occur

ACOUSTIC INPUT

FILTER BANK
(CRITICAL BAND MECHANISM)

NEURAL TRANSDUCTION

ANALYSIS OF INTER-SPIKE
INTERVALS AT EACH CF

COMPARE INTERVALS ACROSS CFs
PICK PROMINENT INTERVALS

EVALUATE CONTEXT
PICK APPROPRIATE INTERVALS

PITCH

FIG. 4.7 A schematic model for the perception of the pitch of complex tones. The model depends upon both place and timing information.

between successive spikes. The interval corresponding to the fundamental, 5 ms, will be present, but other intervals, such as 4.0, 4.5, 5.5 and 6.0 ms, will also occur (Evans, 1978; Javel, 1980).

The next stage in the model is a device which analyses, separately for each CF, the interspike intervals which are present. The range of intervals which can be analysed is probably limited, and varies with CF. At a given CF the device probably operates over a range from about 0.5/CF to 15/CF seconds. This range is appropriate for the time intervals which would occur most often.

The next stage is a device which compares the time intervals present in the different channels, and searches for common time intervals. The device may also integrate information over time. In general the time interval which is found most often will correspond to the period of the fundamental component. Finally the time intervals which are most prominently represented across channels are fed to a decision mechanism which selects one interval from among those passed to it. This device incorporates memory and attention processes, and may be influenced by immediately preceding stimuli, context, conditions of presentation, and so on. The perceived pitch corresponds to the reciprocal of the final interval selected.

Consider how this model deals with a complex tone composed of a few low harmonics, say the 3rd, 4th and 5th harmonics of a 200 Hz (missing) fundamental. In those neurones responding primarily to the 600 Hz component, an analysis of time intervals between successive nerve firings would reveal intervals of 1.67, 3.33, 5.0, 6.67 . . . ms, each of which is an integral multiple of the period of that component. Similarly the intervals in the 800 Hz 'channel' will be 1.25, 2.5, 3.75, 5.0 . . . ms, while those in the 1000 Hz 'channel' will be 1, 2, 3, 4, 5 . . . ms. The only time interval which is in common across all of the channels is 5 ms; this corresponds to the pitch of the missing fundamental. Thus this stimulus will evoke a clear, unambiguous pitch.

Consider next what happens when a small group of high harmonics is presented, say the 12th, 13th and 14th harmonics of 200 Hz. These harmonics will not be resolved in the filter bank, and so essentially only one channel of timing information will be available. Furthermore, the time interval information will be ambiguous, many values closely spaced around 5 ms being present. Thus, while a pitch corresponding to the missing fundamental may be perceived, that pitch will be weak and ambiguous, as is observed psychophysically. This can explain why lower harmonics tend to dominate in the perception of pitch; the temporal information they provide is far less ambiguous, provided that information is combined across channels. The pitch associated with high harmonics can be made more clear by increasing the number of harmonics, since the ambiguities can be reduced by comparing across channels. This also is observed psychophysically.

If a small group of very high harmonics is presented, then they may fail to evoke a sense of musical pitch. This can be explained in terms of the limited range of time intervals which can be analysed at each CF. For harmonics above about the 15th, the time interval corresponding to the fundamental will fall outside the range which can be analysed in the channel responding to those harmonics. This is one factor contributing to the limited existence region of the tonal residue (section 3.A). The other factor is the absolute upper limit for phase-locking. When the harmonics lie above 5 kHz the fine structure of the waveform at the filter output will no longer be preserved in the temporal patterning of neural impulses. Thus the later stages of analysis of interspike intervals will not reveal the regularities necessary to determine the fundamental.

The way in which this model determines the pitch for a group of low harmonics resembles that proposed by Terhardt (1974). In his model each partial gives rise to potential pitches corresponding to subharmonics of that partial, and the perceived pitch is that for which the number of coincidences is greatest. In our model these 'subharmonic' pitches correspond to the interspike intervals evoked by a given partial. For example a 1 kHz tone will evoke intervals of 1, 2, 3, 4, 5 . . . ms, and these correspond to pitches of 1000, 500, 333.3, 250, 200 . . . Hz. The differences between the models are as follows: Terhardt's model requires a learning phase in which the associations between partials and subharmonics are learned, whereas in our model the 'subharmonics' occur automatically in the temporal patterns of neural firing. Secondly, Terhardt's model cannot explain the pitch produced by high, unresolved harmonics, whereas in our model they arise as part of the same process as is used for lower harmonics.

The way that our model deals with the pitch of nonharmonic complex tones depends on the spacing of the components relative to their centre frequency. If the components are widely spaced, and therefore resolvable, the pitch of the complex will be determined in a similar way to that proposed by Terhardt. Say, for example, that components at 840, 1040 and 1240 Hz are presented. The time intervals in the 840 Hz channel will be 1.19, 2.38, 3.57, 4.76, 5.95 . . . ms, all of which are integral multiples of the period, 1.19 ms. Similarly, the intervals in the 1040 Hz channel will be 0.96, 1.92, 2.88, 3.85, 4.8, 5.76 . . . ms, and those in the 1240 Hz channel will be 0.81, 1.61, 2.42, 3.22, 4.03, 4.84 . . . ms. In this case there is no time interval which is exactly the same in all channels, but there is a near coincidence at 4.8 ms, the intervals in the three channels being 4.76, 4.8 and 4.84 ms. The perceived pitch will thus correspond to the reciprocal of 4.8 ms, i.e. 208 Hz. When the components are closely spaced, and therefore unresolvable, then the pitch will be derived from the time interval which is most prominently represented in the pattern of neural impulses evoked by the complex. In this case our model works in the same way as the temporal model outlined in section 2.D. The perceived pitch will correspond to the time interval between peaks in the fine structure of the waveform (at the output of the auditory filter) close to adjacent envelope maxima. The pitch will be ambiguous since several 'candidate' time intervals may be present.

In our model, just as in the other models we have discussed, combination tones may play a role in determining the pitch percept. Their role may be particularly important when the stimulus itself contains only closely spaced components. The combination tones will act like lower partials, and will be more resolvable than the partials physically present in the stimulus.

The pitches of stimuli without spectral peaks, such as periodically interrupted noise, are explained by the model as arising from the time interval information present primarily in the channels with high CFs, where the filter bandwidths are wider. When a filter has a wide bandwidth, the temporal structure of the input will tend to be preserved at the output (see Chapter 1, section 4 and Fig. 1.5). Thus the temporal patterns of firing will reflect the interruption of the noise. However, the time intervals between successive nerve impulses will be much less regular than for a periodic sound, since the exact waveform of the noise varies randomly from moment to moment; the only regularity is in the timing of the envelope, not the fine-structure. Thus the pitch of interrupted noise is weak.

The simple model we have presented does not account for the pitches which arise from a combination of the information at the two ears. However, it can easily be extended to do this by making the following reasonable assumptions. There is a separate filter bank, transduction mechanism and interval analyser for each ear. There is also a device determining interaural time intervals for spikes in channels with corresponding CFs (see Chapter 5). The results of the separate interval analysis for each ear, and of the interaural interval analysis, are fed to a common central interval comparator and decision mechanism.

In summary, the model we have presented can account for the major features of the pitch perception of complex tones, including the 'dominant region', the 'existence region', the pitch of nonharmonic complexes, and pitches produced by binaural interaction. Furthermore, it is consistent with the evidence presented earlier in this chapter that the pitch of pure tones is determined primarily by temporal mechanisms for frequencies up to 5 kHz. Notice, however, that both 'place' and temporal analysis play a crucial role in the model; neither alone is sufficient.

5   THE PERCEPTION OF MUSIC

Since this topic could easily occupy a book of its own, we limit ourselves to discussing certain selected aspects related to the rest of this chapter. The specially interested reader is referred to Ward (1970), who gives a more comprehensive review. Other relevant material will be found in Chapter 6.

A   *Octaves, musical intervals and musical scales*

It has been known for very many years that tones which are separated by an octave (i.e. where the frequencies are in the ratio 2:1) have an essential similarity, and indeed are given the same name (C, D, etc.) in the traditional musical scale. It is also the case that other musical intervals correspond to simple ratios between the frequencies of the tones. For example, a fifth corresponds to a frequency ratio of 3:2, a major third to 5:4 and a minor third to 6:5. When musical notes in these simple ratios are sounded simultaneously, the sound is pleasant, or consonant, whereas departures from simple, integral, ratios, as in certain progressive modern music, tend to result in a less pleasant or even a dissonant sound. This does not always hold for pure tones, a pair of which tend to be judged as consonant as soon as their frequency separation exceeds a critical band (Plomp and Levelt, 1965). However, complex tones blend harmoniously and tend to produce chords only when their fundamental frequencies are in simple ratios. In this situation several of their harmonics will coincide, whereas for non-simple ratios the harmonics will differ in frequency, and produce beating sensations. Thus at least part of the dissonance may be explained in terms of this beating, or interference, of harmonics on the basilar membrane when the harmonics are close together, but not identical, in frequency. This cannot account for the whole of the effect, however; a pronounced dissonance from two mistuned pure tones may be heard when the tones are presented one to each ear. It is of interest, then, to consider why we prefer certain frequency ratios, for both the simultaneous and successive presentation of tones, why octaves sound so similar, and why some sounds are consonant and others dissonant.

One type of theory suggests that we learn about octave relationships and about other musical intervals by exposure to harmonic complex sounds (usually speech sounds) from the earliest moments in life. For example, the first two harmonics in a periodic sound will have a frequency ratio 2:1, the 2nd and 3rd will have a ratio 3:2, the 3rd and 4th 4:3, etc. Thus by exposure to these sounds we learn to associate harmonics with particular frequency ratios. We discussed earlier in this chapter Terhardt's (1972c) suggestion that such a learning process could account for the phenomenon of the perceptual 'stretching' of the octave. If judgements of similarity and of consonance or dissonance also depend upon familiarity, then a learning process will also account for our perception of other musical intervals (Terhardt, 1974).

An alternative theory suggests that we prefer pairs of tones for which there is a similarity in the time patterns of neural discharge. This view was put forward as early as 1898 by Meyer, and has since been supported by Boomsliter and Creel (1961), among others. If it is the case that the pitch of a complex tone results from an analysis and correlation of the temporal patterns of firing in different groups of auditory neurones, then such an analysis would also reveal similarities between different tones when they are in simple frequency ratios. It is certainly the case that both our sense of musical pitch and our ability to make octave matches largely disappear above 5 kHz, the frequency at which neural synchrony no longer appears to operate. Furthermore, the highest note (fundamental) for instruments in the orchestra lies just below 5 kHz. One could argue from this that our lack of musical pitch at high frequencies is a result of a lack of exposure to tones at these frequencies. However, notes produced by musical instruments do contain harmonics above 5 kHz, so that if the learning of associations between harmonics were the only factor involved, there would be no reason for the change at 5 kHz.

It is of interest that the musical scale in general use today does not consist of notes in exact simple ratios. The common scale, the equal temperament (ET) scale, enables musicians to play in any key they choose, whereas with a system involving simple ratios only one key could be used. In the ET scale the octave (which still corresponds to a frequency ratio of 2:1) is divided into

12 equal logarithmic steps, known as semitones. Each successive semitone has a frequency about 5.9% higher than its neighbour. The deviations from a simple ratio scale are small, although they are probably great enough· to produce noticeable increases in the beating of harmonics of simultaneously presented complex tones at several points in the scale.

While simple ratios may be preferable for simultaneously presented tones, it is not clear whether this is the case for tones presented successively. A number of experiments investigating preferred notes in performances on stringed instruments of various kinds have shown that there is no simple answer. Some workers have found preferences for simple ratios, while others have found that the preferred scale corresponds fairly closely to ET, except that notes higher than the tonic or keynote tend to be sharpened relative to that note. Boomsliter and Creel (1963) asked musicians to play familiar tunes on a monochord, a one-stringed instrument with continuously variable tuning. They found that while subjects consistently chose the same tuning for a given note within a given tune, they chose different tunings, for what is ostensibly the same note, in different melodies and in different parts of the same melody. However, Boomsliter and Creel found that the chosen patterns formed a structure of small whole number ratios to the tonic and to additional reference notes linked by small whole number ratios to the tonic. Thus within small groups of notes simple ratios are preferred, although the 'reference' point may vary as the melody proceeds.

Whether or not there is something inherently preferable about simple frequency ratios, it is clear that individual differences and cultural background can influence significantly the musical combinations that are judged to be 'pleasant' or otherwise. Thus, for example, Indian musical scales contain 'microtones' in which the conventional scale is subdivided into smaller units, producing many musical intervals which do not correspond to simple ratios. Indian music often sounds strange to western ears, especially on first hearing, but it clearly does not sound strange to Indians; indeed, the microtones, and the various different scales which can be composed from them, are held to add considerably to the richness of the music and to the variety of moods which it can create.

While there is a psychoacoustic basis for consonance and dissonance judgements, these judgements also display individual differences and follow changes in the cultural norm. Modern classical music, for example, by Stravinsky and Stockhausen, contains many examples of chords which would have been considered dissonant 20 years ago but which are now enjoyed by many people.

B   *Absolute pitch and tone deafness*

Some people have the ability to recognize and define the pitch of a musical tone without reference to a comparison tone. This faculty is called absolute pitch, and is quite rare, probably occurring in less than 1% of the population. It seems to be distinct from the ability which some people develop to judge the pitch of a note in relation to, say, the lowest note which they can sing. Rakowski (1972) investigated absolute pitch by asking observers to adjust a variable signal so as to have the same pitch as a standard signal, for various time delays between the standard and variable tones. He used two groups of subjects, one group having been specially selected for their absolute pitch. For long time delays the subjects without absolute pitch showed a marked deterioration in performance, presumably because the pitch sensation stored in memory was lost. The subjects with absolute pitch seemed able to recall this memory with the aid of their 'imprinted' pitch standards, so that only a small decrement in performance was observed. When the standard tone belonged to the normal musical scale (e.g. $A_2 = 110$ Hz) there was hardly any decrement in performance with increasing time delay. The subjects did not seem able to acquire new standards and never, for example, learned to remember a 1000 Hz tone 'as such'; it was always recalled as being a little lower than C_6. Attempts to improve absolute pitch identification by intensive training have met with some success (Cuddy, 1968), but the levels of performance achieved rarely equal those found in genuine cases of absolute pitch. It seems likely that absolute pitch is a faculty acquired through 'imprinting' in childhood a limited number of standards. Ward (1963a, b; 1970) has suggested that the converse is true; we may all start with a sense of absolute pitch, but the ability is trained out of us because we are reinforced for relative and not absolute pitch judgements. The limited success achieved by training in adulthood tends, at the moment, to favour the idea of some sort of imprinting.

The term 'tone deafness' is a misnomer, since nearly everyone is able to judge that two tones are different in pitch when their frequency difference exceeds a certain amount. Many people, on the other hand, have difficulty in reproducing (i.e. singing) musical notes or sequences of notes, often because the notes fall outside the normal range which they would produce in speaking. It is likely that practice effects, and musical experience in general, have a considerable influence on this ability. A second difficulty commonly experienced by naive listeners is that of assigning a direction to a pitch change; they can often hear that two tones are different, but they cannot decide which is the higher in pitch. These people show a considerable improvement with practice, and it is usually found that listeners who claim to be tone deaf are eventually able to make very fine frequency discriminations. Beckett and Haggard (1973) did, however, find large differences in initial discrimination level between self-assessed musical and nonmusical subjects, and it is of interest why such large differences arise. Very probably both genetic and environmental factors are involved.

6   GENERAL SUMMARY

In this chapter we have discussed how the pitches of simuli are related to their physical properties, and to the anatomical and physiological properties of the auditory system. In principle, there are two ways in which the frequency of a sound may be coded; by the distribution of activity across different auditory neurones and by the temporal patterns of firing within and across neurones. It is likely that both types of information are utilized but that their relative importance is different for different frequency ranges and for different types of sounds.

The neurophysiological evidence in animals indicates that the synchrony of nerve impulses to a particular phase of the stimulating waveform disappears above 4–5 kHz. Above this frequency our ability to discriminate changes in the frequency of pure tones diminishes, and our sense of musical pitch disappears. It is likely that this reflects our use of temporal information in the frequency range below 4–5 kHz.

For complex tones two theories have been popular. One, the temporal theory, suggests that the pitch of a complex tone is derived from the time intervals between successive nerve firings evoked at a point in the cochlea where adjacent partials are interfering with one another. The second theory, the pattern recognition theory, suggests that pitch is derived by a central processor operating on neural signals corresponding to the individual partials present in the complex sound. In both theories, combination tones in the frequency region below the lowest partial may influence the pitch percept.

The pattern recognition theory is supported by the finding that low, resolvable, harmonics tend to dominate in the perception of pitch, and by the finding that a pitch corresponding to a 'missing fundamental' can be perceived when there is no possibility of an interference of partials in the cochlea. This has been demonstrated by presenting partials dichotically, one to each ear, or successively in time. The temporal theory is supported by the finding that (weak) pitches can be perceived when the harmonics are too close to be resolvable, and also when the stimuli have no well-defined spectral structure (e.g. interrupted noise). Thus neither of the theories can account for all of the experimental results.

We have proposed a model which incorporates features of both the temporal and the pattern recognition models. The model assumes that a complex stimulus first passes through a bank of filters (critical bands) with continuously overlapping centre frequencies. The outputs of the filters produce activity in neurones with corresponding CFs. The temporal pattern of activity in each 'channel' is analysed by a device which measures the time intervals between successive nerve impulses. Then a comparator or correlation device searches across channels looking for common time intervals.

The prominent time intervals are fed to a decision device which selects among the intervals. The perceived pitch corresponds to the reciprocal of the interval selected, and will usually be the same as the pitch corresponding to the fundamental component. This model can account for the majority of experimental results presented in this chapter.

Certain aspects of the perception of music may be related to the basic mechanisms underlying pitch perception. There is some evidence, for example, that we prefer musical intervals, or pairs of tones, for which there is a similarity in the time patterns of neural discharge. On the other hand it is clear that early experience, individual differences and cultural background also play a significant role in such judgments.

FURTHER READING

The following contain quite extensive reviews of the perception of pitch, although they come to slightly different conclusions from those reached in this chapter:

de Boer, E. (1976). On the 'residue' and auditory pitch perception. In *Handbook of Sensory Physiology*, Vol. 5 (eds W. D. Keidel and W. D. Neff), Springer-Verlag, Berlin.

Plomp, R. (1976). *Aspects of Tone Sensation*. Academic Press, London and New York.

5 Space perception

1   INTRODUCTION

The ability to localize sound sources is of considerable importance to both humans and animals; it will determine the direction of objects to seek or to avoid, and will indicate the appropriate direction to direct visual attention. The precision of sound localization is remarkable, particularly for brief sounds, or for those occurring in noisy or reverberant surroundings. While the most reliable cues used in the localization of sounds depend upon a comparison of the signals reaching the two ears, there are also phenomena of auditory space perception which result from monaural processing of the signals.

   The term 'localization' refers to judgements of the direction and distance of a sound source. Sometimes, when headphones are worn, the sound image is located inside the head. The term 'lateralization' is used to describe the apparent location of the sound source within the head. Headphones allow precise control of interaural differences and eliminate effects related to room echoes. Thus lateralization may be regarded as a laboratory version of localization which provides an efficient means of studying direction perception.

   While our binaural abilities are important for the accurate localization of sounds, this is not their only function. Using two ears, we are able selectively to attend to sounds coming from a particular direction while effectively excluding other sounds. This ability is particularly important in noisy surroundings, or when there are several sound sources competing for our attention.

   As well as being able to judge the direction of a sound source, we are able, in some cases, to estimate its distance. This ability is particularly developed in blind people, who can use information from echoes and reflections to determine the positions of objects in the environment.

2   THE LOCALIZATION OF PURE TONES AND BINAURAL BEATS

The cues which enable us to localize sounds may vary depending on the nature of these sounds. We consider first steady sinusoidal sounds. Later on we discuss a much more common class of sounds: those which are discontinuous, or contain transients.

Consider a sinusoidal sound source lying to one side of the head. The sound reaching the farther ear will be delayed in time and will be less intense relative to the nearer ear. There are thus two possible cues as to the location of the sound source. However, owing to the physical nature of the sounds, these cues are not equally effective at all frequencies. Low frequency sounds have a wavelength which is long compared with the size of the head, and thus the sound 'bends' very well around the head. This process is known as diffraction, and the result is that little or no 'shadow' is cast by the head. On the other hand, at high frequencies, where the wavelength is short compared with the dimensions of the head, little diffraction occurs. A 'shadow', almost like that produced by a beam of light, occurs. Interaural differences in intensity are negligible at low frequencies, but may be as large as 20 dB at high frequencies. This may easily be illustrated by placing a small transistor radio close to the ear. If that ear is now blocked with a finger, only sound bending around the head and entering the other ear will be heard. The sound will be much less 'tinny', since high frequencies will have been attenuated more than low; the head effectively acts like a low-pass filter. Interaural intensity differences will thus be more important at high frequencies than at low.

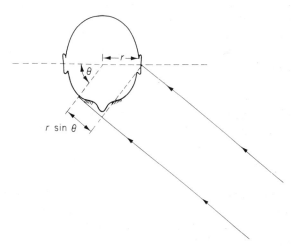

FIG. 5.1 Illustrating the difference in arrival time at the two ears for a distant sound source at an angle θ radians to the observer. If we denote the radius of the head (about 3.5 in or 9 cm) by r, then the path difference d between the two ears is given by

$$d = r\theta + r\sin\theta.$$

For a sound directly to one side of the observer $\theta = \pi/2$ radians and $d = (3.5 \times \pi/2) + (3.5 \times \sin \pi/2) = 9$ in Since sound takes about 30 μs to travel 1 cm, the corresponding time delay is about 690 μs.

If a tone is delayed in one ear relative to the other, then there will be a phase difference between the two ears; thus, if nerve impulses occur at a particular phase of the stimulating waveform, the relative timing of the nerve impulses at the two ears will be related to the location of the sound source. However, for sounds whose wavelength is comparable with, or less than, the distance between the two ears there will be ambiguity. The maximum path difference between the two ears is about 23 cm, which corresponds to a time delay of about 690 μs (see Fig. 5.1). Ambiguities will occur when the half-wavelength of the sound is about 23 cm, i.e. when the frequency of the sound is about 750 Hz. At this point a sound lying to one side of the head will produce waveforms at the two ears which are in opposite phase (phase difference between the two ears of 180°). From the observer's point of view the location of the sound source is now ambiguous, since the waveform at the right ear might be either a half-cycle behind that at the left ear or a half-cycle ahead. Head movements, or movements of the sound source, may resolve this ambiguity, so that there will be no abrupt upper limit in our ability to use phase differences between the two ears. However, when the wavelength of the sound is less than the path difference between the two ears, the ambiguities increase; the same phase difference could be produced by a number of different source locations. For periodic sounds, phase differences will only provide useful cues for frequencies below about 1500 Hz.

In a classic study Stevens and Newman (1936) investigated the localization of tone bursts with smooth onsets and offsets for observers on the roof of a building, so that reflected sounds were minimized. The listeners had to report the direction of the source, in a horizontal plane, to the nearest 15°. Although left–right confusions were rare, a low frequency sound in front was often indistinguishable from its mirror image behind. If these front–back confusions were discounted, then the error rate was low at very low and very high frequencies, and showed a maximum for midrange frequencies (around 3000 Hz for Stevens and Newman's data). These data were taken to indicate two different mechanisms for sound localization, one operating best at high frequencies and one at low. For middle frequencies neither mechanism operates efficiently, and errors are at a maximum.

These results have been broadly confirmed by more recent experiments (Sandel *et al.*, 1955) using anechoic chambers, except that systematic biases have been found in addition to errors; there is a tendency to underestimate the deviation of the source from the median plane when the frequency of the tone is between 1500 and 5000 Hz. When these systematic errors are eliminated, the greatest uncertainty in localization occurs at a frequency of about 1500 Hz. Sandel *et al.* also used an arrangement of two loudspeakers such that the resultant combined tone led in phase at one ear, but had a greater amplitude in the other. They found that the sound was located towards the side with the phase lead for frequencies below about 1500 Hz and towards the side with greater amplitude for frequencies above this. Near 1500 Hz listeners were confused.

These experiments confirm that the extent to which the cues of interaural time and intensity differences are used in the localization of pure tones is strongly related to what would be predicted from the physical nature of these cues. Intensity differences are more important at high frequencies, while phase differences only provided usable cues for frequencies below about 1500 Hz. Experiments using headphones (Mills, 1960) have shown that we are able to detect differences in intensity at the two ears even for low frequencies, and that these differences can produce a sense of location to one side. The smallest detectable difference for low frequencies is, however, larger than would occur in real life except under exceptional circumstances (e.g. holding a telephone close to one ear).

A phenomenon which seems to be closely related to the ability of the auditory system to process phase differences at the two ears is that of binaural beats. These may occur when a tone of one frequency is presented to one ear and a tone of slightly differing frequency is presented to the other ear. The sound appears to fluctuate or warble at a rate corresponding to the frequency difference between the two tones. Notice that binaural beats are quite different from the physical beats which are produced when the two frequencies are mixed in the electrical or acoustical system. Such physical beats or 'uniaural' beats occur because the two frequencies are alternately in phase and out of phase, and thus alternately cancel and reinforce one another; the intensity fluctuates at a rate depending on the frequency difference between the two tones. Binaural beats, on the other hand, depend upon an interaction in the nervous system of the inputs from the two ears, and have been considered to provide a demonstration that the discharges of neurones in the auditory nerve preserve information about the phase of the acoustic stimulus. If neural firings tend to occur at a particular phase of the stimulating waveform, then at some common neural centre the trains of neural firings from the two ears will superimpose differently depending on the relative phase of the stimuli at the two ears. There is thus a neural basis for the subjective fluctuations which occur when the relative phase at the two ears fluctuates, as it does when tones with slightly different frequencies are presented to the two ears.

Since binaural beats differ in their origin from 'uniaural' beats, it is hardly surprising that the two kinds of beats differ subjectively; binaural beats are never as distinct as uniaural beats. In addition, Licklider *et al.* (1950) pointed out that there is a continuum of subjective effects depending on the frequency separation of the two tones. As the frequency separation is slowly increased from zero, the listener may hear a tone that periodically shifts in subjective location, then fluctuates in loudness, then seems 'rough' and finally separates into two subjectively smooth tones. Uniaural beats can be observed over the entire audible frequency range, whereas binaural beats are essentially a low frequency phenomenon. Estimates of the highest frequency for which binaural beats can be observed have varied. The beats are heard most distinctly for frequencies between 300 and 600 Hz, but become progressively more difficult to hear at high frequencies. The exact upper limit depends upon the intensity used and upon the experimental technique, but it is generally agreed that the beats are exceedingly difficult to hear for frequencies above 1000 Hz (Licklider *et al.*, 1950). Uniaural beats are most distinctly heard when the two tones are matched for intensity, and cannot be heard at all when the intensities of the two tones differ greatly. Binaural beats, however, can be heard when there are large differences in intensity at the two ears (Tobias, 1963) and may even be heard when the tone to one ear is below absolute threshold (Groen, 1964). Thus phase-locking seems to occur over a wide range of stimulus intensities.

One interesting feature of binaural beats is that the upper limit of the frequency at which they are perceived is higher for men than for women. Further, the upper limit for women changes with the menstrual cycle, so that just at the onset of menstrual flow the upper limit for women approaches that of men (Tobias, 1965; Haggard and Bates, 1974). These changes are presumably related to hormonal variations and variations in retained body fluid, both of which could affect nerve transmission. It is possible that similar variations in performance will be observed for other kinds of tasks which are influenced by the timing of nerve impulses, e.g. the localization of sounds and the perception of residue pitches. Indeed, the extent to which such variations occur could be used to assess the importance of temporal information in these tasks.

3   THE IMPORTANCE OF TRANSIENTS

All sounds which occur in nature have onsets and offsets, and many also change their intensity or their spectral structure as a function of time. Interaural differences in the time of arrival of these transients provide cues for the localization of these sounds which are not subject to the phase ambiguities which occur for steady tones. Such cues are often eliminated in experiments using pure tones, by turning the tones on and off very slowly, although for pure tones the transient cues may be comparable in effectiveness to the continuously available cues of ongoing intensity and phase differences. Klump and Eady (1956) measured thresholds for the detection of interaural time differences using stimuli delivered via headphones. They compared three types of stimuli: band-limited noise (containing frequencies in the range 150–1700 Hz), 1000 Hz pure tones with gradual rise and fall times, and clicks of duration 1 ms. The first stimulus varies continuously as a function of time, and thus provides transient information which is repeated many times during the presentation time of the stimulus; the pure tone provides only information relating to ongoing phase differences; while the click is effectively a single transient. The threshold interaural time differences were $9\,\mu s$, $11\,\mu s$ and $28\,\mu s$. Thus the greatest acuity occurred for the noise stimulus, with continuously available transient information, but the tone gave performance which was only slightly worse. The single click gave rise to the poorest performance. It is worth noting, however, that the tones in this experiment were of relatively long duration (1.4 s). For tones of shorter duration our acuity is not so great, so that cues related to onset and offset transients (which would be comparable to those provided by the clicks) become relatively more important.

For sounds with ongoing transient disparities, such as bursts of noise, our ability to detect interaural time differences improves with duration of the bursts for durations up to about 700 ms, when the threshold disparity (the smallest detectable time difference at the two ears) reaches an asymptotic level of about $6\,\mu s$ (Tobias and Zerlin, 1959). It is remarkable that such small time differences between the ears are detectable, since the 'jitter' in the instant of initiation of nerve impulses has a standard deviation of about 100 μs at 1 kHz. Tobias (1972) has discussed some of the ways in which this accuracy might be achieved, including the possibility that there is a direct neural pathway from one cochlea to the other. At the present time, however, the neural mechanism by which we discriminate these remarkably small time intervals remains a mystery.

Tobias and Schubert (1959) investigated the relative importance of onset disparities and ongoing disparities in lateralization judgements by pitting one against the other. They presented bursts of noise via headphones, with a particular onset time difference, and determined the amount of ongoing disparity needed to counteract the onset information and recentre the subjective image. They found that small ongoing disparities offset much larger transient onset disparities and that for durations exceeding 300 ms the onset has no effect. Even for short bursts (10 ms) the ongoing disparity has the greater effect. For very short impulsive sounds the importance of onset disparity will be much greater; for brief clicks this will be the only kind of transient disparity. It is worth noting that for high frequency pure tones the ongoing phase differences at the two ears are not processed by the auditory system. However, these tones can still be lateralized on the basis of onset transient disparities.

Stimuli such as noises and clicks contain energy over a wide range of frequencies. Yost *et al.* (1971) attempted to determine which frequency components were the most important, by studying the lateralization of clicks whose frequency content had been altered by filtering. The subjects were asked to discriminate a centred image (produced by identical clicks at each ear) from a displaced image (produced by delaying the click to the left ear only). They found that discrimination deteriorated for clicks which were high-pass filtered, so that only energy above 1500 Hz was present, but was largely unaffected by low-pass filtering. Masking with a lowpass noise produced a marked disruption, while a high-pass noise had little effect. Thus it seems that the discrimination of lateral position on the basis of time delays between the two ears depends largely on the low frequency content of the clicks, although somewhat poorer discrimination is possible with only high frequency components. This result is somewhat surprising at first sight, since the high frequency components in the click contribute to the 'sharpness' of its edges (a low-pass filtered click will have longer rise and decay times) and therefore to the precision with which its timing can be defined. However, the finding ties in rather well with the results obtained with pure tones, showing that we cannot compare phases between the two ears of frequencies above 1500 Hz. When a click is presented to the ear, it produces a waveform, at a given point on the basilar membrane, looking rather like a decaying sinusoidal oscillation (see Fig. 1.11). The frequency of the oscillation will depend on which part of the basilar membrane is being observed; at the basal end the frequency will be high and at the apical end it will be low. For frequencies below 1500 Hz the phases of these decaying oscillations at the two ears can be compared, thus conveying accurate information about the relative timing of the clicks at the two ears. For frequencies above 1500 Hz this 'fine structure' information will be lost; only timing information relating to the envelope of the decaying oscillation will be available at the point of binaural interaction, thus reducing the accuracy with which the clicks can be localized. (See section 6 for further discussion on this point.)

Henning (1974) has provided further evidence for the importance of the amplitude envelope. He investigated the lateralization of high frequency tones which had been amplitude modulated. (See Fig. 3.7 for an illustration of this waveform.) He found that the detectability of interaural delays in the envelope of a 3900 Hz carrier modulated at a frequency of 300 Hz was about as good as the detectability of interaural delays in a 300 Hz pure tone. However, there were considerable differences among individual observers; the interaural delays necessary for 75% correct detections in his forced choice task had values of 20, 50 and 65 μs for three different subjects (all stimuli had 250 ms durations and 50 ms rise–fall times). Henning found that time delay of the envelope rather than time delay of the 'fine-structure' within the envelope determines the lateralization. The signals could be lateralized on the basis of time delays in the envelope even when the carrier frequencies were different in the two ears. Thus it seems that for complex signals containing only high frequency components, listeners extract the envelopes of the signals and compare the relative timing of the envelopes at the two ears. However, lateralization performance is best when the carrier frequencies are identical, and poor lateralization results when the complex waveforms at each ear have no frequency component in common. Thus factors other than the amplitude envelope can affect lateralization performance.

At first sight there appears to be a discrepancy between the results of Henning and the results of Yost *et al.* (1971); Yost *et al.* found extremely poor lateralization for clicks which had been filtered so as to contain only high-frequency components, whereas Henning found relatively good performance for AM tones containing only high frequency components. The crucial difference is one of duration; in Henning's experiment many fluctuations in envelope amplitude occurred during the presentation time of the stimuli, while Yost *et al.* presented only single clicks. When Yost *et al.* presented a train of clicks, they found that performance for high-pass clicks improved with increasing duration. As Henning points out, these results indicate that duration is an important determinant of the detectability of interaural time differences.

It is worth noting that all the experiments described in this section were carried out using headphones. While this does not in any way negate the results, it does mean that cues related to interaural intensity differences have been eliminated. These cues may, in a normal listening environment, have a significant effect on the localization of sounds containing high frequency components. Subjective impressions indicate that sounds containing high frequency components may be easily and accurately located, and at least a part of this ease will be related to the intensity differences at the two ears and to the differences in spectral composition at the two ears which are produced by the low-pass action of the head and by the pinnae (see section 4).

If we ignore, for the moment, the influence of the pinnae, then we may regard the head as a pair of holes separated by a spherical obstacle. If the head is kept stationary, then a given interaural time difference will not be sufficient uniquely to define the position of the sound source in space; there is a cone of confusion (see Mills, 1972, and Fig. 5.2). The particular way that the ears are situated on the head also gives rise to the fact that we are much better at localizing sounds in the horizontal dimension than in the vertical dimension. Ambiguities related to the cone of confusion, or to the location of a sound source in the vertical direction, may be resolved by head movements. If we rotate our heads about a vertical axis by, say, 20°, and this results in a 20° shift in the apparent lateral position of the auditory image in relation to the head, then we locate the sound source in the horizontal plane. If the rotation of the head is accompanied by no change in the auditory image, then the sound is located either directly above or directly below the observer. Intermediate shifts in the location of the auditory image lead to intermediate vertical height judgements (Wallach, 1940). Hirsh (1971) has

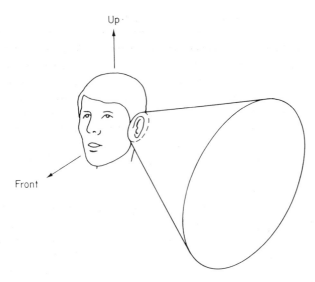

FIG. 5.2 A cone of confusion for a spherical head and a particular interaural time delay. All sound sources on the surface of the cone would produce that interaural time delay. For details of how to calculate the cone of confusion see Mills (1972).

reviewed a number of experiments showing improved localization abilities when head movements are allowed, so that in many cases monaural hearing is as good as binaural hearing (see below for further details). These experiments, and the results of a number of clinical studies, indicate that for hearing aid wearers the ability to localize will be greater for head-worn aids than for body-worn aids (see below for further discussion of this point).

4   MONAURAL LOCALIZATION AND THE ROLE OF THE PINNAE

Several workers have reported that under some conditions the localization of sounds with one ear can be as accurate as that with two, particularly if head movements are allowed (e.g. Freedman and Fisher, 1968). However, most of the experiments on monaural localization have used rather coarse steps in degrees from one sound source (usually a loudspeaker) to the next, so that in many conditions nearly perfect performance was achieved for both monaural and binaural modes; in other words, the coarseness of the measure may well have obscured any superiority in binaural conditions. To overcome these problems, Harris and Sergeant (1971) instructed subjects to keep their heads as still as possible, and determined the minimum audible angle (the smallest detectable change in angular position in the lateral plane, denoted

MAA) for a moving sound source. The subjects listened (1) with both ears open, (2) with one ear plugged, muffed and noise masked. They found that the monaural MAA was as small as the binaural MAA for white noise, but that for tones the monaural MAA was usually larger by a factor of 2 or more. For complex sounds, such as white noise, movements of either the head or the sound source produce changes in the spectral patterning at each ear (see below), and these changes provide cues as to the extent and direction of the movement. Thus for such complex sounds monaural localization can be as good as binaural. For simple stimuli, such as pure tones, the binaural mode is superior, although moderately good localization is still possible in the monaural mode.

While head movements, or movements of the sound source, are clearly important and can help to resolve ambiguities in vertical direction, our abilities at judging vertical direction are far in excess of what would be predicted if only information related to head movements or interaural differences were available. For example, we are able to judge the location of a burst of white noise in the median plane (the locus of points equidistant from the two ears) when the duration of the burst is too short to allow useful information to be gained from head movements.

Many workers have suggested that the action of the pinnae provides for verticality judgements (e.g. Butler, 1969) and for the discrimination of front from back, while others (e.g. Batteau, 1967; Freedman and Fisher, 1968) have suggested that the pinnae are important for localization in every direction. Batteau investigated the action of the pinna using a scaled-up model, with a microphone inserted in the 'ear canal'. He found that the pinna transformed the incoming signal so that the initial signal was followed by a series of time delayed replications. This kind of effect is limited to signals containing high frequency components; only for frequencies above about 6 kHz is the wavelength of the sound sufficiently short to produce strong interactions with the pinna. For these high frequencies the sound enters the ear via a number of different paths: a direct path producing the initial signal, and several paths via the 'corrugations' in the pinna, producing the delayed replications. For lower frequencies the 'corrugations' have a negligible effect on the incoming sound. Batteau suggested that the pattern of delays differed characteristically according to locale, so that the encoding action of the pinna would in principle allow for a unique direction to be assigned to a sound source.

To investigate whether we are actually able to use these time delays, Batteau inserted microphones into casts of actual pinnae held on a bar without a model of the head in between them. The sounds picked up by the microphones were played to the subjects via high fidelity headphones. Thus the subjects had remotely controlled but realistic outer ears! The subjects were able to make reasonably accurate judgements of both azimuth (left–

front–right, etc.) and elevation. When the pinnae were removed from the microphones, judgements were quite erratic. It is noteworthy that with the artificial pinnae in place subjects reported that the sounds were actually localized out 'in space' and not, as is usually the case with headphones, simply lateralized inside the head. This impression persisted even when one microphone was disconnected. Clearly, then, the pinnae are providing some information as to the location of sound sources. In order to demonstrate more clearly that the pattern of temporal delays was the crucial factor, Batteau constructed a set of time delays artificially using a delay line. Signals were fed directly to the ear canal via tubes. The signals conveyed an impression of locale which could be altered by adjusting the pattern of delays. Thus the presence of such time delayed replications seems to be a sufficient condition for the perception of direction.

A number of other experiments have indicated that the pinnae can play a role in sound localization. Freedman and Fisher (1968) investigated the localization of short bursts of white noise presented in an acoustically treated room. They compared three conditions: (1) with subjects listening normally, (2) with sound conducted directly to the ears via 10 cm metal tubes and (3) with casts of pinnae on the ends of the tubes. If head movements were restricted there was no significant difference between (1) and (3), while both produced significantly more accurate localization than did (2). However, if head movements were allowed, there were no differences between the three conditions, all subjects achieving nearly perfect performance. While this experiment demonstrates pinna effects, the accuracy required was not great (22.5°), and the effects were not important when head movements were allowed. It is of interest that in condition (3) the casts were not of the subject's own pinnae. Pinnae differ considerably between people, and it would be of interest to know how far we are able to use, or to learn to use, information from other people's pinnae!

It is clear from these experiments that the encoding action of the pinna can indicate the direction of a sound source. However, the real importance of this coding is still a matter of debate. Most of the experiments investigating monaural localization have used widely spaced loudspeakers, so that acuities of the order of 1–2°, which can be achieved under binaural conditions, could not have been measured. Further, pinna encoding effects can only be of importance when the stimuli contain high frequency components; only for frequencies above about 6 kHz is the wavelength of the sound sufficiently short to produce strong interactions with the pinna. However, some pinna effects have been found for frequencies lower than this. Gardner and Gardner (1973) investigated localization in the median plane for wideband noise and for bands of noise with various different centre frequencies. They found that occlusion of the pinnae cavities (filling them with moulded rubber plugs) decreased localization abilities, the largest effects occurring for wideband noise and for the bands of noise with highest centre frequencies (8 and 10 kHz), although there was still some effect at 3 kHz.

One problem with Batteau's theory of time-delay encoding is that the time delays involved are exceedingly small; 10–300 μs is a typical value given by Batteau. While the auditory system is capable of dealing with such time differences for stimuli presented to opposite ears, it is unlikely that the system could resolve two stimuli arriving at the same ear when they are separated by only 100 μs. However, the time delays described by Batteau would not only alter the temporal structure of the stimuli; they would also modify the effective spectrum of the stimuli reaching the eardrum. Depending on the particular time delays which were present, certain frequency bands would be boosted, while others would be reduced in intensity. This has been confirmed by measurements at the entrance to the ear canal of human observers (Blauert, 1969/1970). The head and pinna together form a filter which is something like a 'comb' filter. Further, the frequency bands which are boosted depend on the direction of sound incidence. Blauert has shown that the perceived direction of the sound source depends upon these boosted bands and that there is relatively little variation between observers in these kinds of judgements. If both ears are stimulated with identical narrowband noise signals, the direction of the sound sensation depends upon frequency only, and not upon the direction of sound incidence. Similar kinds of results have been found by Butler (1971) for the localization of tone bursts with one ear occluded. The perceived direction of the sound source depends on frequency, rather than on the actual location of the sound source. While the effects described by Batteau are limited to frequencies above 6 kHz, effects related to the modification of the spectrum of the stimulus may operate at much lower frequencies than this, because the head, as well as the pinnae, can affect the spectrum. The effects described by Blauert and by Butler were found for frequencies between 500 Hz and 16 kHz. We may conclude that while the presence of time delayed replications is a sufficient condition for the perception of direction, it is not a necessary one. It seems likely that observers are actually processing information relating to the spectrum of the stimulus, and that time delays are only effective by virtue of the spectral changes which they produce.

If the listener is to make efficient use of spectral cues associated with the direction of a sound source, then he must be able to distinguish spectral peaks and dips related to direction from peaks and dips inherent in the character of the stimulus itself. Thus one might expect that a knowledge of the sound source and room conditions may also be important. To some extent, the two ears provide separate sets of spectral cues, so that the difference between the two ears could be used to locate unfamiliar sound sources, but for sound sources in the median plane (i.e. sound sources which are equidistant from the two ears) the cues at the two ears will be almost identical for all locations. Plenge (1972, 1974) has presented evidence that we do, in fact, make comparisons with stored stimulus patterns in judging the location of a sound source. He showed that if subjects were not allowed to become familiar with the characteristics of the sound source and the listening room, then localization was disturbed. In many cases the sound sources were lateralized in the head rather than being localized externally. This was particularly true for sound in the median plane. However, such familiarity does not seem to require an extended learning process. We become familiar with sound source characteristics and room acoustics within a very few seconds of entering a new situation.

5   THE PRECEDENCE EFFECT

In a normal listening environment the sound from a given source, such as a loudspeaker, reaches our ears via a number of different paths. Some of the sound will arrive by a direct path, but a good deal of it will only reach our ears after one or more reflections from the surfaces of the room. In spite of this, we are not normally aware of these reflections, or echoes, and they do not appear to influence our judgements of the direction of the sound source. Thus we are still able accurately to locate a speaker in a reverberant room where the total energy in the reflected sound may be greater than that reaching our ears by a direct path.

Wallach *et al.* (1949) investigated the way the auditory system copes with echoes in experiments using both sound sources in free space and sounds delivered by headphones. In the experiments using headphones pairs of clicks were delivered to each ear (two clicks in each earphone). The delay between the two clicks in a pair, and the time of arrival of the first click in a pair could be varied independently (see Fig. 5.3). The results can be summarized as follows:

1   Two brief sounds that reach an observer's ears in close succession will be heard as a single sound if the interval between them is sufficiently short. The interval over which fusion takes place is not the same for all types of sounds. The upper limit of the interval is about 5 ms for single clicks, but may be as long as 40 ms for sounds of a complex character, such as speech or music.
2   If two brief sounds are heard as fused into a single sound, the location of the total sound is determined largely by the location of the first sound. This is known as the precedence effect.
3   The effect is only shown for sounds of a discontinuous or transient character.
4   The second sound, or echo, can be shown to have a small but demon-

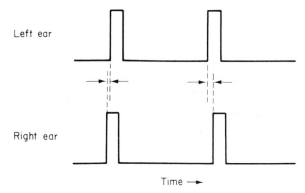

Left ear

Right ear

Time ⟶

FIG. 5.3 The stimulus sequence used by Wallach *et al.* (1949) to investigate the precedence effect. The first pair of clicks arrive at the ears with a small interaural time disparity, indicated by the arrows. The second pair of clicks simulate a room echo and have a different interaural disparity. The whole stimulus sequence is heard as a single sound whose location is determined primarily by the interaural delay of the leading pair of clicks.

strable effect. If the location of the second sound departs more and more from the location of the first sound, it will pull the total sound along with it up to a maximal amount (about 7°) and then it becomes progressively less effective.

5 If the interval between the arrival of the two sounds is 1 ms or less, the precedence effect does not operate; some average or compromise location will be heard.

6 If the second stimulus is made sufficiently intense (15 dB above the first sound), it overrides the precedence factor.

7 The precedence effect is favoured for sounds which are qualitatively similar; if the 'echo' differs greatly from the leading sound, then fusion will not occur.

The precedence effect seems to be essentially a binaural phenomenon; it is the interaural differences in the leading sound which allow an accurate assessment of its location in the presence of echoes. The fusion effect itself also seems to depend on binaural interaction. A simple demonstration of this may be obtained by placing one finger in an ear while listening to a speaker in a reverberant room; immediately the characteristics of the room become more apparent. The sound becomes 'muddy' and booming, and it is difficult to locate the speaker accurately. Batteau (1968) has reported that filling the pinnae with silicone rubber produces an increase in subjective amount of reverberation, possibly indicating that pinna encoding effects are also involved. However, no formal experiments on this topic have been reported.

It is clear that the precedence effect plays an important role in our perception of everyday sounds. It enables us to locate, interpret and identify sounds in spite of wide variations in the acoustical conditions in which we hear them. Without it listening in reverberant rooms would be an extremely confusing experience. Sometimes, on the other hand, the effect can be an inconvenience! An example of this is found in the stereophonic reproduction of music. Contrary to popular opinion, the stereo information on a record is coded almost entirely in terms of intensity differences in the two channels; time disparities are eliminated as far as possible, because these would only provide meaningful information for one particular separation of the loudspeakers. If the sound originates in one channel only, then the sound will be clearly located towards that channel. If the sound is equally intense in both channels, then the sound will be located in the centre, between the two channels, provided that the loudspeakers are equidistant from the listener. If, however, the listener is slightly closer to one loudspeaker than to the other, the sound from that loudspeaker will reach him earlier in time, and if the time disparity exceeds 1 ms, the precedence effect will operate; the sound will appear to originate entirely from the nearer loudspeaker. In a normal room this gives the listener a latitude of about 60 cm on either side of the central position. Deviations greater than this will produce significant changes in the 'stereo image'. Almost all of the sound (except that originating entirely from the farther loudspeaker) will appear to come from the closer loudspeaker. Thus the notion of the 'stereo seat' is quite close to the truth. Recently attempts have been made to broaden the acceptable listening area, using 'omnidirectional' loudspeakers, which radiate sound in all directions rather than beaming it forward. It is claimed that with these loudspeakers the listening position is not critical, but many listeners have complained that they are unable to locate a sound source precisely with these loudspeakers no matter where they sit. Clearly, further research is needed before the benefits, if any, of these loudspeakers can be evaluated. This point is discussed further in Chapter 8, section 3.

6   TIME–INTENSITY TRADING

If identical clicks are presented to the two ears via headphones, then the sound source is usually located in the middle of the head; the image is said to be centred. If now the click in the left ear is made to lead that in the right ear by, say, 100 μs, the sound image will move to the left. However, by making the click in the right ear more intense, it is possible to make the sound image move back towards the right, so that once again the image is centred. Thus it seems possible to trade a time difference at the two ears for an intensity difference.

This finding led to the theory that time differences and intensity differences are eventually coded in the nervous system in a similar sort of way. In particular, it was suggested that the latency of neural responses was shorter to more intense sounds, so that intensity differences were transformed into time differences at the neural level. Thus Deatherage and Hirsh (1957) stated:

> . . . once the frame of reference becomes neural, we would hypothesize that intensity, having made its contribution to neural time, may drop out of consideration, leaving the judgement of localization almost entirely dependent upon results of comparison of neural time.

Many investigators have measured the value of the time–intensity trade, expressed in μs/dB, for different types of stimuli. It is clear that the results are affected by many different variables, including absolute intensity, frequency or frequency band, duration and presence of noise. Thus reported values of the trading function have varied from 1.7 μs/dB for pure tones (Shaxby and Gage, 1932), to 100 μs/dB for pulse trains (Christman and Victor, 1955). Harris (1960) measured the trading relation for clicks which had been high-or low-pass filtered at various cutoff frequencies. He found that low-pass clicks, with cutoff frequencies below 1500 Hz, gave values of about 25 μs/dB, whereas high-pass clicks gave values of about 90 μs/dB. At low sensation levels (20 dB) a discontinuity was apparent at about 1500 Hz, but this disappeared at higher levels. He also noted that when an image is centred by offsetting an intensity difference with a time difference, the variability of the judgements is greater than when sounds equal in intensity are centred. Thus it seems that time differences and intensity differences may not be truly equivalent.

More recently a number of workers have reported that both for tones of low frequency and for clicks observers may report two separate sound images. For tones Whitworth and Jeffress (1961) found that one sound, the 'time image', was little affected by interaural differences in level, and showed a trading ratio of about 1 μs/dB. The other, the 'intensity image', showed a trading ratio of about 20 μs/dB. For clicks Hafter and Jeffress (1968) found ratios of 2–35 μs/dB for the 'time image', and 85–150 μs/dB for the 'intensity image'. Recently Hafter and Carrier (1972) have confirmed that observers are able to detect differences between diotic signals (identical in each ear) and dichotic signals which have been centred by opposing a time difference with an intensity difference. Thus these experiments confirm that time and intensity differences are not truly equivalent. Notice that in a normal listening situation time and intensity differences would not be opposed. Presumably the perceptual mechanism 'expects' them to covary in a physically realistic fashion, and it is only when this does not occur that two sound images are perceived.

Jeffress (1971) has suggested that there are at least two mechanisms underlying localization (and lateralization), one of which is affected by interaural differences in both level and time, operates over the whole of the auditory range and is responsible for the intensity image. The other is little affected by differences in level, but operates on interaural time differences over the frequency range below 1500 Hz. This suggestion of a dual mechanism agrees well with the generalizations made earlier in this chapter. When we discussed the experiments of Yost *et al.* (1971) on the lateralization of filtered clicks, we saw that the most accurate localization was possible when energy was present below 1500 Hz, since in that frequency range the timing of the 'fine-structure' of the waveforms on the basilar membrane can be compared at the two ears. For frequencies above this the fine-structure information will be lost, and only the envelopes of the waveforms on the basilar membrane will be compared. Physiological evidence (Kiang *et al.*, 1965) indicates that changes in the intensity of clicks produce relatively little change in latency for those (lower frequency) fibres which display phase-locking; firings still occur at a particular point of a positive-going deflection on the basilar membrane. However, relatively more responses tend to occur on the first few deflections of the basilar membrane (recall that a click produces a waveform resembling a decaying sinusoidal oscillation), so that the mean latency of neural response, a measure related more to the en-velope of the signal, is shorter. This is illustrated in Fig. 5.4.

There is, then, some physiological support for Jeffress's suggestion of two central mechanisms. One, the time mechanism, will operate on the time differences in firing of phase-locked neural fibres, which are little affected by changes in level. The second, the intensity mechanism, will be affected both by interaural time differences and by differences in the mean latency of neural response to impulsive signals which result from interaural level differences. We may assume that dual localizations in trading experiments result from conflicts between the two systems.

Taken together, the results of trading experiments make it quite clear that there is not a single simple trade between time and intensity. Rather there appear to be two different mechanisms by which time and intensity differences interact. However, it is only in the rather artificial situation of the laboratory that these two mechanisms produce sound images in widely different locations. In real life time and intensity differences will nearly always work in conjunction to provide a single, well-defined sound image.

7   GENERAL CONCLUSIONS ON SOUND LOCALIZATION

We have seen that the human observer is capable of using a great variety of physical cues in determining the location of sound source. Time differences at the two ears, intensity differences at the two ears, changes in the spectral composition of sounds due to head-shadow and pinna effects, and changes in all of these cues produced by head or sound source movements, can all

FIG. 5.4 Poststimulus time (PST) histograms of the response to click stimulation of a single auditory nerve fibre, as a function of click level. Each histogram shows the number of nerve firings occurring at a particular time after the instant of click presentation. The CF of the neurone was 630 Hz. Click level is expressed relative to a high reference level, the higher click levels being at the bottom of the figure. From Kiang *et al.* (1965), by permission of the author and MIT Press.

influence the perceived direction of a sound source. In laboratory studies usually just one or two of these cues are isolated. In this way it has been shown that sometimes a single cue may be sufficient for accurate localization of a sound source. In other experiments one cue has been opposed by another, in order to investigate the relative importance of the cues, or to determine whether the cues are encoded along some common neural dimension. These experiments have shown that, in some senses, the cues are not equivalent, but, on the other hand, they may also not be independent. For real sound sources, such as speech or music, all of the cues described above may be available simultaneously. However, in this situation they will not provide conflicting cues; rather the multiplicity of cues will render the location of the sound sources more sure and more accurate.

8   BINAURAL MASKING LEVEL DIFFERENCES

We pointed out earlier than separation of sound sources was one of the benefits of auditory localization. We will now turn to a group of laboratory experiments which have explored the psychoacoustical basis of such separation in considerable detail. Consider the situation shown in Fig. 5.5a. White noise from the same noise generator is fed to both ears via stereo headphones. Pure tones, also from the same signal generator, are fed separately to each ear and mixed with the noise. Thus the total signals at the two ears are identical. Assume that the level of the tone is adjusted until it is just masked by the noise, i.e. it is at its masked threshold, and let its level at this point be L_0 dB. Provided that the equipment isolates the versions of the noise and of the tone that each ear will receive, we can invert the signal (the tone) in phase at one ear only (this is equivalent to turning the waveform upside-down; see Fig. 5.5b). The result is that the tone becomes audible again. The tone can be adjusted to a new level, L_π, so that it is once again at its masked threshold. The difference between the two levels, $L_0 - L_\pi$ (dB) is known as a masking level difference (MLD), and its value may be as large as 15 dB at low frequencies (around 500 Hz), decreasing to 2–3 dB for frequencies above 1500 Hz. Thus simply by inverting the signal waveform at one ear we can make the signal considerably more easy to detect.

An example which is perhaps even more startling is given in Fig. 5.5c. The noise and signal are fed to one ear only, and the signal is adjusted to be at its masked threshold. Now the noise alone is added at the other ear; the tone becomes audible once again! (Fig. 5.5d). Thus by adding noise at the non-signal ear we make the tone considerably more easy to detect. Further, the tone disappears when it, too, is added to the second ear, making the sounds at the two ears the same. Notice that it is important that the same noise is added to the non-signal ear; the noises at the two ears must be

FIG. 5.5 Illustration of two situations in which binaural masking-level differences (BMLDs) occur. In conditions (a) and (c) detectability is poor, while in conditions (b) and (d), where the interaural relations of the signal and masker are different, detectability is good (hence the smiling faces).

correlated or derived from the same noise generator. Release from masking is not obtained when uncorrelated noise (derived from a second noise generator) is added to the non-signal ear.

The phenomenon of the MLD is not limited to pure tones. Similar effects have been observed for complex tones, clicks and speech sounds. It seems to be the case that whenever the phase or level differences of the signal at the two ears are not the same of those of the masker, our ability to detect and identify the signals will be improved relative to the case where the signal and masker have the same phase and level relationships at the two ears. Such differences will only occur in real situations when the signal and masker are located in different positions in space. Thus one implication of the MLD phenomenon is that the detection and interpretation of signals, including speech, will be improved when the signal and masker are not coincident in space. The MLD is thus seen to be very closely related to the 'cocktail party' phenomenon. However, it appears that the MLD is not merely another aspect of our ability to localize sounds, because the largest MLDs occur with the situation of phase inversion (see above) which only occurs naturally for midfrequency pure tones at highly restricted angular locations. Further, large MLDs occur in situations where the signal and masker are not subjectively well separated in space (see later).

At this point we must introduce some terminology. When the relative phase of the signal at the two ears is the same as the relative phase of the masker, the condition is called homophasic. When the phase relations are opposite, the term 'antiphasic' is used. In general we can describe a particular situation by using the symbols N (for noise) and S (for signal), each being followed by a suffix denoting relative phase at the two ears. A phase inversion is equivalent to a phase shift of 180° or π radians. Thus $N_0 S_\pi$ refers to the condition where the noise is in phase at the earphones and the signal is inverted in phase. In general, this leads to the largest MLDs, although $N_\pi S_0$ is also large.

A number of models have been presented which attempt to account for the MLD phenomenon. In general, these have not attempted explanations at the physiological level, but have rather been 'black box' models, assuming that the auditory system is capable of certain types of processing without specifying exactly how it is done. Before we discuss these models we shall present some of the experimental findings which the models have to explain.

A   The MLD as an empirical phenomenon

One very general finding which has emerged from MLD studies is that the largest effects occur at low frequencies. Effects greater than 2–3 dB are limited to the frequency region below about 1500 Hz, and it is noteworthy that this is also the highest frequency for which we are able to compare phases at the two ears in localizing sounds. Thus it is likely that the MLD depends at least in part on the transmission of temporal information about the stimulus to some higher neural centre which compares the temporal information from the two ears.

A second general feature which has emerged is that for a wideband masker not all of the frequency components are effective; just as was the case for normal masking (see Chapter 3), only those components in a critical band around the signal seem to be effective in masking it. Mulligan *et al.* (1967) presented a tone to one ear only and investigated the effects of various different masking noises at the two ears. They found that so long as the critical band levels at the two ears remained the same, changes in the masker's bandwidth and overall level at one ear, with respect to the other, had no effect on detection. In other words, only changes within the critical band affected the detectability of the tone. A narrow band of noise at the non-signal ear was sufficient to provide release from masking produced by a wider band of correlated noise (derived from the same noise generator) at the other ear, but no release was observed when the noise was uncorrelated.

In addition to improving the detectability of tones, conditions which produce MLDs also favour other aspects of our ability to analyse signals. For example, when speech signals are presented against noisy backgrounds, we may be able to detect that something was said, but not to identify what was said. In such situations a number of workers have shown improved speech intelligibility under antiphasic conditions (e.g. Hirsh, 1950). More recently Gebhardt and Goldstein (1972) measured frequency DLs for tones presented against noise backgrounds and found that, for a given signal-to-noise ratio, antiphasic DLs are substantially smaller than homophasic ones when the signals are close to masked threshold. Thus antiphasic conditions improve our ability to identify and discriminate signals, as well as to detect them.

The relative importance of spatial factors in the MLD was investigated by Carhart *et al.* (1969). They measured thresholds for spondees and mono-syllables in the presence of four competing maskers, a situation which mirrors the 'cocktail party' phenomenon quite closely. Two of the maskers were modulated white noise and two were whole sentences. They used several different listening conditions, including homophasic, antiphasic and those where the signal or the maskers were delayed at one ear relative to the other. In these latter conditions the different maskers were sometimes given opposing time delays, so that some would be located towards one ear and some towards the other. Sometimes the signal was subjectively well-separated in location from the masking sounds, and under these conditions subjects reported the task of identifying the spondees to be easier. However, the largest MLDs were obtained for the antiphasic condition, where there is no clear separation in the subjective locations; rather the sound images are located diffusely within the head. Thus escape from masking and lateralization/localization seem, to some extent, to be separate capacities.

Recently it has been reported that MLDs occur for both forward and backward masking (Small *et al.*, 1972; Dolan and Trahiotis, 1972). Substantial MLDs (4–5 dB) are found for silent intervals between the signal and the masker of up to 40 ms. Thus it seems that detailed aspects of the waveforms at the two ears (such as phase) are retained in the auditory system until interaction between the signal and masker occurs.

9   MODELS TO EXPLAIN MLDs

Although several models have been proposed to account for the MLD, none is completely successful in explaining all aspects of the experimental data. We shall discuss the two models which have been the most influential in this area, and follow this with a more general discussion.

A   *The Webster–Jeffress model*

Webster (1951) pointed out that a narrowband noise resembles a sinusoid whose amplitude and phase vary slowly from moment to moment. The band of noise which is effective in masking the tone, the critical band, may also be thought of in this way. Adding a tonal signal to this noise will yield a resultant which generally will differ in phase and amplitude from the original noise. If, for example, adding the signal at one ear advances the signal-plus-noise in phase, adding the signal reversed in phase at the other ear will retard it. This is illustrated in Fig. 5.6a. The effects may be illustrated graphically at one instant in time by a vector diagram (Fig. 5.6b). The noise is represented by a vector whose length denotes the amplitude and whose angle denotes the phase. The signal is denoted by a second vector, whose length again denotes amplitude, but which generally differs in phase from the noise by an angle α. The figure shows the case where an antiphasic signal is added to a narrow band of noise in phase at the two ears. It may be seen that the resultant leads in phase at one ear and also has a greater amplitude at that ear. With a noise masker and a tonal signal the phase angle of addition, α, will vary constantly, so that the differences in level and phase at the two ears will vary from moment to moment. In some cases one ear will lead in time but the other will receive the more intense stimulus.

According to the Webster–Jeffress model, binaural detection is based upon the differences in phase and level at the two ears which result from the addition of the signal to the band of frequencies in the noise which contribute to the masking of the signal. Thus the cues for detection will be similar to those involved in the ordinary localization and lateralization of binaural signals.

Jeffress and his colleagues (e.g. McFadden *et al.*, 1972) have described a series of experiments on MLDs where the phase angle between the signal and noise, α, was controlled, thus controlling the relative magnitude of the interaural time and level differences. They used a rather special stimulus situation, where both signal and masker were the same narrow band of noise. When α is 0°, the signal is added to the masker in one ear and subtracted in the other. There is no interaural phase difference, but the level difference is maximal. For this condition substantial MLDs (up to 15 dB) occurred for frequencies of 250, 1000 and 2000 Hz. When α is 90°, the signal

(a)

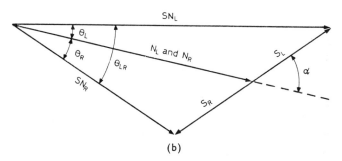

(b)

FIG. 5.6   In (a) oscilloscope traces of the signals presented to the left ear (upper) and right ear (lower) are shown. For the first part of the trace only a narrowband noise, identical in the two channels, is present. Then a tonal signal, reversed in phase in one channel relative to the other, is added. Note the resultant phase and amplitude shift between the two channels. In (b) the situation at one instant in time is represented by a vector diagram. The in-phase narrowband noise is represented by N_L and N_R. The signal in the left ear is denoted by S_L, and the signal in the right ear, which is opposite in phase, by S_R. The phase angle of addition, α, would vary randomly from moment to moment. Note that the resultant in the left ear, SN_L, differs from the resultant in the right ear, SN_R, in both amplitude and phase. From Jeffress (1971), by permission of the author.

vectors are at right-angles to the masker vector, so that the interaural phase difference is a maximum, but there is no interaural level difference. For this condition large MLDs were found for frequencies of 250, 500 and 1000 Hz, but not for 2000 Hz. For α between 90° and 180° the ear that is leading in time will receive the weaker stimulus. Thus time and intensity will be in opposition. Substantial MLDs were still found, although the subjects were sometimes not able to lateralize the signal clearly to one side. This inability to lateralize is probably not due to a cancellation of time and intensity; as we discussed earlier, the subjects will tend to hear two sound images, so that responses are inconsistent.

Jeffress (1971) has summarized these results as follows:

> Detection thus appears to be an aspect of lateralization. The signal is detected because it is heard as a displacement from the noise in the median plane. Even when time and level are in opposition there is movement away from the median plane, a movement which is detectable although ambiguous in direction.

Subjects differ in their sensitivity to the two cues, time and level differences, and at 2000 Hz only level differences can be used.

Clearly, this model, when applied to the particular stimuli used by Jeffress, does explain the data rather well. However, the use of the same stimulus as both a signal and masker is a rather special case. For a tonal signal presented against a wideband random noise, the phase angle, α, will vary randomly from moment to moment. Thus the subjective lateral position of the signal-plus-noise (the noise here referring to those components in a critical band around the tone) will also vary randomly from moment to moment. This does not fit in with observers' reports. Rather, if the tone can be faintly heard, it will be lateralized fairly precisely in one position. Thus for the $N_0 S_\pi$ condition, the noise will generally be lateralized in the middle of the head, whereas the tone will be heard towards one side. For their narrowband signals and maskers McFadden *et al.* (1971) state that "the phenomenology associated with detecting an S_π signal is that during a signal-plus-masker trial, there is a slight movement or shift in the auditory 'image'". If the model applied equally well to a tonal signal in wideband noise, then a part of the sound image should be heard as fluctuating in position. This does not seem to be the case.

The model also cannot explain the finding of MLDs in forward and backward masking. In order for the vector addition of signal and masker to occur, these must be present simultaneously. Thus the model deals rather well with some specific stimulus situations, but fails to account for the data in others.

B   *Durlach's equalization and cancellation model*

This mathematical model, presented by Durlach (1963), has four basic components, which are illustrated in Fig. 5.7. First, the stimulus in each ear is assumed to be filtered, by a mechanism analogous to the critical band. Then the total output from one filter is transformed relative to that at the other filter in such a way that the masking components become the same in both channels (the E process). The signal in one channel is then subtracted from that in the other (the C process), thus eliminating the masking signal. If

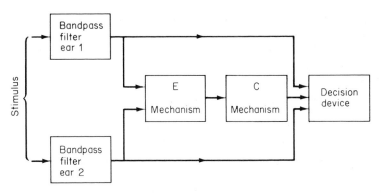

FIG. 5.7 Illustration of the major components in Durlach's (1963) equalization and cancellation model of binaural processing.

the interaural relations of the signal are different from those of the masker, then some of the signal will remain after the C process, so that if precision is perfect, the signal-to-noise ratio is improved by an infinite amount. The output from the EC mechanism is fed to a decision device which also receives inputs directly from the bandpass filters. It is assumed that the subject's detection performance is determined by the largest signal-to-noise ratio at the inputs to the decision device. The ratio at the binaural input (from the EC mechanism), divided by the ratio at one of the monaural inputs, is called the 'EC factor', and describes the change in masked threshold produced by the binaural processing.

Clearly, human observers do not show infinite MLDs. In order to account for this, it is assumed that the EC process is performed imperfectly, so that there will be a residue of noise at the output of the C mechanism. The imperfections are assumed to be of two types: (1) those resulting from a random jitter independent of stimulus configuration, and representable as random errors in the amplitude and time alignment of the signals at the input to the C mechanism; (2) those resulting from 'atypical' stimuli that require atypical E transformations in response. Examples of the second type might be broadband masking signals that differ by an interaural phase shift rather than an interaural time shift, or signals that differ by an interaural time shift greater than the time it takes a sound to travel around the head.

It is assumed that there are a number of possible modes of operation of the EC mechanism, but that a selector mechanism chooses that mode which gives the best 'EC factor'. It is usually assumed that the types of operation which the E mechanism can perform are those which would be involved in the localization or lateralization of sounds, namely shifts in time and shifts in intensity. For a tone a phase shift is equivalent to a time shift, and for a narrowband noise this is also approximately true. Thus for the $N_\pi S_0$ condition the appropriate E process will be a shift in time of the noise components around the tone. Since a narrowband noise resembles a sinusoid, a shift in time equal to half a period of the sinusoid will be equivalent to inverting the phase.

A problem arises when we consider antiphasic conditions for wideband signals, such as speech sounds, in wideband maskers. If, for example, the noise is inverted in one ear with respect to the other, a shift in time will only cancel the noise components in certain frequency regions, while in other frequency regions the noise will actually be increased. Further, such a shift in time will tend to cancel the signal components in certain frequency regions. Since substantial MLDs do occur under these conditions, we must assume either that different time shifts are used in different frequency bands, or that the E mechanism is capable of a rather strange and demanding operation—that of inverting a waveform. It would seem reasonable that if such complicated transformations are required of the E mechanism, then the MLDs would be *smaller* than those found in the case where, for example, the masker in one ear is simply delayed in time with respect to the other. However, this does not seem to be the case. The experiments of Carhart *et al.* (1969) which we described above clearly showed that the largest MLDs are found in antiphasic conditions, rather than in conditions where the maskers were simply time delayed.

The main advantage of Durlach's model is that, with certain simple assumptions, it allows detailed quantitative predictions to be made about the outcome of experiments, some of which are as yet undone. We shall not attempt to describe these here, or to relate in detail the experimental findings to the predictions. The interested reader is referred to Durlach (1972). As with the Webster–Jeffress model, the EC model explains certain aspects of the data rather well, but fails in other cases. To some extent the models are complementary, each one being able to explain some of the results which do not fit the other. The EC model provides the best fit to data on the detection of signals in wideband maskers, whereas the Webster–Jeffress model provides the better explanation for narrowband signals and maskers. Neither model can satisfactorily explain the finding of MLDs in forward and backward masking, although the EC model could be extended to do this.

10   GENERAL DISCUSSION

Although the models we have described are by no means the only explanations of MLDs that have been published, they are fairly typical of work in this area. The main difference in the models is in their emphasis; the Webster–Jeffress model is more concerned with explanations in terms of the characteristics of the signals themselves, whereas the EC model is more concerned with the types of operation that the observer might be able to perform in detecting binaural signals. Neither model is completely satisfactory in providing a description of the subjective experiences that accompany binaural detection. As Durlach (1972) has said of the EC model, "although the primary purpose of the model is to describe objective performance and not the subjective experience, it would obviously be more satisfactory if the model seemed less artificial when compared with this experience".

A second limitation of the models is that they were designed only to account for detection performance, and not for the improvements that occur in the discrimination of above-threshold signals. Durlach (1972) has pointed out that the EC model can be extended to account for binaural phenomena other than improved detection, but as yet neither the EC model nor the Webster–Jeffress model can account for the improved intelligibility of speech sounds which occurs under antiphasic conditions.

The results we have been discussing have certain implications for the design and fitting of hearing aids. Firstly, head movements play a significant role in our ability to localize sounds and to understand speech in noisy environments (Hirsh, 1971). For this to benefit the hearing aid wearer, the aid must be mounted on the head, not the body. Secondly, binaural cues improve sound localization and allow the MLD effect to operate. Thus, for a person deaf in both ears, two head-worn hearing aids are needed. Two hearing aids will also avoid the loss of signal due to head shadow effects. Thirdly, the use of two hearing aids will enable the precedence effect to operate, so that the listener will be less susceptible to room echoes. Fourthly, if the pickup is actually mounted in the outer ear, advantage can be taken of the encoding effects of the pinna. The extent to which these factors are important will vary with different types of deafness, and will also depend on the quality of the hearing aid. Attempts to demonstrate the 'cocktail party' effect using conventional hearing aids have proved difficult (Kuyper and de Boer, 1969), although significant improvements in intelligibility do result if signals are fed to the hearing aids via high quality microphones (Kuyper, 1972). It is likely that the advantages to be gained from MLD effects will not be fully realized with conventional hearing aids unless their low frequency response is considerably improved. Similar limitations would presumably apply to the use of pinna encoding effects, except that here an extended high frequency response would be required, which is often not utilizable by the subject requiring an aid.

For many patients head-worn aids are not practicable, because the high level of amplification required can only be provided by a body-worn aid. However, for such patients significant advantages can be gained by using two separate hearing aids, one feeding each ear. Byrne and Dermody (1975) showed that localization of sound with binaural body-worn hearing aids was far superior to localization with monaural body-worn aids. Heyes and Ferris (1975) presented similar results, although they found that postaural aids produced better localization than body worn aids, and that a single postaural aid was about as good as a pair of chest-mounted aids. They concluded that "a single chest-mounted aid is so poor that for those hearing-aid users for whom sound localization is important, for example, the blind, its provision should be regarded as a last resort".

11   THE INFLUENCE OF VISION ON AUDITORY LOCALIZATION

Many everyday experiences indicate that auditory localization can be influenced by conflicting visual cues. At a cinema the loudspeakers are usually placed behind the screen, in its centre (except where stereo or multichannel sound is used), yet the sound still appears to come from the actor's mouth as he moves about the screen. Similarly, the loudspeaker in a television set is usually located to one side of the screen, but the sound does not appear to be 'detached' from the visual image.

A number of experiments in recent years have shown that exposure to conflicting auditory and visual cues for a period of time may lead to an after-effect in which the localization of sounds is systematically displaced. This does not indicate that the whole of our capacity for auditory localization is learned; indeed the ability to locate sounds seems to be present very early in life, so that a sharp click may elicit an appropriate orienting response from a baby a few minutes after birth (Peiper, 1963). However, it may be the case that connections between the 'frames of reference' for auditory space and for spaces in other modalities (visual, vestibular and kinaesthetic) may be modifiable to some extent.

Young (1928) and later Willey *et al.* (1937) attempted to distort auditory space using a pseudophone, by which a tube from each ear is led to a trumpet on the opposite side of the head. With this arrangement, sounds from the left are heard as coming from the right, and vice versa. Although the listeners were able to learn to respond appropriately, no genuine auditory reorientation appeared to take place, even after a week of exposure. Held (1955) used an electronic pseudophone which displaced the interaural axis by 22° about the vertical axis of the head. After wearing this for a day, listeners were tested with the pseudophone set to give no displacement. They reported that a single sound source produced two images, one near the normal position and one displaced from it in the opposite direction to the original direction of rotation of the pseudophone. More recently Kalil and Freedman (1967) found that after wearing a pseudophone which displaced a sound 15° to the right of a visible source, subjects heard a sound presented straight in front of them (from a concealed source) as displaced a few degrees to the left. Freedman, Wilson and Rekosh (1967) have reported similar effects for subjects exposed to discordant auditory and kinaesthetic cues. Weerts and Thurlow (1971) suggested that the after-effects might arise from asymmetrical auditory stimulation. However, they found that subjects who are exposed to a sound coming from straight ahead, but who turn their eyes 20° to the side towards a visible loudspeaker, show a shift in the localization of the sound during presentation, and also a corresponding after-effect. Thus substantial effects can be produced under conditions of symmetrical auditory stimulation. Among subjects who turned their heads to the side, the largest effects were found for those who expected to hear the sound coming from the visible source. Subjects who did not turn their eyes, but were led to expect that the sound would appear to come from a loud-speaker 20° to one side, showed no significant shift. Thus the results cannot be simply explained in terms of 'suggestion'. Weerts and Thurlow carried out a number of further experiments in an attempt to isolate the cause of the shifts in localization. They found that part, but not all, of the shift during the exposure period can be understood in terms of a shift in perceived head direction. When subjects were asked to indicate their head direction with a flashlight pointer, they showed a slight shift, whether their eyes were open or closed. The after-effects were shown not to be due to a change in physical or perceived eye or head position, or to a shift in felt arm position (when using a pointer). Further, the effects are not due to some distortion of the visual fields, since essentially the same results were obtained for subjects blindfolded during the test conditions. Thus the most likely explanation of these results does seem to be a sort of 'recalibration' of auditory space on the basis of visual information.

Some experiments of Wallach (1940) also indicate the importance of visual orientation in auditory localization. His subjects had their heads fixed in the vertical axis of a cylindrical screen which rotated about them. The screen was covered in vertical stripes, and after watching the movement of these for a few moments, the observer would perceive himself as in constant rotation and the screen as at rest. A stationary sound source was then activated straight ahead of the observer. Since the observer in this situation perceives himself as moving, he has to interpret the sound source as lying directly above or below him. If the sound source is at a constant azimuth (e.g. 20° to the left of the observer), the sound source cannot be interpreted as lying above the observer, since interaural differences of time and intensity now exist. Instead the source is perceived as rotating with the listener at an elevation which is approximately the complement of the constant azimuth (in this case at an elevation of about 70°). Thus our interpretation of auditory spatial cues is strongly influenced by our perceived visual orientation. Or, more correctly, the highest level of spatial representation involves an integration of information from the different senses.

12   THE PERCEPTION OF DISTANCE

Just as was the case for judgements of lateral position, there are a number of cues which we can use in judging the distance of a sound source. For familiar sounds, intensity may give a crude indication of distance from the listener. Over moderate distances the spectrum of a complex sound source may also be changed, owing to the absorbing properties of the air; high frequencies are attenuated more than low. However, judgements will again depend on familiarity with the specific situation (Coleman, 1962, 1963). In addition to these cues, the curvature of the wavefront can indicate the distance of a sound source. When this is nearby, the wavefront will be strongly curved, whereas a distant source will produce a plane wavefront. The curvature of the wavefront influences interaural differences in intensity and time, so that a combination of the information from these two could provide a cue as to distance. The fact that time and intensity fail to trade completely (see section 6) indicates that the time and intensity information is preserved separately in the nervous system, so that in principle judgements of distance could be made. Further, in real life many different time–intensity combinations will occur, depending on the distance of the sound source, but we never perceive two sound 'images'. Thus everyday experience indicates that we combine the information from time and intensity differences to produce a single sound image at a well-defined distance. As yet, however, it has not been clearly demonstrated, in a laboratory situation, that we are able to use interaural time and intensity combinations in judging distance.

So far we have discussed the cues which could be used to judge the distance of a sound source in free space. Normally we listen in rooms with reflecting walls, so that the ratio of direct to reflected sound, and the time delay between direct and reflected sound, provide cues as to distance. Von Békésy (1960) showed that altering these ratios produced the impression of sounds moving towards or away from the listener. The work of Wallach *et al.* (1949) on the precedence effect (section 5) showed that we exhibit little direct awareness of room echoes; rather these are fused with the leading sound. It seems that we are still able to use information related to echoes, in spite of this perceptual fusion.

We may conclude that, just as was the case for judgements of the direction of sound sources, judgements of distance may depend on a multiplicity of cues. Intensity, spectral changes, curvature of the wavefront and reflected sounds may all influence judgements of distance, but some of these depend strongly on familiarity with the sound source and the listening environment. In general, localization of sounds in depth is relatively inaccurate, and errors of the order of 20% are not uncommon for unfamiliar sound sources.

13   OBSTACLE DETECTION AND THE BLIND

It is well known that many blind people, and some sighted people, are able to detect the presence of obstacles in the environment and to judge their distance. However, such people are not often able to explain how they do this, and the descriptions which are used, such as 'feeling the objects on my face', are not particularly helpful. Supa *et al.* (1944) carried out a series of experiments to determine the cues involved in what they called 'facial vision'. In an initial experiment they found that blindfolded normal subjects could learn to avoid objects after a short learning period, but that blind subjects could normally detect objects at greater distances. Both normal and blind subjects could distinguish between the first perception of an object at a distance and the 'near approach' to it.

There have been two types of cues suggested as the basis for facial vision. These are cutaneous sensation due to air currents and auditory sensation based on the reflection of sound from obstacles. Supa *et al.* attempted to eliminate each of these cues in turn; cutaneous cues were removed by covering the skin with veils and sleeves while auditory cues were removed by plugging the ears or by using a background masking noise. They concluded that stimulation of the face and other areas of the skin is neither a necessary nor a sufficient condition for obstacle detection, whereas aural stimulation is both necessary and sufficient.

These experiments were extended by Cotzin and Dallenbach (1950). They used a sound source, whose movement could be controlled by a listener, with a microphone suspended above it at about ear height. The sound picked up by the microphone was fed to the listener via an earphone, and he was required to report when an obstacle was detected. Both wide-band noise and pure tones were used as stimuli. The authors concluded that: (1) changes in pitch (or in a pitch-like quality for the noise) are a sufficient condition for the detection of an obstacle; (2) changes in loudness are neither necessary nor sufficient; (3) high frequencies (around 10 kHz) are necessary for obstacle detection; and (4) the bases of obstacle detection are pitch changes resulting from a Doppler shift (a change in apparent frequency when the observer and the sound source are in relative motion; an example is the change in pitch of a train whistle as the train approaches and passes a stationary observer).

The pitch changes Cotzin and Dallenbach suggested as a basis for obstacle detection will only occur when the observer is moving. However, other auditory cues may be available to signal the presence and distance of an obstacle. Wilson (1967) has pointed out that, in the neighbourhood of an obstacle, sound reaches the observer both directly and by reflection from the obstacle. Interference between these signals introduces a series of maxima and minima in the spectrum, the frequencies of which depend on the path difference. For a sound containing a wide range of frequencies a pitch is heard (sometimes called the 'reflection tone') which becomes higher as the obstacle is approached. Thus the value of this pitch, and its rate of change as the obstacle is approached, will provide cues as to the distance of the object. In addition, the spectrum of the reflected sound will be modified according to the size of the obstacle; a large object will reflect both high and low frequencies, whereas a small object will only reflect high frequencies. Thus spectral changes in the reflected sound will provide at least a crude estimate of the size of the object. Further changes in spectrum may result if the obstacle absorbs certain portions of the spectrum, or if it introduces frequency dependent phase shifts. Thus a crude form of obstacle recognition may even be possible. Tests using blind subjects have shown that objects subtending an angle as small as 3.5° can be detected, and that changes in distance of the order of 20% and in area of the order of 30% can be discriminated (Kellog, 1962). Kellog also investigated the discrimination of discs covered with different types of material. He found that some materials could be discriminated with high accuracy (plain wood and velvet could be discriminated 99.5% of the time) while others, such as painted wood and glass, could not be discriminated at all. In general, discrimination was good between 'soft' and 'hard' materials, but, surprisingly, denim cloth and velvet could be distinguished with 86.5% accuracy. Rice (1967) found that some subjects could distinguish between a circle, a square and a triangle of the same surface area with an accuracy of about 80%. In order to achieve these discriminations most subjects emitted both normal vocal sounds and clicking and hissing sounds.

In an attempt to make the auditory correlates of objects and their spatial relationships simpler, and to provide more detailed information, a number of aids for the blind have been developed. One of these consists of a 'torch' which projects a beam of noise into the environment and which can be pointed by the observer so as to scan different objects in the environment. A development of this (Kay, 1966) projects a beam of ultrasonic vibrations, whose reflections are picked up by a receiver on the 'torch' and recoded to provide an audible output through an earpiece. The device is designed so that bleeps are heard whose pitch is directly related to distance from the objects producing the reflections. Because of its very high frequency, the ultrasonic beam behaves almost like a beam of light, so that the device can be used to pick up the silhouette of an object. A possible problem, however, is that the sensory display provided is not consistent with the displays resulting from normal auditory space perception, and facility in use may require long learning. No doubt, further studies of the cues used in obstacle detection will suggest the development of other aids for the blind.

14   GENERAL CONCLUSIONS

In this chapter we have discussed the cues and the mechanisms involved in the localization of sounds. Our acuity in locating sounds is greatest in the horizontal dimension, fairly good in the vertical direction and least good in the depth (distance) dimension. For each of these dimensions we are able to use a number of distinct cues, although the cues may differ depending on the type of sound and on the mode of presentation. The multiplicity of cues provides a certain redundancy in the system, so that even under very difficult conditions (reverberant rooms or brief sounds) we are still capable of quite accurate localization.

Binaural processing, using information relating to the differences of the signals at the two ears, contributes to our ability to localize sounds, and may also improve our ability to detect and analyse signals in noisy backgrounds. This is illustrated by laboratory studies of the binaural masking level difference (MLD), and by the 'cocktail party' phenomenon. Binaural processing also helps us to suppress room echoes, and to locate sound sources in reverberant rooms.

Our judgements of auditory location may be influenced by visual or kinaesthetic stimulation. Such stimulation may also lead to after-effects in which the apparent position of a sound source is slightly displaced from its 'true' position. These effects may indicate that there is some 'plasticity' in the relations between auditory, visual and kinaesthetic space, so that a 'recalibration' of auditory space can occur on the basis of information from other modalities.

Blind people, and blindfolded normal subjects after some practice, are able to detect obstacles in the environment, and to make crude estimations of their distance and of their size and nature. This ability depends upon the reflections of sound from the obstacles, although subjects are not always aware of this. Again, a number of possible cues may be used in this situation, but the most important one is probably the 'reflection tone' which results from the interference of direct and reflected sound, and whose pitch depends on path difference.

FURTHER READING

The following chapter by Mills gives a clear, but slightly dated review of sound localization:

Mills, A. W. (1972). Auditory Localization. In *Foundations of Modern Auditory Theory*, Vol. 2 (ed. J. V. Tobias), Academic Press, New York.
An extensive review of data and models related to binaural hearing can be found in:
Durlach, N. I. and Colburn, H. S. (1978). Binaural phenomena. In *Handbook of Perception*, Vol. 4 (eds E. C. Carterette and M. P. Friedman), Academic Press, New York.
Colburn, H. S. and Durlach, N. I. (1978). Models of binaural interaction. In *Handbook of Perception*, Vol. 4 (eds E. C. Carterette and M. P. Friedman), Academic Press, New York.

6 Auditory pattern and object perception

1 INTRODUCTION

So far we have described several attributes of auditory sensation such as pitch, subjective location and loudness, which can be related in a reasonably straightforward way to the physical properties of stimuli. In many cases we have discussed the neural code which may underly the perception of these attributes. In everyday life, however, we do not perceive these attributes in isolation. Rather, the auditory world is analysed into discrete sound sources or auditory objects, each of which may have its own pitch, timbre, location and loudness. Sometimes the source may be recognized as familar in some way, e.g. a particular person talking, and often the 'object' perceived may be identified, e.g. a particular spoken word. In this chapter we will discuss four related aspects of auditory object and pattern perception. Firstly, we will discuss the factors involved in the identification of a single object from among a large set of possible objects. Secondly, we will discuss some of the cues we use to analyse a complex mixture of sounds into discrete sources. Thirdly, we will discuss the perception of sequences of sounds. Finally, we will describe the general 'rules' which govern the perceptual organization of the auditory world.

2 OBJECT PERCEPTION AND IDENTIFICATION

Many of the attributes of sensation we have described so far, such as pitch and loudness, may be considered as unidimensional: if we are presented with a large variety of sounds with different pitches it is possible to order all of the sounds on a single scale of pitch going from low to high.* Similarly, sounds differing in loudness can be ordered on a single scale going from quiet to loud. Our ability to identify one object from among a large set of objects depends upon there being several dimensions along which the objects vary. When a set of stimuli vary along a single dimension we can only

*Actually this is a slight over-simplification: see Shepard, R. N. (1964). Circularity in judgments of relative pitch. *J. Acoust. Soc. Am.* **36**, 2346–2353.

name the individual stimuli in the set when their number is less than about 5–6. For example, Pollack (1952) investigated the ability of subjects to name musical tones with different pitches, as a function of the number of possible tones. He found that they could only do this reliably when the number of possible tones was less than 5–6. This was true whether the tones were spread over a wide frequency range of several octaves, or were concentrated in a relatively narrow range, say one octave (subjects with absolute pitch do better in this task). In order for us to be able to identify more stimuli than this, extra dimensions are required. In hearing the extra dimensions arise in two main ways. Firstly, complex stimuli will contain more than one frequency component, so that the patterning of spectral energy as a function of frequency will be important. Secondly, auditory stimuli typically vary with time, and the temporal patterning can be of crucial importance to perception. Auditory space, or location, can sometimes provide extra dimensions, for example, by indicating the size of an object, but usually it defines where, rather than what, an object is. Thus auditory pattern or object perception depends primarily on structures in frequency and time, of which music and speech represent advanced forms.

A   *Time-invariant patterns and timbre*

If a single frequency component is presented, then the sound pattern can be described by just two numbers, specifying frequency and intensity. However, almost all of the sounds which we encounter in everyday life are considerably more complex than this, and contain a multitude of frequencies with particular levels and relative phases. The distribution of energy over frequency seems to be one of the major determinants of the quality of a sound or its timbre. Timbre has been defined by the American Standards Association (1960) as "that attribute of auditory sensation in terms of which a listener can judge that two sounds similarly presented and having the same loudness and pitch are dissimilar". Differences in timbre enable us to distinguish between the same note played on, say, the piano, the violin and flute. Timbre as defined by the ASA depends upon more than just the frequency spectrum of the sound; fluctuations over time can play an important role, and we will discuss the effects of these in section 2.B. For the purpose of this section we can adopt a more restricted definition suggested by Plomp (1970): "Timbre is that attribute of sensation in terms of which a listener can judge that two steady complex tones having the same loudness, pitch and duration are dissimilar".

Unlike pitch or loudness, which may be considered as unidimensional, timbre is multidimensional; there is no single scale along which we can compare or order the timbres of different sounds. Thus we need some way of describing the spectrum of a sound which takes into account this multidimensional aspect, and which can be related in a psychologically realistic way to the subjective timbre. A crude first approach is to look at the overall distribution of spectral energy. For example, complex tones with strong lower harmonics (below the 6th) sound mellow, whereas tones with strong harmonics beyond the 6th or 7th sound sharp and penetrating. However, a much more quantitative approach has been described by Plomp and his colleagues (Plomp *et al.*, 1967; Plomp, 1970). They used a technique which is similar to factor analysis, and which allows the determination of the principle dimensions of variation in a set of stimuli. Firstly, a spectrum is characterized with a set of numbers representing the amplitudes in some 18 third-octave frequency bands. This relatively broadband analysis achieves a basic economy consistent with the frequency-analysing power of the peripheral auditory system; critical bands are roughly one third-octave in width over a fairly wide frequency range. A representative sample of spectra is then obtained (e.g. the vowels of a language spoken by a set of speakers with subjectively different voices). The level in each third-octave band will vary as a function of vowel or speaker, but the levels in different bands will not be entirely independent, particularly for bands of adjacent frequency. Thus the information about the vowel or speaker conveyed by the levels in the 18 third-octave bands is redundant, or partially duplicated. This redundancy can be eliminated by statistical procedures that yield the chief higher order dimensions underlying the differences between sounds in the sample chosen. Each higher order dimension will be a weighted function of each of the original 18 amplitude dimensions. Different sets of higher order dimensions will be obtained according to whether we emphasize the differences between different vowels or the differences between different speakers.

This procedure results in a reduction in the number of dimensions needed to account for the differences between the different spectra in the set. In general, the more the number of dimensions is reduced, the less satisfactorily are those differences accounted for. Three dimensions are sufficient to account for about 82% of the total variation. Thus, with a reasonably small error, each vowel can be represented as a point in a three-dimensional space. If we take into account variations between different speakers, or between the same speaker on different occasions, the representation of each vowel becomes a 'blob' of a certain volume in this three-dimensional space.

Consider now the subjective significance of these higher order dimensions. To investigate this, Pols *et al.* (1969) also carried out perceptual analyses of their vowel stimuli, using a technique based on triadic comparison. In this method the subject has to decide, for each possible group of three stimuli, which pair is most similar and which pair is least similar. On the basis of these judgements a multidimensional perceptual space can be constructed for the different vowel sounds. (The exact method by which this is done is rather complex. The interested reader is referred to Shepard, 1962, and Kruskal, 1964.) Each vowel is represented as a point in the multidimensional space, and the greater the distance between these points the more dissimilar are the vowels judged to be. As was the case for the physical analysis, the number of dimensions can be reduced at the expense of a loss of 'goodness of fit'. When Pols and co-workers compared the three-dimensional physical configuration with the three-dimensional perceptual configuration, they found a close correspondence; the correlation coefficients for the three dimensions were 0.992, 0.971 and 0.742. When six dimensions were used, the correlation coefficients were even higher. Pols and co-workers summed up these results as follows:

> From this remarkable correspondence, it can be concluded that the subjects used for their perceptual judgements information comparable with that present in the physical representation of these signals. The perceptual differences between the stimuli, to be considered as timbre differences, appear to be qualified by their differences in frequency spectra.

It should not be assumed that the dimensions derived by Pols and co-workers represent *the* chief mode of functioning of a *fixed* set of pattern analysers, or that the number of dimensions involved in timbre judgements is necessarily small. It is likely that the number of dimensions required is limited by the number of critical bands required to cover the audible frequency range. This would give a maximum of 23 dimensions, or, if we exclude very high and very low frequencies, about 15. For a restricted class of sounds, however, a much smaller set of dimensions may be involved. It appears to be generally true, both for speech and nonspeech sounds, that the timbres of steady tones are determined primarily by their frequency spectra.

B   *Time-varying patterns*

Although differences in static timbre may enable us to distinguish between two sounds which are presented successively, they are not always sufficient to allow the absolute identification of an 'auditory object', such as a musical instrument. One reason for this is that the frequency spectrum of the sound may be markedly altered by the transmission path. In practice, the recognition of a particular timbre, and hence of an 'auditory object', may depend upon several other factors. Schouten (1968) has suggested that these include: (1) Whether the sound is periodic, having a tonal quality for repetition rates between about 20 and 20 000 per second, or irregular, and having a noiselike character; (2) Whether the waveform envelope is constant, or fluctuates as a function of time, and in the latter case what the fluctuations are like; (3) Whether any aspect of the sound (spectrum, periodicity or envelope) is changing as a function of time; (4) What the preceding and following sounds are like.

The recognition of musical instruments, for example, depends quite strongly on onset transients and on the temporal structure of the sound envelope. The characteristic tone of a piano depends upon the fact that the notes have a rapid onset and a gradual decay. If a recording of a piano is reversed in time, the timbre is completely different. It now resembles that of a harmonium or accordion, in spite of the fact that the longterm average spectrum is unchanged by time reversal. In addition, many instruments have noiselike qualities which strongly influence their subjective quality. A flute, for example, has a relatively simple harmonic structure, but synthetic tones with the same harmonic structure do not sound flutelike unless each note is preceeded by a small 'puff' of noise. In general, tones of standard musical instruments are poorly simulated by the summation of steady component frequencies, since such a synthesis cannot produce the dynamic variation with time characteristic of these instruments. Thus traditional electronic organs (pre 1965), which produced only steady tones, could produce a good simulation of the bagpipes, but could not be made to sound like a piano. Modern synthesizers shape the envelopes of the sounds they produce, and hence are capable of more accurate and convincing imitations of musical instruments.

3   INFORMATION USED TO SEPARATE AUDITORY OBJECTS

It is hardly ever the case that the sound reaching our ears comes from a single source. Usually the sound arises from several different sources, but we have little difficulty in assigning the different frequency components in the sound to their appropriate sources. Our ability to do this is far greater than we might expect from simple studies of masking, and the critical band. In this section we will consider some of the physical cues which are used to achieve this perceptual separation. In section 5 we will consider the perceptual rules which can be derived from this, and the rules which govern the perception of auditory sequences. The physical cues which we will describe are not completely independent of one another, and no single one of them always works perfectly. The ways in which the cues are used will provide pointers to the rules governing perceptual organization.

A   *Fundamental frequency*

When we listen to two steady complex tones together (e.g. two musical instruments or two vowel sounds), we do not generally confuse which harmonics belong to which tone. Rather we hear each tone as a separate source, even though the harmonics may be interleaved, and sometimes overlapping. We can do this only if the two tones have different fundamental frequencies. Broadbent and Ladefoged (1957), in an experiment using synthetic vowels, showed that the normal percept of a single fused voice occurs only if all the harmonics have the same fundamental frequency. If the harmonics are split into two groups, with different fundamental frequencies, then two separate sounds are heard. This result can be explained by extending the model of pitch perception presented in Chapter 4, section 4. We assume that the pitch of a complex tone results from a correlation or comparison of time intervals between successive nerve firings in different auditory neurons. Only those 'channels' which show a high correlation will be classified as 'belonging' to the same sound. This simple extension is not entirely satisfactory, since, when two complex tones are presented, there will be many channels in which the responses are influenced by harmonics from both tones. In these channels the temporal pattern of firing may be dominated by one harmonic, or may reflect the presence of more than one harmonic. Apparently, the auditory system is capable of partitioning the temporal information within a channel, assigning part to one tone and part to the other. We do not know how this is achieved. However, it is even more difficult to see how such an analysis could be achieved by a mechanism operating only on the spatial pattern of neural activity.

B   *Onset disparities*

Rasch (1978) investigated the perceptual ability to separate two complex tones in a masking procedure. One of the tones was treated as a masker and the level of the other (the higher in pitch) was adjusted to find the point where it was just detectable. When the two tones started at the same time, and had exactly the same temporal envelope, the threshold of the variable tone was between 0 and −20 dB relative to the level of the masking tone. Thus when a difference in fundamental frequency is the only cue, the maximum difference in level for which the higher tone will still be heard is 20 dB. Rasch also investigated the effect of starting the high tone just before the low tone. He found that threshold depended strongly on onset asynchrony, reaching a value of −60 dB for a delay of 30 ms. Thus, when the high tone starts 30 ms before the low tone, it can be heard much more easily, and with much greater differences in levels between the two tones.

Although the percept of his subjects was that the high tone continued throughout the low tone, Rasch showed that this percept was not based upon sensory information received during the presentation time of the low tone. He found that identical thresholds were obtained if the high note terminated immediately after the onset of the low tone. It appears that the perceptual system 'assumes' that the high tone has continued, since there is no evidence to the contrary. This effect is related to the continuity phenomenon which we described in Chapter 3, section 5, and we will discuss it further in this chapter, section 5.

Rasch showed that if the two notes have simultaneous onsets but different rise times, this also can give very low thresholds for the high tone, provided that tone has the shorter rise time. Under these conditions, and those of onset asynchronies up to 30 ms, the notes sound as though they start synchronously. Thus we do not need to be consciously aware of the onset differences for the auditory system to be able to exploit them in the perceptual separation of complex tones. Rasch also pointed out that the onset differences used in his experiments correspond roughly with the asynchronization of simultaneous notes found in performed music. This supports the view that the asynchronies are an important factor in the perception of the separate parts or voices in polyphonic music.

One modern-day example of the role of onset differences in aiding perceptual separation comes from electronic organs which have a synthesizer section. If the same note is played on the synthesizer section (set to, say, piano) and on the more conventional section (set to, say, violins), then the two notes will remain perceptually separate even though they have exactly the same fundamental frequency. The main reason for this is that the shape and rise time of the envelope at onset will be different for the two notes.

C *Contrast with previous sounds*

The auditory system seems particularly well-suited to the analysis of changes in the sensory input. The perceptual effect of a change in a stimulus can be roughly described by saying that the preceding stimulus is subtracted from the present one, so what remains is the change. The changed aspect stands out perceptually from the rest. Alternatively we might say that steady stimulation results in some kind of adaptation. When some aspect of a stimulus is changed, that aspect is freed from the effects of adaptation, and thus will be enhanced perceptually. While the underlying mechanism is a matter of debate the perceptual effect certainly is not.

A powerful demonstration of this effect may be obtained by listening to a stimulus with a particular spectral structure and then switching rapidly to a white noise stimulus. A white noise heard in isolation may be described as 'colourless'; it has no well-defined pitch and has a neutral sort of timbre. However, when a white noise follows immediately after a stimulus with spectral structure, the noise sounds 'coloured'. The coloration corresponds to the *inverse* of the spectrum of the preceding sound. For example, if the preceding sound is a noise with a bandstop or notch, the white noise has a pitchlike quality, with a pitch value corresponding to the centre frequency of the notch (Zwicker, 1964). The white noise may be given a speechlike quality if the preceding sound has a spectrum which is the inverse of that of a speech sound, such as a vowel (Summerfield *et al.*, 1981).

A second demonstration of the effects of a change in a stimulus can be obtained by listening to a steady complex tone with many harmonics. Usually this will be heard with a single pitch corresponding to the fundamental component, and the individual harmonics will not be separately perceived. However, if one of the harmonics is changed in some way, either by altering its relative phase or its level, then that harmonic will stand out perceptually from the complex as a whole. For a short time after the change is made a pure-tone quality will be perceived, but the perception of the harmonic will gradually fade, until it merges with the complex once more. Notice that a *decrease* in level of a harmonic can produce this effect; the direction of the change is not crucial. Our ability to hear out harmonics when they change in some way is in excess of what would be expected on the basis of the critical bandwidth, or on the basis of direct studies of this ability for steady, unchanging, complex tones (see Chapter 3, section 2.E). This illustrates the powerful nature of the change detection mechanisms.

Change detection is obviously of importance in assigning sound components to their appropriate sources. Normally we listen against a background of sounds which may be relatively unchanging, such as the humming of machinery, traffic noises, and so on. A *sudden* change in the sound is usually indicative that a new source has been activated, and the change detection mechanisms enable us to isolate the effects of the change and interpret them appropriately.

D   *Correlated changes in amplitude or frequency*

In section 3.B we described the work of Rasch (1978) showing that the perceptual separation of two complex tones could be enhanced by introducing an onset asynchrony. The threshold of detection of the higher of the two notes could be markedly reduced if that note started 30 ms before the lower note. Rasch also showed that, even when the two notes started synchronously, it was possible to enhance their perceptual separation by frequency modulating the upper note. This modulation was similar to the vibrato which often occurs for musical tones, and it was applied so that all the components in the higher note moved up and down in synchrony. Rasch found that the modulation could reduce the threshold for the higher tone by 17 dB. Thus, when two complex tones are presented simultaneously, their perceptual separation can be enhanced if the components of one or the other are frequency modulated in a coherent way. A similar enhancement of perceptual separation can be produced by amplitude modulation of one of the tones.

Modulations in frequency or in amplitude can be effective not only in separating different groups of components, but also in producing a perceptual fusion of components. This may occur even when those components do not have a harmonic relationship. For example, if we present a steady complex sound containing many components with randomly distributed frequencies, a single noiselike sound will be heard, with a certain timbre. A subgroup of components in the complex can now be made to stand out perceptually from the rest by making them vary in a coherent way in either frequency, amplitude or both. This group will be perceived as a prominent 'figure' against a steady background, and both the figure and the background will have a timbre different from that of the original, unvarying sound.

The fusion of components which vary in a coherent way can also affect the perception of a single harmonic complex tone. Say, for example, we present the 3rd, 4th and 5th harmonics of a 200 Hz fundamental, namely 600, 800 and 1000 Hz. This complex may be perceived in two ways. We may listen in an analytic mode, hearing the pitches of one or more individual components (Chapter 3, section 2.E) or we may listen in a synthetic mode, hearing a single pitch corresponding to the missing fundamental (Chapter 4, section 2.B). The analytic mode is more likely if the complex is presented continuously, or if we build up the complex by adding one tone at a time. However the synthetic mode is more likely if all the components in the complex are turned on and off together; the coherent behaviour of the components causes them to be fused into a single percept.

E   *Sound location*

It is a matter of everyday experience that components coming from the same direction will tend to be assigned to a single source, whereas those coming from different directions will be assigned to different sources. Thus the cues used in sound localization will also help in the analysis of complex auditory inputs. We described in Chapter 5 a phenomenon that was related to this, namely the binaural masking level difference (BMLD). The phenomenon can be summarized as follows: whenever the phase or level differences of a signal at the two ears are not the same as those of a masker, our ability to detect the signal will be improved relative to the case where the signal and masker have the same phase and level relationships at the two ears. The practical implication is that a signal will be easier to detect when it is located in a different position in space from the masker. Although most studies of the BMLD have been concerned with threshold measurements, it seems clear that similar advantages of binaural listening can be gained in the identification and discrimination of signals presented against a background of other sound.

An example of the use of binaural cues in separating an auditory 'object' from its background comes from an experiment by Kubovy *et al.* (1974).

They presented eight continuous sinusoids to each ear. The sinusoids had frequencies corresponding to the notes in a musical scale and each component had the same phase in the two ears. By shifting the phase of one of the sinusoids, relative to its counterpart in the opposite ear, that component could be displaced in subjective space from the rest, and was heard to stand out perceptually. A sequence of phase shifts in different components was clearly heard as a melody. This melody was completely undetectable when listening to the input to one ear alone. Thus differences in relative phase at the two ears can allow an auditory 'object' to be isolated in the absence of any other cues.

4   THE PERCEPTION OF TEMPORAL PATTERNS

A   *The perception of rhythm*

Just as sounds can be patterned according to the amount of energy in different frequency regions, so also can they be patterned according to how they vary as a function of time. Many of the auditory sequences occurring naturally are rhythmic, so that one might reasonably expect that the perceptual mechanisms are designed to make use of these rhythms (Sturgess and Martin, 1974). If an auditory pattern is rhythmic, then certain elements in the pattern are temporally redundant, so that once early elements of the pattern are heard, later elements, and possibly the end of the pattern as well, can be anticipated.

A number of workers have investigated the 'perceptual organization' or subjective grouping of repeating sequences of two elements (e.g. a high pitched buzz and a low pitched buzz). Royer and Garner (1966, 1970) required subjects to give verbal reports of the way such sequences were perceived. They found that subjects usually organized the pattern beginning at specific elements. These elements, termed preferred start points, either began a run of identical elements or were chosen to produce a pattern ending in a run of identical elements (HHHLHLHL or LHLHLHHH). If the temporal patterns were made more complex by the addition of features such as temporal pauses or intensity accents, organization could be either by these features or by the pattern structure of the elements. If the pattern structure was made to conflict with the pause organization by inserting a temporal pause before a nonpreferred start point (HHLHLHLH HHLHLHLH . . .) the pause organization was dominant. These experiments indicate a powerful subjective tendency for such patterns to be perceived as organized wholes. The physical characteristics which determine the organization are arranged in a hierarchical manner, timing being the most important characteristic. Handel (1973) has confirmed that if repeating patterns are segmented by temporal pauses, the pattern perception is based on the structure of the temporal grouping rather than on the structure of the pattern elements. In other words, the exact timing of the elements is more important in determining the subjective rhythm than is the patterning of the elements themselves (produced by pitch variations in this case).

B   *Auditory streaming*

In all the experiments on temporal patterning that we have described so far, the rate of presentation of elements was relatively slow (3–4 elements per second), and all the elements in the pattern were perceived as being part of a single pattern. When we listen to fast tone sequences (say 10 per second), this does not always happen. The tones are not grouped simply according to their physical temporal order, but according to their attributes, e.g. their pitches. This has been called rhythmic fission. Van Noorden (1971) investigated this phenomenon using a tone sequence where every second B was omitted from the regular sequence ABABAB . . ., producing a sequence ABA ABA. . . He found that this could be perceived in two ways, depending on the frequency separation of A and B. For small separations a single rhythm, resembling a gallop, is heard. For larger separations two separate tone sequences can be heard, one of which (A A A) is running twice as fast as the other (B B B). Van Noorden found that for some conditions either fusion or fission could be heard, according to the instructions given and the set of the subject.

Bregman and Campbell (1971) called the fission of the sound into perceptually separate tone sequences 'primary auditory stream segregation'. Bregman (1978) has suggested that each stream corresponds to an auditory 'object', and that stream segregation reflects the attribution of different components in the sound to different sources (section 5). Components are more likely to be assigned to separate streams if they differ widely in frequency, or if there are rapid jumps in frequency between them.

Dowling (1968, 1973) has shown that stream segregation may also occur when successive tones differ in intensity or in spatial location. He presented a melody composed of equal-intensity notes, and inserted between each note of the melody a tone of the same intensity, with a frequency randomly selected from the same range. He found that the resulting tone sequence produced a meaningless jumble. Making the interposed notes different from those of the melody, either in intensity, frequency range, or spatial location, caused them to be heard as a separate stream, enabling subjects to pick out the melody.

A number of composers have exploited the fact that stream segregation occurs for tones widely separated in frequency. By playing a sequence of tones in which alternate notes are chosen from separate frequency ranges, an instrument such as the flute, which is only capable of playing one note at a time, can appear to be playing two themes at once. Many fine examples of this are available in the works of Bach.

C   Judgement of temporal order

A phenomenon which is probably related to that of stream segregation occurs in judgements of the temporal order of sounds. Ladefoged and Broadbent (1960) reported that extraneous sounds in sentences were grossly mislocated, so that a click might be reported as occurring a word or two away from its actual position. Surprisingly poor performance was also reported by Warren *et al.* (1969), for judgements of the temporal order of three or four unrelated items, such as a hiss, a tone and a buzz. Most subjects could not identify the order when each successive item lasted as long as 200 ms, and naive subjects required that each item lasted at least 700 ms to identify the order of four sounds presented in an uninterrupted series of repeated sequences. These durations are well above those which are normally considered necessary for temporal resolution in speech and music. (Winckel, 1967, reported that the temporal order of musical notes is resolvable down to about 50 ms per note.) Further, it is known that for smaller numbers of items the threshold duration for discrimination is much smaller; Hirsh (1959) found that for pairs of unrelated items durations as small as 20 ms still allowed correct order discrimination.

The poor order discrimination described by Warren *et al.* is probably related to the phenomenon of stream segregation. The sounds they used do not represent a coherent class, except that they are all nonspeech. They have different waveform and spectral characteristics, and, as for tones widely differing in frequency, they do not form a single auditory stream. Items in different streams appear to float about with respect to each other in subjective time, in much the same way as a click superimposed on speech. Thus temporal order judgements are difficult. It should be emphasized that the relatively poor performance reported by Warren *et al.* is found only in tasks requiring absolute identification of the order of sounds, and not in tasks which simply require the discrimination of different sequences. Further, with extended training and feedback subjects can learn to distinguish between *and* identify orders within sequences of nonrelated sounds lasting only 10 ms or less (Warren, 1974). For sequences of tones the component durations necessary for correct order identification may be as low as 2–7 ms (Divenyi and Hirsh, 1974). To explain these effects Divenyi and Hirsh suggested that two kinds of perceptual judgements are involved. At longer component durations the listener is able to hear a clear sequence of steady state sounds, whereas at shorter durations a change in the order of components introduces qualitative changes that are capable of being discriminated by the trained listener. Similar explanations have been put forward by Green (1973) and Warren (1974).

Bregman and Campbell (1971) investigated the factors that make temporal order judgements for tone sequences difficult. They used naive subjects, so that performance presumably depended on the subjects actually perceiving the sounds as a sequence, rather than on their learning the overall sound pattern. They found that in a repeating cycle of mixed high and low tones subjects could discriminate the order of the high tones relative to one another, or of the low tones among themselves, but they could not order the high tones relative to the low ones. The authors suggested that this was because the two groups of sounds split into separate perceptual streams, and that judgements across streams are difficult. In a further investigation of this effect Bregman and Dannenbring (1973) used tone sequences in which successive tones were connected by frequency glides. They found that these glides reduced the tendency for the sequences to split into high and low streams, while at the same time order perception was easier. Conditions using partial glides also showed decreased stream segregation, although the partial glides were not quite as effective as complete glides. Thus complete continuity between tones is not required to reduce stream segregation; a frequency change 'pointing' towards the next tone allows the listener to follow the pattern more easily.

The effects of frequency glides, and other types of transitions, in preventing stream segregation or fission are probably of considerable importance in the perception of speech. Speech sounds may follow one another in very rapid sequences, so that the glides and partial glides observed in the acoustic components of speech may be a strong factor in maintaining the speech as a unified stream (see Chapter 7).

5   GENERAL PRINCIPLES OF PERCEPTUAL ORGANIZATION

Bregman (1978), and Bregman and Pinker (1978) have suggested that it is useful to make a distinction between two concepts in hearing: source and stream. A *source* is some physical entity which gives rise to acoustic pressure waves, for example a violin being played. A *stream*, on the other hand, is the percept of a group of successive and/or simultaneous sound elements as a coherent whole, appearing to emanate from a single source. For example, it is the percept of hearing a violin being played. A great many different sorts of physical cues may be used to derive separate perceptual streams corresponding to the individual sources which give rise to a complex acoustic input. Bregman and Pinker (1978) describe this acoustic factoring as *parsing*; the acoustic information is parsed to form separate streams in the same way that visual information falling on the retina is parsed to form objects and backgrounds. The parsing has two aspects: "the grouping together of all the simultaneous frequency components that emanate from a single source at a given moment, and the connecting over time of the changing frequencies that a single source produces from one moment to the next".

The Gestalt psychologists (e.g. Koffka, 1935) described many of the factors which govern perceptual organization, and, as we shall see, their descriptions and principles apply well to the way physical cues are used to achieve the parsing of the acoustic input. The Gestalt psychologists viewed these principles as the consequence of fields of force in the brain. This now seems unlikely, and we shall instead take the view that the 'rules' of perceptual organization have arisen because, on the whole, they tend to give the right answers. That is, use of the rules generally results in a grouping of those parts of the acoustic input that arose from the same source, and a segregation of those that did not. No single rule will always work, but it appears that the rules can generally be used together, in a coordinated and probably quite complex way, in order to arrive at a correct interpretation of the input. In the following sections we will outline the major principles or rules of perceptual organization. We should note that all of these apply both to vision and hearing, and that they were generally described first in relation to vision.

A   Similarity

This principle is that elements will be grouped if they are similar. In hearing, similarity will usually imply similarity of timbre, pitch, loudness, or subjective location. We have already seen examples of this principle in studies of the perception of tone sequences. If we listen to a rapid sequence of pure tones, say 10 tones per second, then tones which are closely spaced in frequency, and therefore similar, will form a single perceptual stream, whereas tones which are widely spaced form separate streams.

In the case of complex tones the basis of 'similarity' is not so clear. Van Noorden (1975) investigated the perception of sequences of complex tones each of which was composed of a group of harmonics of a missing fundamental. When the (missing) fundamentals were different, but the harmonics fell in the same frequency region, fusion occurred; the tones formed a single perceptual stream. When the (missing) fundamentals were the same, but the harmonics fell in different frequency regions, fission took place; the harmonics in different frequency regions formed separate perceptual streams. Thus for sequences of complex tones it appears that pitch does not provide the basis for similarity; tones with the same (missing) fundamental, and therefore the same pitch, do not necessarily form a single stream, whereas tones with similar timbres do, even if the pitches are different. This demonstration of van Noorden is not entirely clear-cut, however, since some of the complex tones he used contained only a few high harmonics, and hence had a rather weak, ambiguous pitch (see Chapter 4).

A final example of grouping on the basis of similarity comes from a study by van Noorden (1975) of the perception of a sequence of tones with the same frequency but with an intensity which alternated between two values. When there was a large difference between the two intensity values, the sequence of loud tones formed a separate perceptual stream from the soft tones, and attention could be directed either to the loud tones or the soft tones. When the tones were similar in intensity, a single stream was perceived with a tempo twice that of either the loud or the soft tones. Thus similarity in loudness can form the basis of perceptual grouping.

B   Good continuation

This principle exploits a physical property of sound sources, that changes in frequency, intensity, location or spectrum tend to be smooth and continuous, rather than abrupt. Hence a smooth change in any of these aspects is taken to indicate a change within a single source, whereas sudden changes indicate that a new source has been activated. Again, we have already seen examples of this in the perception of tone sequences. Bregman and Dannenbring (1973) showed that the tendency of a sequence of high and low tones to split into two streams was reduced when successive tones were connected by frequency glides. Such glides are commonly found in speech sounds (see Chapter 7), and probably help to hold the speech together as a single perceptual stream.

A second example comes from studies using synthetic speech (see Chapter 7). In such speech large fluctuations of an unexpected kind in the fundamental frequency (and correspondingly in the pitch) give the impression that a new speaker has stepped in to take over a few syllables from the primary one. However, it appears that, in this case, the smoothness of the pitch contour is not the sole factor which determines whether an intrusion will be perceived. A single speaker's fundamental frequencies cover a range of about one octave, but the intrusion effect is observed for much smaller jumps than this, provided they are inconsistent with the changes in the fundamental required by the linguistic and phonetic context. Thus it appears that the assignment of incoming spectral patterns to particular speakers is done on the basis of fundamental frequency, but in a manner which requires a knowledge of the 'rules' of intonation; only deviations which do not conform to the 'rules' are interpreted as a new speaker.

Darwin and Bethell-Fox (1977) have reported an experimental study of this effect. They synthesized spectral patterns which changed smoothly and repeatedly between two vowel sounds. When the pitch of the sound patterns was constant they were heard as coming from a single source, and the speech sounds heard included glides (l as in let) and semivowels (w as in we). When a discontinuous, steplike pitch contour was imposed on the patterns, they divided into two perceptually distinct speech sources, and the speech was perceived as containing predominantly stop consonants (e.g. b as in be, and d as in day). Apparently a given group of components can only be perceived as part of one stream (section 5.D). Thus the perceptual segregation produces illusory silences in each stream during the portions of the signal attributed to the other stream, and these silences are interpreted, together with the gliding spectral patterns in the vowels, as indicating the presence of stop consonants (see Chapter 7). It is clear that the perception of speech sounds can be strongly influenced by stream organization.

C   *Common fate*

The different frequency components arising from a single sound source usually vary in a highly coherent way. They will tend to start and finish together, to change in intensity together, and to change in frequency together. This fact is exploited by the perceptual system, and gives rise to the principle of common fate: if two or more components in a complex sound undergo the same kinds of changes at the same time, then they are grouped and perceived as part of the same source. This is a powerful principle, and it gives rise to perceptual abilities far in excess of what would be expected from studies using steady stimuli.

There are two examples of common fate which we have described, and which are of importance in the perceptual analysis of sounds such as speech and music. The first concerns the role of the onsets of sounds. Components will be grouped together if they start syncronously; otherwise they will form separate streams. The onset asynchronies necessary to allow the separation of two complex tones are not large, about 30 ms being sufficient. The asynchronies which are observed in performed music are typically as large as, or larger than this, so that when we listen to polyphonic music we are easily able to hear separately the melodic line of each instrument.

Our second example concerns modulations; components which are amplitude- or frequency-modulated in a synchronous way will be grouped together. Again, this has its counterpart in performed music. The notes produced by musical instruments are often amplitude- or frequency-modulated (tremolo, vibrato), and this helps us to assign the appropriate harmonics to each instrument. Although our examples have both been drawn from the perception of music, very similar considerations apply to the case where several people are talking at once. The components from any single voice will start and finish together, and, at least over short periods of time, will vary together in amplitude and frequency. This contributes to our ability to hear out one voice from a mixture of voices.

D *Belongingness*

Broadly speaking, this principle is that a single component in a sound can only be assigned to one source at a time. For certain types of stimuli the perceptual organization may be ambiguous, there being more than one way to interpret the sensory input. When a given component might belong to one of a number of streams, the percept may alter depending on the stream within which that component is included.

An example is provided by the work of Bregman and Rudnicky (1975). They presented a long tone sequence which contained within it a group of four tones. Two of the tones, labelled X, had the same frequency, but the middle two, A and B, were different. The four-tone sequence was either XABX or XBAX. The listeners had to judge the order of A and B. This was difficult because the AB pair occurred quickly, and because A and B were perceived as part of a longer four-tone pattern, including the two 'distractor' tones, labelled X. However, by moving another stream of tones, called 'captor' tones, near to the frequency of the distractor tones, it was possible to capture the distractors into a separate perceptual stream, leaving the tones AB in a stream of their own. This made their order easy to judge. It seems that the tones X could not be perceived as part of both streams. When only one stream is the subject of judgement and hence of attention, the other one may serve to remove distractors from the domain of attention.

E *Closure*

In everyday life the sound from a given source may frequently be temporarily obscured by other sounds. While the obscuring sound is present there may be no sensory evidence which can be used to determine whether the obscured sound has continued or not. Under these conditions the obscured sound tends to be perceived as continuous; it will be heard as such. The Gestalt psychologists called this process 'closure'. One example of this occurs when reception of FM radio is disturbed by ignition noise from passing traffic. The interference is perceived as a series of clicks or a buzz *superimposed* on the continuous speech or music signal. In fact, what happens is that the interference temporarily captures the response of the radio, so that while each interfering click is present nothing at all of the desired signal gets through. The perceptual system fills in the missing parts of the signal.

A laboratory example of this phenomenon is the continuity effect described in Chapter 3, section 5. When a sound A is alternated with a sound B, and B is more intense than A, then A may be heard as continuous, even though it is interrupted. The sounds do not have to be steady. For example, if B is noise, and A is a tone which is gliding upwards in frequency, the glide is heard as continuous even though certain parts of the glide are missing. Notice that for this to be the case, the gaps in the tone must be filled with noise. In the absence of noise, discrete jumps in frequency will be clearly heard.

The continuity effect will also work for speech stimuli alternated with noise. In the absence of noise to fill in the gaps, interrupted speech sounds hoarse and raucous. When noise is presented in the gaps, the speech sounds more natural and continuous (Miller and Licklider, 1950). For connected speech at moderate interruption rates the intervening noise actually leads to an improvement in intelligibility (Dirks and Bower, 1970). This may be because the abrupt switching of the speech produces misleading cues as to which speech sounds were present (Chapter 7). The noise serves to mask these misleading cues.

It is clear from these examples that the perceptual filling in of missing sounds does not take place solely on the basis of evidence in the acoustic waveform. Our past experience with speech, music, and other stimuli must play a role, and the context of surrounding sounds is obviously important. We should note, however, that the filling in will only occur when one source is perceived as masking or occluding another. This percept must be based on acoustic evidence that the occluded sound has been masked. Thus, if a gap is not filled by a noise, or other sound, the perceptual closure will not occur; a gap will be heard.

F   *The figure–ground phenomenon and attention*

Several times in this chapter we have referred in passing to the role of attention. It seems that we are not generally capable of consciously attending to every aspect of the auditory input (or indeed of other sensory inputs); rather certain parts are selected for conscious analysis. In principle, we might think it possible to attend to and compare any arbitrary small group of elements in a complex acoustic signal. However, this does not appear to be the case. Rather it appears that the complex sound is analysed into streams, and we attend primarily to one stream at a time. This attended stream then stands out perceptually, while the rest of the sound is less prominent. The Gestalt psychologists called the separation into attended and unattended streams the figure–ground phenomenon. At a crowded cocktail party we attend to one conversation at a time, and the other conversations form a kind of background. Similarly, when we listen to a piece of polyphonic music, we attend primarily to one melodic line at a time. We can, of course, switch attention from one conversation to another, or from one melodic line to another, and we may have some awareness of the other voices, but it appears that one stream at a time is selected for a complete conscious analysis. Neisser (1967) has suggested that attention may be brought to bear *after* the preliminary analysis into streams has occurred. The 'preattentive' processes involved thus place constraints upon attention: it is difficult to attend simultaneously to, or to make relative judgements about, elements which form parts of two separate perceptual streams.

Although the formation of auditory streams places constraints upon attention, we should not view this as an entirely one-way process; attention may also influence the formation of streams. For example, when we listen to a sequence of alternating tones, with an interval of about seven semitones between the tones, we may hear either fission or fusion depending on our attentional 'set' (van Noorden, 1975). We can listen selectively, trying to hear either the upper tones or the lower tones, or we can listen comprehensively, trying to hear all the tones together. The associated percepts seem to be mutually exclusive. When we listen without any particular set, we may hear first one percept and then the other. The change over occurs at irregular intervals, and appears spontaneous. This is an example of a perceptual reversal, resulting from an ambiguity in the interpretation of the sensory input (see section 5.D).

We may interpret the importance of changes in stimuli (section 3.C) in the context of the figure–ground phenomenon. Whenever some aspect of a sound changes, while the rest remains relatively unchanging, then that aspect is drawn to the listener's attention: it becomes the figure, while the steady part forms the background. This is of practical value since events of significance in the world are usually associated with a change of some kind. Our sensitivity to change provides a way of directing our attention to new and potentially important events in the environment.

Finally, we should note that our ability to direct attention to one stream among a number, and indeed to form the stream in the first place, does not depend only upon information available in the acoustic waveform. The Gestalt rules themselves constitute a form of knowledge, but other sources of information or knowledge may also be involved. An example of this comes from the 'cocktail party' phenomenon, our ability to attend selectively to one conversation among many. It turns out that we can follow a conversation more successfully if the *subject matter* of that conversation is different from that of the other conversations. Clearly, this involves relatively high level processes. We shall discuss this point further in Chapter 7.

6   GENERAL CONCLUSIONS

In everyday life the sound reaching our ears generally arises from a number of different sound sources. The auditory system is usually able to parse the acoustic input, so that the components deriving from each source are grouped together and form part of a single perceptual stream. Thus, each source may be ascribed its own pitch, timbre, loudness and location, and sometimes a source may be identified as familiar.

The identification of a particular sound source depends on the recognition of its timbre. For steady sounds the timbre depends primarily on the distribution of energy over frequency. The perceptual differences in the timbres of sounds can be represented as distances in a multidimensional space. This space correlates highly with that derived from a physical analysis of the sound using filters whose bandwidths approximate the critical bandwidths of the ear. The time structure of sounds can also have an influence on their timbres, with onset transients being particularly important.

Many different physical cues can be used to achieve the perceptual separation of the components arising from different sources. These include differences in fundamental frequency, onset disparities, contrast with previous sounds, changes in frequency and intensity, and sound location. No single cue is effective all the time, but used together they generally provide an excellent basis for the parsing of the acoustic input.

When we listen to rapid sequences of sounds, the sounds may be perceived as a single perceptual stream, or they may split into a number of perceptual streams, a process known as primary auditory stream segregation, or fission. Fission is more likely to occur if the elements making up the sequence differ markedly in frequency, amplitude, location or spectrum. Such elements would normally emanate from more than one sound source. When two elements of a sound are grouped into two different streams, it is more difficult to judge their temporal order than when they form part of the same stream.

The general principles which govern the perceptual organization of the auditory world correspond well to those described by the Gestalt psychologists. The principle of *similarity* is that sounds will be grouped into a single perceptual stream if they are similar in pitch, timbre, loudness or subjective location. The principle of *good* continuation is that smooth changes in frequency, intensity, location or spectrum will be perceived as changes in a single source. whereas abrupt changes indicate a change in source. The principle of *common fate* is that if two components in a sound undergo the same kinds of changes at the same time, then they will be grouped and perceived as part of a single source. The principle of *belongingness* is that a given element in a sound can only form part of one stream at a time. The principle of *closure* is that when parts of a sound are masked or occluded, that sound will be perceived as continuous, provided that there is no direct sensory evidence to indicate that it has been interrupted.

Usually we attend primarily to one perceptual stream at a time. That stream stands out from the background formed by other streams. Stream formation places constraints upon attention, but attention may also influence the formation of streams. Stream formation may also depend upon information not directly available in the acoustic waveform.

FURTHER READING

This is an area in which comparatively little work has been done, and there is no authoritative text. The following provide some useful additional material:

Bregman, A. S. (1978). The formation of auditory streams. In *Attention and Performance* Vol. 7 (ed. J. Requin), Lawrence Erlbaum, New Jersey.

Bregman, A. S. and Pinker, S. (1978). Auditory streaming and the building of timbre. *Can. J. Psychol.* 32, 19–31.

Kubovy, M. and Pomerantz, J.R. (1981). *Perceptual Organization*, Lawrence Erlbaum, New Jersey.

7 Speech perception

1 INTRODUCTION

In this chapter we shall be concerned with the problem of how the complex acoustical patterns of which speech is composed are transformed at the perceptual level into linguistic units. The details of this process are still not fully understood, in spite of an increasing volume of research over the past 30 years or so. What has become clear is that speech perception does not proceed via simple transformations from physical cues directly available in the acoustic waveform. This has been illustrated both by perceptual studies and by attempts to build machines which recognize speech (see Hyde, 1972). A given speech sound is not represented by a given, fixed acoustic pattern in the speech wave; instead the pattern representing it will vary according to the preceding and following sounds, in a complex manner. This has led to a particular kind of theoretical orientation, according to which speech perception is an active process which involves reference to articulatory mechanisms. This idea has had a widespread influence. A similar theory was described in Chapter 4 in relation to the perception of 'residue' tones. For such tones, which are composed of a number of harmonics of a fundamental tone, the pitch corresponds to the (missing) fundamental. Thurlow (1963) suggested that this pitch was mediated by vocal activity; the subject produces a matching signal whose fundamental frequency is adjusted so that its harmonics coincide with those of the externally presented tone. The perceived pitch will correspond to that fundamental frequency. According to Thurlow, the vocal activity could be overt or subliminal, or involve only auditory imagery.

Certain theories of speech perception have been advanced which, in their basic assumptions, are similar to Thurlow's theory. Firstly, they emphasize that speech perception is a process involving active matching. Secondly, they emphasize that reference to articulation is involved, although the reference may take place entirely in the nervous system, in terms of the neural commands corresponding to articulation, and may not involve actual muscular movements. And, finally, they state that the perception will correspond to the internally generated matching stimulus rather than to the stimulus which was actually presented. One of the aims of this chapter will be to present the reader with some of the reasons why such theories have been felt to be necessary and to discuss why they have had such an important place in the development of theories of speech perception; Thurlow's mediation hypothesis has had relatively little influence on theories of pitch perception, whereas 'active' theories of speech perception have generated a tremendous amount of discussion and experimental work. A second aim of the chapter will be to assess the extent to which such theories are supported by recent experimental evidence.

It is clear that for connected discourse speech perception does not depend solely on cues present in the acoustic waveform. The linguistic context is also of considerable importance. A word or part of a word which is highly probable in the context of a sentence will be 'heard' when the acoustic cues for that word are minimal or even completely absent. For example, Warren (1970b) has shown that when an extraneous sound (such as a cough) completely replaces a speech sound in a recorded sentence, listeners believe they hear the missing sound. This phenomenon is probably related to the continuity effect described in Chapter 6; when a weak sound is alternated with a louder sound of similar frequency, the weak sound appears continuous even though it is, in fact, pulsating. The effect reported by Warren has been shown to depend on similar factors; the listeners only 'hear' the missing sound if the cough is relatively intense and contains frequency components close to those of the missing sound. This kind of filling-in process is obviously of importance when we are listening in noisy environments, and it illustrates the importance of non-acoustic cues in speech perception. On the other hand, we are able to recognize words spoken in isolation, provided they are clearly articulated, so that linguistic context is not a *necessary* requirement for the perception of speech.

It is far beyond the scope of this book to give more than a brief description of certain selected aspects of speech perception. We shall not emphasize the aspects of speech recognition related to semantic cues (the meaning of preceding and following words), syntactic cues (grammatical rules) and circumstantial cues (speaker identity, subject matter, etc.), although these may be of considerable importance, especially in noisy environments. We shall concentrate rather on the processing of cues in the acoustic waveform. The study of these cues has been greatly aided by the use of speech synthesizers. These devices allow the production of acoustic waveforms resembling real speech to a greater or lesser extent; the closeness of the resemblance depends upon the complexity of the device and the trouble to which the experimenter is prepared to go. However, in contrast to real speech, these waveforms have controlled and precisely reproducible characteristics. Using a speech synthesizer, the experimenter can manipulate certain features of the speech waveform, leaving all the other characteristics unchanged, and so he can investigate what aspects of the waveform determine how it will be perceived. The results of such experiments have been instrumental in the formulation of theories of speech perception.

2   THE NATURE OF SPEECH SOUNDS

The most familiar units of speech are words, which can often be broken down into somewhat smaller units—that is, into syllables. However, linguists generally consider that even syllables can be analysed in terms of sequences of smaller units—the speech sounds or phonemes. To clarify the nature of phonemes, consider the following examples. The word 'bit' is composed of three phonemes, an initial, a middle and final element. We use each of these phonemes when we discriminate 'bit' from 'pit', 'bet' and 'bid'. Thus, for the linguist, the phonemes are the basic units of sound that in any given language differentiate one word from another. On their own they do not symbolize any concept or object (many are not even pronounceable in isolation), but in relation to other phonemes they distinguish one word from another, and in combination they form syllables and words. Not all linguists or psychologists would accept that it is appropriate to consider phonemes as 'the basic units' of speech, and indeed a few would deny that the phoneme has any perceptual reality as a unit (e.g. Warren, 1976). However, the analysis of speech in terms of phonemes has been widespread and influential, and we shall, for the purposes of discussion, continue to use the concept. When a letter is used to represent a phoneme this is indicated by a slash (/) before and after the letter.

The simplest view of speech perception would hold that speech is composed of a series of sounds or acoustic features, and that each feature, or set of features, corresponds to a particular phoneme. Thus the speech sounds would have a one-to-one correspondence with the phonemes, and a sequence of speech sounds would be perceived as a sequence of phonemes, which would then be combined into words and phrases. This view has been seriously challenged, largely as a result of experiments using synthetic speech conducted at the Haskins Laboratories, in the USA. To understand this challenge we must consider in more detail the characteristics of speech sounds.

Figure 7.1 illustrates how the phonemes of English can be classified according to the way in which they are produced by the articulatory apparatus. The section which follows outlines the relationship between the manner of production and the acoustic characteristics of the speech. Speech sounds are produced by the vocal organs, namely the lungs, the windpipe, the larynx (containing the vocal cords), the throat or pharynx, the nose and nasal cavities, and the mouth. The part of this system lying above the larynx is called the vocal tract, and its shape can be varied extensively by movements of various parts such as the tongue, the lips and the jaw. The glottis is an opening at the upper part of the windpipe, between the vocal cords, and it can affect the flow of air from the lungs by opening or closing. The term 'glottal source' refers to the sound energy produced by the flow of air past the vocal cords as they open and close quite rapidly in a periodic or quasi-periodic manner. This produces a periodic complex tone with a relatively low pitch, whose spectrum initially contains energy at harmonics covering a wide range of frequencies. This spectrum is subsequently modified according to the shape of the vocal tract. Speech sounds produced while the vocal cords are vibrating are said to be voiced. For some speech sounds the vocal cords do not vibrate, but remain open. Such sounds are said to be voiceless, and they arise from turbulence at a constriction of the vocal tract above the glottis (e.g. /s/ as in 'sit').

The speech sounds produced by a constriction are classified into a number of different types. A fricative consonant is characterized by a turbulent noise, and may consist of that noise alone (as in /s/), or may consist of that noise together with a glottal source (/z/). Stop consonants are characterized by a sudden rapid closing and opening of a complete constriction somewhere in the vocal tract. This stops the flow of air for a short time, with a consequent reduction or cessation of acoustic energy, after which the airflow and energy abruptly resume. As for fricatives, stops may be voiced (as in /p/ or /b/) or voiceless (as in /t/ or /d/). Affricatives are like a combination of stop and fricative; they are characterized by turbulence together with a momentary obstruction to the flow of air through the vocal tract. An example is /dʒ/ as in 'judge'. Nasals, such as /m/ and /n/, are produced by allowing air to flow through the nasal passages. These different classes of speech sounds differ from each other in the *manner* in which they are produced. In addition, there are, within each class, differences in the *place* of production (the place where a constriction generates sound energy, e.g. teeth, lips, roof of the mouth, etc.). All of these differences will be reflected in the acoustic characteristics of the speech wave, as revealed by the speech spectrum. However, for consonants the spectra will not be static, but will change as a function of time. Vowels, on the other hand, may have relatively stable spectra, at least for short periods of time. For further details of the relationship between articulation and the acoustic characteristics of speech, the reader is referred to Fant (1960).

Speech, then, is an example of *par excellence* of auditory patterns which vary in frequency, in amplitude and in time. In order to display these variations simultaneously a device known as the speech spectrograph is used. This consists of a large number of filters, each responsive to a particular narrow band of frequencies. The outputs of the filters as a function of time are used to produce a display known as the speech spectrogram. In this display the amount of energy in a given frequency band is plotted as a

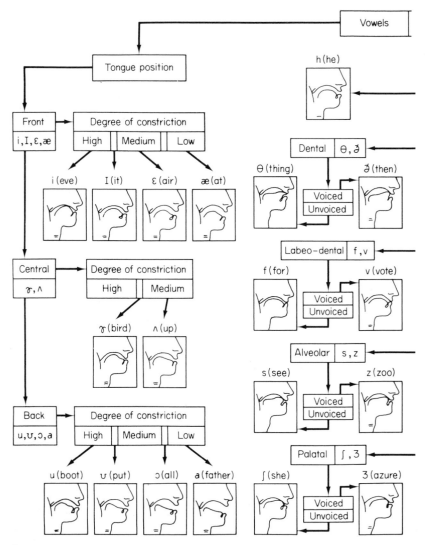

* In the above classification /e/ (hate), /o/ (obey) are considered as diphthongs and /tʃ/ (chew) and /dʒ/ (jar) are considered as stop-fricative combinations

FIG. 7.1 Classification of phonemes according to their manner and place of production. Adapted from figures in Potter *et al.* (1947).

function of time. Frequency is represented on the ordinate, time along the abscissa, and intensity by the darkness of the line used. A typical example is given in Fig. 7.2. Very dark areas indicate high concentrations of energy at particular frequencies, while very light areas indicate an absence of energy.

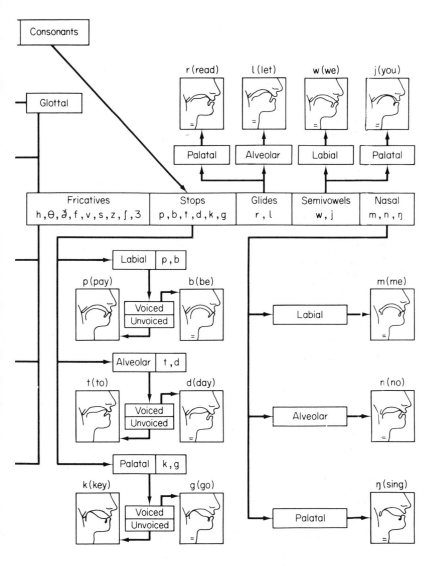

Many speech sounds, and particularly vowel sounds, show peaks in the spectral energy at particular frequencies, known as formant frequencies. The frequencies of the formants are determined by the shape of the vocal tract, which behaves as a filter modifying the glottal source. The formants

FIG. 7.2 A speech spectrogram for the utterance 'I can see you'. Notice the concentration of energy at particular frequencies (formants), except for the /s/ sound, and the lack of silent intervals between successive words. The vertical striations correspond to individual periods of vocal cord vibration, and their spacing depends on the rate of this vibration.

are numbered, the one with the lowest frequency being called the first formant, the next the second, and so on. Vowel sounds may be characterized in terms of their formant frequencies and the amount of energy at each of these formants. As many as six formants may be observed in a speech spectrogram, but the first three are the most important for the purpose of identifying the vowel. There are, of course, other ways of analysing vowel sounds, as we saw in Chapter 6 (cf. the dimensional analysis approach by Plomp and his colleagues), but analysis in terms of formants has been by far the most common and most influential technique.

A marked characteristic of speech sounds is that there are often rapid changes in the frequency of a given formant or set of formants. These changes, known as formant transitions, have been found to be important acoustic cues for the perception of consonants. Speech sounds may be either periodic (voiced), in which case they will have a pitch, or noiselike (voiceless), in which case there will be no well-defined pitch, although timbre variations, based on frequency spectrum, may occur. Vowels, and some consonants, are periodic, and will be similar to the complex tones discussed in Chapter 4. Although they are composed of harmonics, the individual harmonics are usually not resolved in a speech spectrogram, and perceptually the peaks in the spectral envelope (formants) rather than the frequencies of individual harmonics are the important factors in determining what phoneme is present. Speech sounds such as the 's' in 'hiss' have a noiselike character and display a continuous spectrum, usually with a much smoother distribution of energy over frequency.

The speech spectrogram of a complete sentence may show a number of time intervals where there is little or no spectral energy. However, these silent intervals do not always correspond to 'spaces' between words, but often occur during the speech sounds representing a particular word. Thus in explaining speech perception we have to specify not only how the acoustic elements in the speech sound are 'decoded' into individual phonemes, but also how the sequence of sounds is segmented into individual words and syllables.

3 SPEECH PERCEPTION—THE CASE FOR A SPEECH MODE

In what is now a classic paper Liberman *et al.* (1967) gave a number of reasons for thinking that phonemes not only *were* not but *could* not be efficiently communicated by sounds that stand in a one-to-one correspondence with the phonemes. One of their arguments concerned the rate at which speech sounds occur. In rapid speech as many as 30 phonemes per second may occur, and it was argued that this would be too fast for resolution in the auditory system; the sounds would merge into an unanalysable buzz. We saw in Chapter 6 that listeners can, in fact, learn to identify sequences of sounds when the individual items are as short as 10 ms (corresponding to a rate of 100 items per second), but that at these short durations the listeners do not perceive each successive item separately but rather learn the overall sound pattern. It is likely that for continuous speech something similar applies. Even if there are acoustic cues in a one-to-one correspondence with the phonemes, these cues will not be perceived as discrete acoustic events. Rather the listener will recognize the sound pattern corresponding to a group of phonemes, such as those corresponding to a whole syllable, or even a word.

One of the most important arguments of Liberman *et al.* concerned the nature of the acoustic cues which underly the perception of particular phonemes. They used as an example the phoneme /d/ as in 'dawn'. A major cue for the perception of /d/ is a transition in the second formant. Indeed, Liberman *et al.* suggested that the second formant transition was a major cue for most consonant sounds, and was "probably the single most important carrier of linguistic information in the speech signal". Consider the highly simplified spectrographic patterns shown in Fig. 7.3. When these are converted into sound, the first formant transition (the change in frequency of the lowest formant at the beginning of the sound) provides a cue for the class

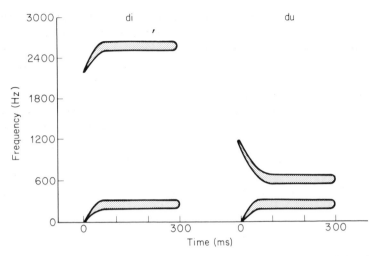

FIG. 7.3 Highly simplified spectrographic patterns which are perceived as /di/ and /du/ when they are converted into sound. From Liberman *et al.* (1967), by permission of the authors and the American Psychological Association.

of voiced stops /b, d, g/. Some other aspect of the sounds determines which of these three is actually heard. The sounds illustrated are actually identified as /di/ and /du/ when presented to listeners. On the basis of a number of perceptual experiments using such synthetic speech sounds, Liberman *et al.* concluded that the second formant transitions in the patterns are the cues for the perception of /d/ as opposed to /b/ or /g/. Notice that although listeners identify each of these sounds as beginning with the phoneme /d/, the acoustic cues at the beginning of the sounds are vastly different for the two examples presented. In the case of /di/ the transition rises from about 2200 to 2600 Hz; in /du/ it falls from 1200 to 700 Hz. Thus the same phoneme can be cued, in different contexts, by acoustic features that are vastly different.

A related argument concerns the nonexistence of clear boundaries between successive phonetic segments. There is no way to cut the patterns shown in Fig. 7.3 so as to recover /d/ segments that can be substituted one for the other, or even to obtain some piece that will sound like /d/ alone. If the right-hand half of the syllable is progressively removed, we hear either /d/ plus a vowel, or a nonspeech sound. According to Liberman *et al.*, this is because "the formant transition is, at every instant, providing information about two phonemes, the consonant and the vowel—that is, the phonemes are being transmitted in parallel". An alternative view would be that since the /d/ phoneme cannot exist alone, it is not a 'unit' of speech.

Liberman *et al.* argue that the kind of context-dependent restructuring seen for the acoustic cues signalling the /d/ phoneme occurs quite generally for consonant sounds. Thus it is rarely possible to find invariant acoustic cues corresponding to a given consonant phoneme. For steady state vowels the frequency positions of the formants do provide more or less invariant cues, but vowels are rarely steady state in normal speech. Usually vowels are articulated between consonants at rather rapid rates, so that "vowels also show substantial restructuring—that is, the acoustic signal at no point corresponds to the vowel alone, but rather shows, at any instant, the merged influences of the preceding or following consonant". The general conclusion is that a single acoustic cue may carry information in parallel about successive phonemes. This reduces the rate at which discrete sounds must be perceived, but at the expense of a complex relation between cue and phoneme. Phoneme perception therefore requires a special decoder. Liberman *et al.* refer to those phonemes whose acoustic cues show considerable context-dependent restructuring as 'encoded', while those phonemes for which there are relatively invariant acoustic cues are called 'unencoded'. They suggested that the perception of encoded phonemes should differ from the perception of unencoded phonemes and from the perception of non-speech sounds.

One piece of evidence for a 'speech mode' in auditory perception is the phenomenon of categorical perception. For an acoustic signal varying along a single dimension, such as frequency, we are normally able to discriminate many more stimuli than we can identify absolutely (see Chapter 6, section 2). However, for encoded phonemes it is found that listeners discriminate very little better than they can identify absolutely. Changes in the acoustic signal which do not change the phoneme identity are perceived with difficulty, or not at all, by the subject, while those acoustic changes which produce a change in phoneme identity are, of course, easily discriminated. Consider, for example, some simplified synthetic speech signals in which the second-formant transition is varied in relatively small, acoustically equal steps through a range sufficient to produce the three phonemes /b/, /d/ and /g/. One does not hear a series of small changes in the acoustic signal, but "essentially quantal jumps from one perceptual category to another" (Liberman *et al.*, 1967). Thus we do not hear changes within one phoneme category, but only changes from one phoneme to another. This is called categorical perception. In order to demonstrate categorical perception both identification and discrimination tasks must be performed. The identification task establishes the boundaries between phonetic categories. The discrimination task is usually of the ABX type. Three successive stimuli are presented, and the listener is required to state whether the last stimulus is the same as the first or the second. For the ideal case of categorical perception discrimination would be high across category boundaries, but would drop to chance level for pairs of stimuli falling within one category. In practice the situation is rarely as straightforward as we have described here, but whenever discrimination of acoustic changes is good across phoneme boundaries and poor within phoneme categories, this is taken as evidence of categorical perception. The situation with steady state vowels is very different. Small physical changes in the acoustic stimulus are perceived as such, so that one vowel may be heard to shade into another, and many intraphonemic variations are heard. Liberman *et al.* suggest that this is because vowels are much less encoded than speech sounds, so that they may be perceived in the same manner as nonspeech sounds. However, vowel sounds in rapidly articulated speech do show restructuring, and there is evidence (Stevens, 1968) that perception of certain vowels in their proper dynamic context is more nearly categorical than is found for steady state vowels.

Although categorical perception has been considered to reflect the operation of a special speech decoder, there is some evidence that categorical perception can occur in a nonliguistic mode. Locke and Kellar (1973) obtained identification and discrimination functions for triads consisting of three simultaneous pure tones, using both musicians and nonmusicians as subjects. Of the three tones in the triad, only the middle tone was varied, in small steps over a range sufficient to produce a chord of A minor (440, 523 and 659 Hz) at one end of the range, and a chord of A major (440, 554 and 659 Hz) at the other end. Categorization was considerably more prominent among the musicians; they tended to recognize the triads as either A minor or A major. Further, the discrimination curves for musicians did parallel predictions from categorization more closely than did the curves for non-musicians. In other words, the discrimination performance of musicians was better for frequency changes which altered the identity of the chord.

A second example of categorical perception for nonspeech stimuli is provided by the work of Miller *et al.* (1976). They presented a low-level noise stimulus whose onset could occur at various times in relation to the onset of a more intense buzz stimulus (a filtered squarewave). The stimuli terminated simultaneously. In one part of the experiment subjects labelled single stimuli with either of two responses; 'no noise' or 'noise'. In the other part of the experiment subjects were required to discriminate among stimuli differing in relative noise onset time. They found that labelling shifted abruptly around a noise lead time of about 16 ms, so that when the noise onset occurred more than 16 ms before that of the buzz the label 'noise' was applied. Otherwise the label 'no noise' was applied. They found further that discrimination was best for pairs of stimuli which lay on either side of the 16 ms boundary. This resembles the categorical perception found for synthetic speech stimuli.

These demonstrations of categorical perception for nonspeech stimuli indicate that the phenomenon is not unique to speech, and that its explanation does not depend on the existence of a special speech decoder. We will return to this point later in the chapter.

A different line of evidence indicating that speech perception is different from the perception of nonspeech is provided by studies establishing the regions in the brain that play a role in the perception of speech and non-speech sounds. These studies are based on the assumption that the crossed neural pathways from the ear to the brain (i.e. from the right ear to the left cerebral cortex, and vice versa) are generally more effective than the un-crossed pathways. If competing stimuli are presented simultaneously to the two ears (e.g. two different spoken messages), then speech stimuli presented to the right ear are better identified than those presented to the left, while the reverse is true for melodies (Broadbent and Gregory, 1964; Kimura, 1964). This suggests that encoded speech signals are more readily decoded in the left cerebral hemisphere than in the right. Studies of deficiencies in speech perception and production for people with brain lesions have also indicated that the left hemisphere plays a primary role in speech perception (Kimura, 1961).

A third line of evidence is provided by studies of the perception and identification of sounds which vary in the extent to which their acoustic characteristics approach those of speech. House *et al.* (1962) required sub-jects to learn to associate members of various ensembles of acoustic stimuli with buttons on a response box. They found that stimuli with spectral and temporal properties similar to those of speech are not learned more readily than simpler stimuli unless they are actually identified by the listener as speech. Thus, as Stevens and House (1972) have put it,

> . . . although one can imagine an acoustic continuum in which the sounds bear a closer and closer relation to speech, there is no such continuum as far as the perception of the sounds is concerned—the perception is dichotomous. Sounds are perceived either as linguistic or as nonlinguistic entities.

Overall, then, the evidence for some special kind of speech-processing mechanism is quite strong. We tend to perceive speech sound categorically, so that most speech sounds are perceived as having a particular identity, and not as being 'in between' two classes of speech sound. There is good evidence that particular parts of the brain are specialized for dealing with speech. And when we are presented with speechlike sounds, there is a perceptual dichotomy: either the sounds are perceived as speech or they are not. Stevens and House (1972) suggested that "the listener need not be set for speech prior to his hearing the signal; his prepared state is triggered by the presence of a signal that has appropriate acoustic properties". Very probably there is a strong involuntary component to this 'triggering' of the speech mode; no matter how hard we try, it is impossible to hear speech in terms of its acoustical characteristics, i.e. as a series of hisses, whistles, buzzes, etc. Rather we perceive a unified stream of speech sounds.

4   MODELS OF SPEECH PERCEPTION

There are no models of speech perception that are sufficiently accurately specified to allow rigorous experimental testing, but two theoretical approaches have had a considerable influence on the direction and emphasis of research in speech perception. These two approaches are those of the Haskins Laboratory investigators and of Stevens and his colleagues at the Massachusetts Institute of Technology. Both groups have been strongly influenced by the problem of the complex relationship between acoustic cues and perceived phonemic segments and by the problem of segmenting the speech wave into syllables and words.

The approach of the Haskins group has been called the 'motor theory' of speech perception. They proposed that speech perception requires a special decoding mechanism which proceeds by reference to articulatory processes. The basic idea is that somewhere in the nervous system the neural signals corresponding to the sensory input are brought into correspondence with internally generated neural signals which would have produced the articulatory movements leading to that sensory input. Early versions of this model, such as that presented by Liberman (1957), assumed that the patterns generated by the listener were actually produced as covert articulatory responses, whose proprioceptive feedback was compared with the stored speech. In later versions this viewpoint has been somewhat modified, since there is clear evidence that speech may be perceived in the absence of any measurable articulatory response on the part of the listener. Thus Liberman *et al.* (1963) suggested that "the neural commands themselves, or rather their equivalents in the central nervous system, might be used to provide the reference system in terms of which the decoding (of speech) is carried out".

Notice that the emphasis is on an active matching process rather than on a direct translation of the acoustic stimulus into speech. Liberman *et al.* (1967) set forward a number of reasons for believing that speech perception proceeds via production rather than via a straightforward auditory decoder.

Firstly, they suggested that since the listener is also a speaker,

> . . . it seems unparsimonious to assume that the speaker-listener employs two entirely separate processes of equal status, one for encoding language and the other for decoding it. A simpler assumption is that there is only one process, with appropriate linkages between sensory and motor components.

This argument is somewhat dubious since one might argue that the processes involved in the motor theory approach are excessively complex and unwieldy, and would result in an inherently slow mechanism. Further, it is not at all clear how the patterns of neural activity corresponding to articulatory commands would be transformed so that they could be compared with the neural traces corresponding to the stored speech signal. Such a transformation would have to take into account all of the complex processing of the auditory stimulus which occurs in the peripheral auditory system, and we have seen that for a wideband signal this is by no means simple.

A second argument of Liberman *et al.* derives from observations of electromyographic (EMG) signals from the speech musculature. These have led to the conclusion that the perceptions of a listener in response to speech are more closely related to the patterns of articulation that produce those speech signals than to the acoustic signals themselves. Thus the patterns of muscular movement which produce a given speech sound may lie more nearly in a one-to-one correspondence with the perception of that sound than the acoustic signals. Again, however, this does not necessarily favour a motor theory. It may well be the case that when a speaker 'decides' to say a particular speech sound, the neural commands corresponding to that sound are more or less invariant. The fact that the acoustic consequences of those neural commands are not invariant is merely a result of that particular way that the articulatory apparatus works. Thus the higher correlation between production and perception than between acoustic signals and perception does not necessarily imply the mediation of production in perception. It merely reflects the fact that the acoustic consequences of a sequence of muscular movements vary according to the order in which those movements are strung together.

The theoretical approach of Stevens and his colleagues is similar in spirit to that of the Haskins group, but is considerably more specific. It has been called the analysis by synthesis model. According to this model, the peripheral patterns of neural activity corresponding to speech sounds are subject to a preliminary analysis, and are also held in a temporary store. Sometimes this preliminary analysis provides sufficient information for phonetic information to be passed on immediately to higher levels of processing. Often, however, the analysis is insufficient, in which case the listener makes a hypothesis as to the nature of the speech sounds. This hypothesis allows the listener to generate patterns, either at the muscular level or at the neural level, corresponding to the articulations which would actually be necessary to produce the hypothesized sounds. These patterns can then be compared with the patterns in the temporary store. The comparison either confirms that the hypothesized utterance is correct or generates an error message which can be used as the basis for further hypotheses. Provided that the error message carries useful new information, no more than two or three hypotheses will be necessary before the utterance is 'correctly' perceived. Notice that this model requires that there be at least a few invariant cues, so that a reasonable initial hypothesis can be generated, otherwise an infinity of bad guesses might result. We may consider the analysis by synthesis model as a more detailed and slightly modified form of the motor theory suggested by the Haskins group. Just as for the motor theory, a major problem for the model is to explain how the two types of patterns could be compared. The generated pattern is a set of neural commands which if executed would result in the articulation of a particular phoneme or word. The stored pattern is some kind of neural representation or memory trace corresponding to the acoustic pattern. Clearly, some very complex transformations would be necessary before any comparison could occur.

One of the strongest arguments in favour of 'active' theories of speech perception was their ability to explain the phenomenon of categorical perception, although, as we shall see, other explanations have now emerged. As we described earlier, the perception of certain speech sounds is discontinuous, even when the acoustic signal is varied continuously. It turns out that the corresponding articulations are also discontinuous. Consider an example given by Liberman *et al.* (1967):

> With /b, d, g/, we can vary the acoustic cue along a continuum, which corresponds, in effect, to closing the vocal tract at various points along its length. But in actual speech the closing is accomplished by discontinuous or categorically different gestures: by the lips for /b/, the tip of the tongue for /d/, and the back of the tongue for /g/.

Thus the categorical perception of these speech sounds can be explained by assuming that they are decoded with reference to articulation and that the articulation is itself categorical.

Unfortunately for the 'active' theories of speech perception, this explanation has been made implausible by the discovery that nonspeech sounds may be perceived categorically (see the experiments by Locke and Kellar, 1973, and Miller *et al.*, 1976, described earlier in this chapter, and the discussion by Lane, 1965). There are several possible alternative explanations, and we will describe two of them here. The first suggests that the differences in perception which are observed for 'encoded' consonants and relatively 'unencoded' vowels may be explained in terms of differences in the extent to which the acoustic cues can be retained in acoustic memory (see later, and also Darwin and Baddeley, 1974 and Pisoni, 1973). The acoustic cues corresponding to the consonant parts of speech sounds are generally at a much lower intensity than those for vowel sounds. In addition, the cues for consonants fluctuate more rapidly and last for a shorter time than those for vowels. Consequently, the acoustic cues for consonants will be much more ephemeral in acoustic memory. It may be that by the time these acoustic cues have been processed in the identification of the phoneme they are lost from auditory memory. Thus further discrimination within phoneme categories, will not be possible. However, for speech sounds such as vowels, the acoustic cues will be retained in acoustic memory for longer periods of time, so that additional discriminations, based upon these stored cues, can be made. As was mentioned earlier (see section 3), the triggering of the 'speech mode' is probably involuntary. Thus the initial processing of cues in acoustic memory, when we are presented with speech sounds, will always relate to the linguistic properties of those sounds. It is only after this initial analysis that discrimination of the cues in a nonlinguistic mode is possible. Those cues which are efficiently stored in acoustic memory will then give rise to continuous perception, whereas if the cues corresponding to a given phoneme are lost, only discrimination based on the prior categorization will be possible. We should note that the ABX design used to test for categorical perception inevitably confounds perception with memory.

A second possible explanation for categorical perception is that categories and boundaries in speech have evolved in order to exploit the natural sensitivities of the auditory system (Stevens, 1981). Thus the boundaries which separate one speech sound from another will tend to lie at a point along the acoustic continuum where discrimination is optimal. Demonstrations of categorical perception using synthetic speech stimuli typically use a series of stimuli which vary in 'acoustically equal steps'. However, the definition of 'acoustically equal' is somewhat arbitrary. For example, if the dimension being varied is frequency, it is not clear whether the steps should have an equal size on a linear scale or a logarithmic scale. Similarly, it is not clear whether the steps should be defined in absolute terms, or relative to some baseline frequency. The latter would be more in accord with Weber's law, but it has seldom been done in speech research. Similar difficulties apply to the choice of equal steps in time. Thus steps which are physically equal on some arbitrary scale may not be equal in psychoacoustic terms. It may be that at category boundaries 'physically equal' steps are actually larger than average in perceptual terms.

In summary, the evidence put forward by Liberman *et al.* (1967) in favour of a motor theory approach can be interpreted in other ways. Although the evidence for a special mode of speech perception is quite strong, the evidence that this special mode operates by reference to articulation is weak. Indeed, a number of workers have presented arguments against a motor theory approach. For example, Fant (1973) says: "The alternative view I would like to propose here is that if the auditory analysis in the hearing process has proceeded so far as to allow the proposed articulatory matching, the decoding could proceed without an articulatory reference". Perhaps one of the most crucial pieces of evidence has been presented by Lenneberg (1962). He described the case of a patient who had an organic defect which prevented the acquisition of the motor skill necessary for speaking a language. Nevertheless, the patient could understand speech and possessed all the grammatical skills necessary for a complete understanding of language. Here, then, is a clear case of someone who cannot speak, but can understand speech. Of course, modern versions of the motor theory assume that mediation takes place not via articulations themselves, but via the neural commands corresponding to those articulations. Thus, in theory, it is not necessary for a listener to speak in order to understand speech. However, it is difficult to understand how a person who had *never* spoken could learn to associate speech sounds with the appropriate neural commands. Similar cases have been reported by Fourcin (1975).

Although we have been arguing that speech perception need not operate by reference to articulation, this does not mean that the listener perceives speech solely by the registration of individual acoustic features. On the contrary, it is likely that the perceptual system uses information not directly available in the acoustic waveform, in order to arrive at a correct interpretation of the speech signal. If a given speech element is exceedingly probable in the context of the utterance as a whole, then that element will be 'heard' when the acoustic cues are minimal or even completely absent. Even for words spoken in isolation, factors related to word probability may affect recognition especially under noisy listening conditions. Broadbent (1967) reported that common words tend to be detected at lower signal-to-noise ratios than rare words, or to be detected more often at the same signal-to-noise ratio. He called this the word-frequency effect, and discussed four models to explain the effect. He concluded in favour of a model based on signal detection theory (see Chapter 3), which has been proposed and elaborated by Morton (1964). According to this model, a listener has an internal 'dictionary' of word units, such that when a unit is caused to be 'fired', a word corresponding to that unit is perceived. Two separate factors determine whether or not a given unit will fire. The first factor is the sensory evidence relating to the acoustic features specifying the word. The second factor is the response bias of the unit—a measure of its 'readiness' to fire—which will be affected by such factors as word probability and context. Thus the dictionary unit corresponding to a given word will fire on the basis of less sensory evidence when that word is highly probable, either because of context or because it is a common word.

This model accounts well for the influence of non-acoustic factors in speech perception, and it would be capable of rapid operation: a dictionary unit would fire 'automatically' on presentation of the appropriate sensory evidence, provided that the sensory evidence were sufficient to exceed the threshold of the unit at that time. However, the model is inadequate in many respects. It does not say how the sensory evidence would be processed in extracting acoustic features indicative of any particular word. In other words, the problem of non-invariance between acoustic cue and perceived phoneme remains. We should note that this problem persists even if units of greater length, such as the syllable or word, are considered. Further, the system does not allow for a re-analysis of the sensory data if the 'wrong' dictionary unit fires. Subthreshold excitation of other dictionary units does not result in any output from the system. Finally, the output of the system is in terms of the identity of words and not in terms of their perceptual attributes. Thus it is not clear how these attributes (man's voice or woman's, accent, direction of sound, loudness, etc.) would be linked to the outputs of the dictionary unit system. This could be a serious problem in situations where several people are talking at once.

Recently it has been suggested that the role of encoded or overlapping cues in speech perception has been somewhat overemphasized (Fischer-Jørgensen, 1972). Cole and Scott (1974) have noted that speech perception involves the simultaneous identification of at least three qualitatively different types of cues: invariant cues, context-dependent cues (e.g. frequency transitions) and cues provided by the waveform envelope. In a review of the literature on consonant phonemes—traditionally considered as highly encoded speech sounds—Cole and Scott conclude that *all* consonant phonemes are accompanied by invariant features, i.e. by acoustic cues which accompany a particular phoneme in any vowel environment. In some cases the invariant information is sufficient uniquely to define the consonant, while in other cases the invariant features limit perception to a possible pair or triplet of phonemes. They show, further, that transitional cues are also present in all consonant–vowel syllables. In other words, any given syllable contains both invariant and transitional cues. The transitional information may sometimes be necessary to discriminate between a pair of phonemes which have been signalled by invariant cues.

Stevens (1980) and Blumstein and Stevens (1979) have pointed out several of the acoustic features which may be used to distinguish between different phonemes in natural, as opposed to synthetic, speech. Some examples of these features are given in Fig. 7.4, which shows several representations of the acoustic attributes of the utterance 'the big rabbits'. The true consonants, such as /p d m s z/, are characterized by a rapid change in spectrum over a time interval in the range 10–30 ms. An example of this is shown in the top left of the figure for the consonant /b/. Vowels and glides, on the other hand, are characterized by much slower changes in the spectrum. Thus, rapidity of spectrum change is the crucial property for distinguishing these classes of sounds.

A second feature is the abruptness of amplitude change accompanying a consonant. A rapid amplitude change together with a rapid spectrum change is indicative of the stop consonants /p t k b d g/. These rapid amplitude changes may be seen in the lower part of Fig. 7.4 for the /b/ and /t/ sounds. A third feature, that of voicing, serves to distinguish between certain pairs of speech sounds. For example, the voiced consonant /b/ is distinguished from the unvoiced consonant /p/ by the presence of a low frequency periodicity during the closure interval. This may be seen in the central part of Fig. 7.4 by the faint vertical striations in the low frequency region just prior to the release of the /b/ sounds. For the voiceless consonant /p/ this low-level periodicity does not occur, and there is also a period of time following consonantal release when there is noise before the onset of vocal fold vibration; this is known as the voice onset time (VOT). Thus voiced and unvoiced consonants are distinguished by the presence or absence of low frequency periodicity during the closure interval, and by the value of the VOT.

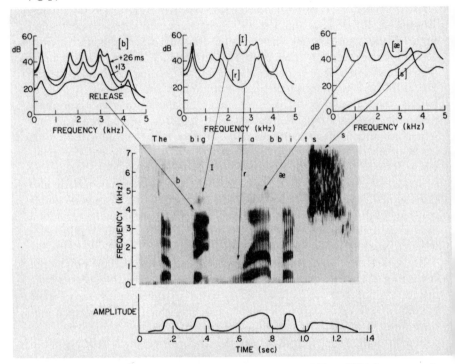

FIG. 7.4 Several representations of the utterance 'The big rabbits'. The middle shows a speech spectrogram like that in Fig. 7.2. At the top are spectra sampled at various points during the utterance. At the bottom is the variation in over-all amplitude with time. The spectra have been 'pre-emphasized', by boosting the high frequencies relative to the low frequencies. From Stevens (1980), by permission of the author and *J. Acoust. Soc. Am.*

For stop consonants a fourth feature is the gross shape of the spectrum sampled at the release of the consonant. This can serve to define the place of articulation of the consonant. For example, the spectra for /p/ and /b/ are spread out or diffuse in frequency, and are flat or falling, as may be seen in the top left of Fig. 7.4. The spectra for /d/ and /t/ are spread out, but are rising, while the spectra for /g/ and /k/ show a distinctive rather narrow peak in the midfrequency range, with other spectral peaks being smaller and well separated from the central peak. Blumstein and Stevens (1980) have shown that sounds with onset spectra having these general shapes will be categorized

appropriately by human listeners. Notice that the features identifying place
of articulation and voicing, when taken together, serve to define uniquely
any stop consonant. Thus the phonemes described by Liberman *et al.* (1967)
as being highly 'encoded' do seem to be indentifiable from relatively invariant acoustic cues.

The bottom part of Fig. 7.4 shows the variation of overall amplitude with
time during the utterance. However, there is considerably more detail
present than is indicated by this smoothed outline. Imagine that we plot the
speech waveform in terms of pressure variations as a function of time. Such a
plot could be obtained as a display on an oscilloscope if the pressure
variations were converted into voltage variations by means of a microphone.
The envelope is the curve produced by drawing a smooth line passing
through the peaks in the waveform; it is a kind of 'outline' of the waveform.
A typical example is given in Fig. 7.5, for the utterance 'I'm a waveform'.

FIG. 7.5 A photograph of an oscilloscope display showing the envelope of the utterance 'I'm a
waveform'.

Notice that for much of the time the envelope shows peaks which are fairly
regularly spaced. This indicates that the speech sounds are periodic and
involve the vibration of the vocal cords (i.e. they are voiced sounds). The
time intervals between these peaks in the envelope are the same as the
corresponding periods of vibration for the vocal cords. The part of the

envelope corresponding to the 've' in wave and the 'f' in form does not show these periodic peaks, because of the noiselike nature of these sounds, and it also has a lower amplitude. Variations in amplitude, and therefore in loudness, also occur during the voiced parts of the speech.

Clearly, then, the waveform envelope gives us information about fluctuations in amplitude as a function of time. Both amplitude and duration have been demonstrated to be of considerable importance in determining the so-called prosodic features of speech (those concerned with intonation and stress). Even a period of silence can provide cues for stress, enabling us to distinguish between such phrases as 'lighthouse keeper' and 'light house-keeper'. However, such cues are only useful if they are evaluated in relation to duration and amplitude cues from adjacent syllables; speech rates and average intensities vary considerably, so that a measurement of amplitude or duration taken in isolation would have little significance. Thus our use of amplitude and duration cues in determining prosodic features indicates that information relating to the waveform envelope can be retained in storage for relatively long time periods.

There is good evidence that the waveform envelope also provides information about the phonemic composition of speech. Many experiments have shown that features such as duration, short periods of silence, relative amplitude and pitch can influence the perception of particular phonemes. All of these features can be extracted from the waveform envelope. An indication of the amount of information which may be carried in the waveform envelope is provided by an experiment of Katz and Berry (1971). They imposed upon a white noise 'carrier' the waveform envelopes of various speech stimuli. They found quite good intelligibility scores for this 'speech-modulated' white noise, although words in sentences were discriminated better than words in isolation, and vowels were discriminated better than consonants. Thus to some extent the auditory system is able to decode speech stimuli on the basis of time–amplitude variations alone. The ability to extract information from the waveform envelope is not, of course, unique to speech; we saw in Chapter 4 that periodically interrupted white noise has a pitch corresponding to the envelope repetition rate, and in Chapter 5 that the envelope of high frequency, amplitude modulated tones can be used in the lateralization of such sounds.

It is clear that in the perception of speech the human listener makes use of a great variety of types of information which are available in the speech wave. Many different cues may be available to signal a given speech element (phoneme), but the cues may not be constant and may differ in relative importance from utterance to utterance. Thus many kinds of context-dependent variations in the acoustic cues occur, and accurate speech recognition will depend upon the listener's ability to allow for the context and compute its effects. The multidimensional nature of the acoustic cues allows for a high level of redundancy in the speech wave; there may be several different acoustic cues for a given phoneme, of which just one or two might be sufficient for recognition. This redundancy can be used to overcome the ambiguities inherent in the speech, to lessen the effects of interfering stimuli, to compensate for distortions in the signal (for example, when the speech is transmitted over a telephone line), and to allow for poor articulation on the part of the speaker. At a higher level, errors made in identifying a speech sound from its acoustic pattern can be corrected by the listener's knowledge of the kinds of speech signals which can be produced by the human vocal tract, by reference to linguistic rules, by the 'sense' of the message, and by knowledge of the characteristics of the speaker, e.g. accent or sex.

5   THE RESISTANCE OF SPEECH TO CORRUPTING INFLUENCES

One way to assess the degree of redundancy in the speech wave is to eliminate or distort certain features and to determine the effect of this on the intelligibility of the speech. The results of such experiments have indicated that speech is, in fact, remarkably resistant to many kinds of quite severe distortions. Most of the experimental data have been obtained using articulation testing methods: a speaker reads a list of syllables, words or sentences to a listener, or group of listeners, and the percentage of items correctly recorded by the listener(s) is called the articulation score.

One factor which can affect speech intelligibility is the amount of background noise. For satisfactory communication the average speech level should exceed that of the noise by 6 dB (i.e. the S/N ratio should be +6 dB). When speech and noise levels are equal (0 dB S/N ratio), the word articulation score reaches about 50%. However, speech may be intelligible at negative S/N ratios (where the speech level is below that of the noise) for connected speech, particularly if the listener is familiar with the subject matter, or if the speech and the noise come from different directions in space (this is an example of the BMLD phenomenon which was discussed in Chapter 5). In many practical situations the noise is intermittent rather than continuous. This decreases the effectiveness of the noise in masking the speech by an amount depending on the on–off ratio of the noise and the interruption rate. At high interruption rates (above about 200 per second) the noise has effects similar to those of continuous noise. At rates between 1 and 200 per second it is possible to patch together the bits of speech heard between the noise, so that the noise is not a very effective masker. At very slow interruption rates whole words or groups of words may be masked, while others are heard perfectly. Thus articulation scores drop once more.

A second factor which may affect speech intelligibility is a change in frequency spectrum. Many transmission systems (e.g. a telephone line) pass only a limited range of frequencies, and some of the first investigations of speech intelligibility were conducted by engineers of the Bell Telephone Laboratories, in an attempt to assess the importance of frequency range. Experiments using filters with variable cutoff frequencies have shown that no particular frequency components are essential for speech recognition. For example, if all frequency components above 1800 Hz are filtered out, using a low-pass filter, then the syllable articulation score is about 67%, while normal conversation is fully intelligible. However, speech is equally intelligible if instead we use a high-pass filter to remove all frequency components below 1800 Hz. Experiments using bandpass filters have shown that, over a fairly wide range of centre frequencies, a surprisingly narrow band of frequencies is sufficient for satisfactory recognition. For example, a band of frequencies from 1000 Hz to 2000 Hz is sufficient to give a sentence articulation score of about 90%. Clearly, then, the information carried by the speech wave is not confined to any particular frequency range. This fits in very well with our notion of speech as a multidimensional stimulus, with many acoustic cues for any given phoneme.

A third kind of disrupting influence which commonly occurs is peak-clipping. If an amplifier or other part of a transmission system is overloaded, then the peaks of the waveform may be flattened off, or clipped. In severe cases the clipping level can be only 1 or 2% of the original speech wave's peak values, with the result that the original speech wave, with its complex waveshape, is transformed into a series of rectangular pulses. This severe distortion does degrade the quality and naturalness of speech, but it has surprisingly little effect on intelligibility; word articulation scores of 80 or 90% can still be obtained.

We see, then, that speech is intelligible under a wide variety of conditions where we might have expected rather poor performance. It remains intelligible in the presence of large amounts of background noise, or when we remove all but a small part of the speech spectrum, or when we destroy time–amplitude variations in the waveform by peak-clipping. Once again we are led to the conclusion that no single aspect of the speech wave is essential for speech perception. Thus the speech wave is highly redundant. Each of the disruptions which we have described will destroy some of the cues carried in the speech waveform, but the remaining cues are sufficient to convey the message. This is, of course, of great practical advantage. If speech perception depended on a near-perfect transmission of sound from speaker to listener, then speech communication is most real situations would become extremely difficult, and devices like the telephone would have to be much more elaborate and costly than they are. Nature has designed the speech communication process so that it can operate under a great variety of adverse conditions.

6   GENERAL CONCLUSIONS

We have seen that speech is a multidimensional stimulus varying in a complex way as a function of both frequency and time. Although the speech wave can be described in terms of amplitude and time, this does not seem to be the most appropriate description from the point of view of the auditory system. Neither is a description in terms of static spectra satisfactory. The representation which best fits the perceived nature of speech, and which is in accordance with the known functioning of the auditory system, uses the dimensions of intensity, frequency and time, as in the speech spectrogram. This shows how the short-term spectrum of the speech varies as a function of time.

A basic problem in the study of speech perception is to relate the properties of the speech wave to the linguistic units of which speech is composed. It is still not clear whether the basic unit of perception is the phoneme or the syllable. A description in terms of phonemes achieves a considerable economy in terms of the number of separate sound patterns which have to be analysed and remembered by the listener, since the number of phonemes is much less than the number of possible syllables. However, this type of economy may not be important in human perception. The ease and consistency with which the phonetician can describe an utterance in terms of phonemic units also argues for the phoneme as a unit of perception. On the other hand, for rapid connected speech the psychoacoustic evidence indicates that the individual phonemes would occur too rapidly to be separately perceived in correct temporal order. Thus the recognition of the overall sound pattern corresponding to a longer segment, such as a syllable, is indicated.

A second problem is that of finding cues in the acoustic waveform which would unambiguously signal a particular linguistic unit. This is a particular problem for certain consonants. While it is possible to find a number of relatively invariant cues for consonants in single words or syllables articulated clearly in isolation, these cues are not so apparent in rapid connected speech. In many cases a phoneme will only be correctly identified if information obtained over a whole syllable or even over a group of several words is utilized. The complex relationship between the speech wave itself and the linguistic units of which speech is composed has been one of the central problems in speech perception, and has had a powerful influence on the development of theories of speech perception.

There is good evidence that speech is a special kind of auditory stimulus, and that speech stimuli are perceived and processed in a different way from nonspeech stimuli. The evidence derives from studies of categorical perception, the phenomenon that speech sounds can be discriminated only when they are identified as being linguistically different; from studies of cerebral asymmetry, which indicate that certain parts of the brain are specialized for dealing with speech; and from the speech–nonspeech dichotomy, the phenomenon that speechlike sounds are either perceived as speech or as something completely nonlinguistic. Examples of this latter effect may occur when listening to faulty synthetic speech which only poorly approximates real speech. This will often be heard as a confusing mixture of buzzes, puffs of noise, whistles, etc., but the listener may suddenly switch into the 'speech mode' when the cacophony becomes intelligible speech.

The complex and variable relationship between the acoustic waveform and the phoneme has led to the development of a number of 'active' models of speech perception, in which speech is decoded by reference to articulatory processes. In one form of these models preliminary analysis of the speech wave, together with any available contextual information, is used to generate a hypothesis about the nature of the utterance. This hypothesized utterance is then checked against the stored neural representation of the speech signal, and if a match is achieved, then that utterance is perceived. In order for such a comparison to be possible, the stored speech and the hypothesized utterance must be transformed so that they are in comparable forms, which in itself would be a highly complex task. An inherent disadvantage of such a system is that in the absence of contextual cues it might be necessary to generate many different hypotheses before a satisfactory match was achieved, so that the process would be intrinsically slow. In fact, we can recognize words spoken in isolation rapidly and easily. At the present time there is no compelling evidence in favour of the active approaches, although it is generally accepted that speech perception involves decoding processes of considerable complexity.

It is clear that speech perception involves processing at many different levels and that separate information at each level may be used to resolve ambiguities or to correct errors which occur at other levels. The initial analysis of speech sounds into phonemes (or syllables) can be checked and readjusted by a stored knowledge of phonetic constraints, i.e. by a knowledge of the kinds of ways in which one phoneme can follow another. Our knowledge of syntactics (grammatical rules) and semantics (word meanings) allows further adjustments and corrections, while situational cues such as speaker identity and previous message content provide yet further information. It is quite possible that the processing of speech does not occur in a hierarchical way from one level to the next, but that there are extensive links between each level. Thus the information at any level may be re-analysed on the basis of information from other levels. Even some details of the speech wave itself may be retained for a short time in 'echoic memory' so that re-analyses may be made.

The multidimensional nature of speech sounds, and the large amount of independent information which is available at different levels of processing, produce a high level of redundancy in speech. This is reflected in the finding that speech intelligibility is relatively little affected by severe corrupting influences. Speech can be accurately understood in the presence of large amounts of background noise, or when it is severely altered by filtering, interruption or peak-clipping. Thus speech represents a highly efficient way of communicating under difficult conditions.

FURTHER READING

The following articles give reviews of speech perception from a slightly different viewpoint to that of this chaper:

Stevens, K. N. and House, A. S. (1972). Speech Perception. In *Foundations of Modern Auditory Theory*, Vol. 2 (ed. J. V. Tobais), Academic Press, New York.

Darwin, C. J. (1976). The perception of speech. In *Handbook of Perception*, Vol. 7 (eds E. C. Carterette and M. P. Friedman), Academic Press, New York.

Studdert-Kennedy, M. (1976). Speech Perception. In *Contemporary Issues in Experimental Phonetics* (ed. N. J. Lass), Academic Press, New York.

8 New developments, practical applications and future outlook

1 INTRODUCTION

It is the purpose of this chapter to describe a few of the practical applications of auditory research and to suggest some possible future developments. In addition, some recently discovered auditory 'effects' will be described, not because of their immediate practical relevance, but because they may provide important insights into the functioning of the auditory system.

2 ADAPTATION EFFECTS AND CHANNELS

In recent years a great deal of work on sensory systems has centred around the concept of 'channels' or groups of neurones responsive to particular properties of stimuli. This has been particularly true of the visual system, where there is evidence for channels 'tuned' to orientation, colour, spatial frequency, movement, and so on. The evidence for these channels comes from two quite separate sources, neurophysiological data and psychophysical data. As an example of the former, cells in the visual cortex have been found which respond best to lines of a particular orientation. The psychophysical evidence comes largely from studies of adaptation effects. The basic idea behind this has been well expressed by Mollon (1974): "If one suspects that a particular attribute of the stimulus is subject to a specialised analysis, then the principle is to try to fatigue, or 'adapt', selectively the neural mechanism tuned to detect that particular attribute". This fatigue or adaptation will then be revealed as an after-effect of some kind, such as an elevation of threshold for the detection of that particular attribute of the stimulus.

In the auditory system one type of organization by channels is well-known and widely accepted, namely the tonotopic organization; different neurones respond selectively to particular frequency components of stimuli, and any single neurone in the auditory nerve will respond optimally to only a relatively narrow range of frequencies. Thus it is quite common to use the phrase 'high frequency channels' to refer to that group of neurones having high characteristic frequencies. However, at the level of the auditory cortex the tonotopic organization appears to be much less well-defined, and many neurones will not respond to steady pure-tones at all (see Chapter 1, section 7). It is thus quite possible that cortical neurones are 'tuned' to more complex properties of stimuli than pure-tone frequency, and recent psycho-physical evidence has tended to support this view. In the auditory cortex of the cat some neurones respond selectively to tones whose frequencies are changing in a particular direction or at a particular rate, or to tones which are modulated in frequency, so as to have a warbling quality (see Fig. 3.7 for an illustration of the waveform of such sounds). Kay and Matthews (1972), using adaptation techniques, have presented evidence showing that channels tuned for the detection of such modulation may exist in the human auditory system. They presented an adapting tone whose frequency was sinusoidally modulated at a particular rate (say 8 times per second), and immediately after cessation of this stimulus they measured the ability to detect frequency modulation in a tone that was much more weakly modulated (i.e. in which the swing in frequency was not so great). They found that when the rate of modulation of the test tone was close to that of the adapting tone, the sensitivity was considerably reduced. The frequency deviation in the modulated test tone had to be increased to about three times the pre-exposure threshold to be detectable immediately after exposure to the adapting tone. Further, the effect was 'tuned' to modulation rate, so that when the modulation rate of the test tone was one-half or two times that of the adapting tone, the effect was very small. The effects were observed for modulation rates of the adapting tone from 1 per second up to 80 per second, although the largest effects occur around the middle of this range.

Kay and Matthews showed that the adaptation did not depend critically on the adapting and test tones having the same 'carrier' frequency, although this did have some effect. They showed, further, that the detectability of frequency modulation at a rate of 8 per second was not affected by prior exposure to a tone that was *amplitude* modulated at a rate of 8 per second. Thus it is not simply the rhythm of the stimulus which is important. They concluded that the channels indicated by these experiments are not con-cerned with modulation periodicity *per se* or with signal spectrum or carrier frequency, but with instantaneous frequency changes. However, rate of frequency change cannot be the critical factor, since the rate of change of frequency (in Hz/s) is considerably different for the adapting stimulus and the test stimulus on which it has a maximal effect. It seems that the periodicity of the frequency changes is the crucial factor in adapting these channels, but the changes must be glides in frequency rather than instantaneous changes; the detectability of a sinusoidal modulation in frequency is not affected by prior exposure to a square-wave modulation (abrupt changes between one frequency and another).

Kay and Matthews (1972) suggested that these channels could be concerned with the extraction of certain features in speech signals, but it is difficult to see exactly what these features would be. Although frequency changes are commonly observed in speech, they are rarely of the periodic nature which these channels would require for activation. Some work of Gardner and Wilson (1979) suggests a slightly different interpretation of these channels. They exposed listeners to tones which were swept repeatedly either upwards or downwards in frequency. The threshold for single upward sweeps was increased by a factor of two to three following exposure to repetitive upward sweeps, but was unaffected by exposure to downward sweeps or to tone bursts of a constant frequency. Similarly the threshold for single downward sweeps was affected only by exposure to downward sweeps. Thresholds for modulated tones, like those used by Kay and Matthews, were elevated by exposure to both up-sweeps and down-sweeps, and to a lesser extent by tone bursts. Gardner and Wilson suggested that their results indicated the existence of channels specifically tuned either to upward sweeps in frequency, or to downward sweeps in frequency. Such sweeps are commonly observed in speech stimuli (see Chapter 7).

Other workers have attempted to investigate more directly the possibility that there are channels tuned for detecting particular features of speech sounds (Bailey, 1973; Eimas and Corbit, 1973; Eimas *et al.*, 1973). These workers have exploited the phenomenon of categorical perception which occurs for speech sounds (see Chapter 7). Bailey (1973) generated a series of synthetic speech stimuli which were identical except for the first 40 ms. The frequencies of the second and third formants were changed during this initial period, so as to produce a /ba/ sound at one end of the series and a /da/ sound at the other (see Fig. 8.1). As we have noted previously, in identifying stimuli from such a series the listeners' responses do not change gradually with changes in the physical stimulus, but change abruptly at some point in the range. Bailey chose an adapting stimulus from one end or the other of the series and presented it to the subject 40 times. He then presented test stimuli chosen to lie around the point on the continuum where the identification normally switches from one syllable to the other. He found that after adaptation to /ba/ an intermediate stimulus was more likely to be perceived as /da/, and vice versa. Other workers have demonstrated similar effects for physical variables such as voice onset time: the time between the initial burst of sound and the onset of vibration of the vocal cords.

These experiments have clearly demonstrated the operation of some form of feature-analysing mechanism in speech perception, although there is still considerable debate as to the exact nature of this mechanism. Eimas and his colleagues have interpreted their results in terms of linguistic feature detectors, arguing that the adaptation is phonetic rather than auditory. They showed that adaptation effects are not obtained if the adapting stimulus is

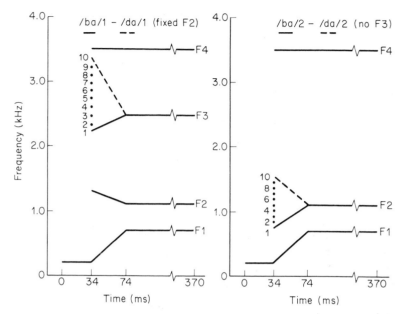

FIG. 8.1   Schematic spectrograms of the stimulus sets used by Bailey (1973). In the left-hand half of the figure F2 is fixed and F3 varies. In the right-hand F2 varies and F3 is absent. In both cases the variation is sufficient to produce a clear perception of /ba/ at one end of the range and /da/ at the other. From Bailey (1973), by permission of the author.

simply the first 50 ms of the syllable /da/, an acoustic pattern which contains all the necessary information to distinguish /ba/ from /da/, but which is not heard as speech. Thus, at least in this case, the adapting stimulus must be perceived as speech if it is to have an adapting effect on a test speech sound.

The conclusion that the adaptation is phonetic is not supported by some experiments of Bailey (1973). He exploited the phenomenon that the distinction between different speech sounds may be carried by many separate cues in parallel. In the case of the /ba–da/ series, changes in both the second formant (F2) and the third formant (F3) provide cues which on their own are sufficient for discrimination (see Fig. 8.1). Bailey constructed two synthetic /ba–da/ series, one with a fixed F2 and all cues in F3, the other with no F3 and all cues in F2. He found cross-adaptation from the F2 cues series to the fixed F2, but none from the F3 cues series to no F3. On the basis of this experiment, and an additional experiment using a fixed third formant, Bailey concluded:

When the cues in the adapter and test syllables are carried by different formants, and are hence spectrally well-separated, very little effect of adaptation is observed. This implies that the cues used here to convey the place distinction in these initial consonants are *independently* extracted, rather than being processed as a combined spectral pattern by a higher-level linguistic feature detector.

Clearly, the issue of auditory versus phonetic detectors is not yet resolved, and it may well be that both types of detectors exist. If phonetic detectors do indeed exist, then this would provide good evidence that the analysis of speech into phonemes is reasonable from a perceptual point of view, but proof of the existence of such detectors would not help us to understand the mechanism by which the complex and variable acoustic cues of speech are decoded into phonemic units. Many curious features of the adaptation process remain to be explained. For example, Bailey (1974) has shown that the adaptation effect is well developed after only eight adapter repetitions, equivalent to about four seconds exposure to the repeated speech sound. If the effect were the result of fatiguing a particular group of neurones, one would expect a longer build-up than this. Cooper (1974) has shown that adaptation to a particular speech sound may not only affect perceptual boundaries, but also produce correlated shifts in the production of speech sounds. This may indicate a link between the perception and production of speech, as is hypothesized in the motor theory of speech perception (Chapter 7). Research on contingent after-effects in vision has shown that the effects are in many ways more like conditioning than sensory adaptation, and this may well be the case for auditory feature detectors. Thus while these effects are fascinating, and possibly of considerable importance, their exact significance must remain in some doubt.

3   PSYCHOACOUSTIC CONSIDERATIONS IN CHOOSING YOUR HI-FI

The last few years have seen a considerable expansion in the sale of sound-reproducing equipment, while at the same time manufacturers have been competing with one another in their efforts to produce 'better' amplifiers, loudspeakers, and so on. Unfortunately, the criterion for 'better' has not usually been clearly defined, and in most cases there has been little effort to investigate the extent to which improvements in technical specification actually produce *audible* improvements. There is, of course, the problem of defining the objectives of high fidelity reproduction. One aim which has often been put forward is that the sound reproduced in the listening room should be the same for the listener as if he had actually had a good seat at a concert. In most practical situations this aim is unrealistic. Firstly, the echoes and reverberations in a concert hall contribute to the listening experience in a way which cannot be accurately simulated in a normal listening room (although reasonable approximations may be possible using multichannel reproduction). It is only in an anechoic chamber that is feasible to recreate exactly the sound field that a listener would experience at a live concert (see section 5). Secondly, the peak sound levels occurring at a concert may be high compared with the levels which are practicable or even tolerable in a domestic situation.

In practice recorded sounds may actually be 'better' than sounds heard at a live performance, for a number of reasons. Recording engineers typically use a large number of microphones and a tape recorder with many independent (but synchronized) channels. The engineer is able to position each microphone so as to capture the sound of a particular instrument or group of instruments, and several different types of microphones may be used in order to optimize the recording for each instrument. Sometimes four or five microphones are used to record the drums alone. The final published recording is obtained by 'mixing down' from, say, 24 channels to two (for stereo) or four (for quadraphonic reproduction). At the stage of mixing down, the engineer and the producer have the option of manipulating the recorded signals in many ways so as to achieve the desired sound quality. For example, the sound spectrum in any of the channels may be altered by banks of filters, so as to produce subtle alterations in timbre or to compensate for the acoustics of the recording room. Cymbals may be made 'crisper', bass notes 'deeper', voices more or less 'breathy', and so on. Reverberation may be added, in controlled amounts and with controlled characteristics, and the impression of the location of different instruments may be controlled by manipulating the amount of sound from each channel which is fed to each of the final channels. In addition, several different recordings of a given piece of music may be taken, and the best sections from each recording spliced together, to give a final performance which is as nearly perfect as possible; even single notes may be spliced in if a musician makes a mistake.

It is generally acknowledged that modern recorded music, reproduced on high quality equipment, can have advantages over live music in terms of clarity and the definition of individual instruments. Further, many pieces of recorded music could not be produced at a live performance, since they rely on techniques of superimposition of separate recordings and on electronic manipulations which can only be performed in a recording studio. It makes sense, then, to define the object of high fidelity as the reproduction of sounds corresponding as closely as possible to the intention of the record producer. Thus the emphasis is on accuracy or fidelity of reproduction.

Any high fidelity reproduction system contains several different components, each of which may alter or distort signals in various ways. The most common system probably involves a record player (pickup, arm and turntable), an amplifier and a set of loudspeakers (usually two). Each of these will distort the signal in some way, and for any particular type of distortion the performance of the chain as a whole will be determined by the performance of its weakest link. It is usually true that much more distortion arises in the transducers of the system (the pickup and the loudspeakers) than in the amplifier; even a cheap amplifier will perform far better than any loudspeaker. Thus audible improvements in a system are much more likely to result from changes in loudspeakers than they are from changes in amplifiers. In the following paragraphs we shall consider in turn each of the major components in a sound-reproducing system, emphasizing those aspects of performance which are likely to be most important in how the system *sounds*.

A   Amplifiers

As was mentioned above, the basic performance of even a moderately priced amplifier is likely to be so good that improvements in technical specification would make little audible difference. Nevertheless, some aspects of performance are worth considering. The necessary power output of an amplifier can only be determined in relation to the loudspeakers with which it will be used. Loudspeakers vary considerably in the efficiency with which they convert electrical energy into sound energy; horn loudspeakers may have efficiencies of 30% or more, while 'acoustic suspension' loudspeakers may convert less than 1% of the electrical energy into sound. Thus it is nonsense to say, as one manufacturer has done, that an amplifier produces 'forty-four watts of pure sound'. In fact, even one acoustic watt, in a normal-sized room, would correspond to an extremely loud sound. There are many loudspeakers available which produce high sound levels (in excess of 90 dB SPL) with quite moderate electrical inputs, say 1 W. In other words, given loudspeakers of reasonable efficiency, it is quite unnecessary to spend a lot of money on a high power amplifier. Additionally, it is worth remembering that a doubling of power (which might mean a doubling in price) produces only a 3 dB change in sound level, which is only just noticeable. Unfortunately, manufacturers have not yet standardized their methods of specifying loudspeaker efficiencies, but a common way is in terms of the electrical input (in watts) required to produce a sound level of 90 dB SPL at a distance of 1 m from the loudspeaker. Sometimes the level specified is 96 dB SPL, in which the case the power required will be four times that needed to produce a level of 90 dB SPL.

One aspect of amplifier performance which is commonly quoted is frequency response. This is measured by using as input to the amplifier a sine wave of constant amplitude but variable frequency. Ideally the output of the amplifier should not vary as a function of frequency, so that all frequencies are amplified to an equal extent. In practice there will be a limit to the range of frequencies which the amplifier will reproduce, and the frequencies at which the output of the amplifier has fallen to one-half power (the 3 dB points) are used to define this range. Modern amplifiers easily out-perform loudspeakers in this respect, and most cover the entire audible range of frequencies (say 20–20 000 Hz) without appreciable fluctuations in output.

Some manufacturers have gone to extremes in this respect, presumably to impress unsuspecting customers, and quote frequency responses such as 5–100 000 Hz. It is quite unnecessary, and indeed undesirable, for an amplifier to cover such a wide frequency range. Very low frequency components produced by record warps may be of high amplitude, and may overload the amplifier if they are reproduced at full power. In addition, such components can produce very large excursions of loudspeaker cones, which may easily damage them. Frequency components between 20 and 100 kHz will not be audible, but if amplified they may contribute to audible distortion and may present quite a high power input to the high frequency unit (tweeter) of a loudspeaker system. Thus the power capacity of both the amplifier and tweeter in reproducing audible frequencies will be limited by the extent to which that power is being wasted in reproducing inaudible high frequencies. In conclusion, the frequency response of an amplifier is rarely a limiting factor in performance, but beware of amplifiers which have frequency responses extending very far beyond the audible range.

Most amplifiers distort signals to some extent. Usually the distortion is specified in terms of the extent to which frequency components are present at the output which were not present at the input of the amplifier. Unfortunately, distortion is not usually specified in a way which allows an easy estimate of its audibility. The most common method is to specify harmonic distortion. A pure tone of a particular frequency is used as input to the amplifier. If the amplifier distorts the signal, the output will not be exactly sinusoidal, but will be a periodic waveform of the same repetition rate as the input. This periodic waveform can be expressed as a fundamental component (of frequency equal to that of the input sinusoid) and a series of harmonics. The total amplitude of the second and higher harmonics, expressed as a percentage of the amplitude of the fundamental, is called the harmonic distortion, and its value may vary from 0.05% or less for a high quality amplifier to 3% for a cheap amplifier. The *audibility* of harmonic distortion is not predictable from this simple percentage, because audibility depends upon the distribution of energy among the different harmonics. If the energy of the distortion products is mainly in the second and third harmonics, then these harmonics will be masked to some extent by the fundamental, and if the signal is a piece of music, they will in any case be masked by the harmonics which are normally present in the input signal. If, on the other hand, the distortion produces high harmonics, then these will be much more easily audible, and subjectively more objectionable. It is not usually possible to determine from the manufacturer's specification what form the harmonic distortion takes, but test reports often mention whether crossover distortion is present. Crossover distortion is manifested by 'kinks' in the output waveform where it changes from positive to negative voltage, or vice versa. It is common in transistor amplifiers but very rare in valve amplifiers. The distortion products produced by this distortion are mainly high harmonics, and so this type of distortion may be detected even at levels as low as 0.1%. In an amplifier in which crossover distortion is absent levels of harmonic distortion of 2–3% would not normally be noticed.

A different way of measuring distortion is to apply two tones of differing frequency to the amplifier input and to measure the levels of other frequencies at the output of the amplifier. Again the levels of the distortion products are usually expressed as a percentage of the level of the primary tones. Each tone will, of course, produce its own harmonic distortion products, but, in addition, there will be frequency components produced by the nonlinear interaction of the two tones. If the frequencies of the two input tones are f_1 and f_2, then 'combination' products will be produced with frequencies such as $f_1 - f_2, f_1 + f_2, 2f_1 - f_2, 2f_1 + f_2$. This type of distortion is called intermodulation distortion. Once again, it is difficult to predict the audibility of a given percentage of intermodulation distortion in a normal listening situation, since the figures quoted by a manufacturer depend upon the exact frequencies and relative levels of the tones chosen for the test. In general, intermodulation distortion is more easily audible than harmonic distortion, but levels of less than 0.5% are unlikely to be detected.

Studies of the audibility of distortion in recorded music have given widely differing results, with some authors claiming that harmonic distortion of about 5% is not detectable (Jacobs and Wittman, 1964). Unfortunately, the *type* of distortion has not normally been specified in these experiments, so that no generalizations can be made. One fairly consistent finding has emerged, however; the wider the range of audible frequencies produced by the equipment, the lower is the level of distortion which can be detected or tolerated. Thus if very good loudspeakers with a wide frequency range are used, the level of distortion in the amplifier must be lower than if loudspeakers with a limited frequency range are used.

In summary, with loudspeakers of moderate quality there is no point in spending a lot of money on an amplifier in order to achieve levels of harmonic or intermodulation distortion less than about 0.5%. However, this only applies if crossover distortion is at very low levels. If very high quality loudspeakers are used, then it may be worth considering an amplifier with slightly lower distortion levels. In practice most listeners would not notice 3% harmonic distortion, provided that the distortion was concentrated in the lower harmonics.

One other aspect of amplifier performance is worth a brief mention. All amplifiers add a certain amount of undesired noise to the signal. This noise usually takes the form of a low frequency hum (related to the frequency of the alternating current supply) and a high frequency hiss. The performance of an amplifier in this respect is usually specified as the ratio of the output power with a relatively high level input signal to the output power due to hum and noise alone. The ratio is normally expressed in decibels, a typical figure being 60 dB. Of course, at a given setting of the amplifier volume control the noise level is constant, but the signal level may vary considerably. Thus, when the signal is at a low level, the signal-to-noise ratio may be much less than 60 dB. The range of levels over which the signal may vary is called the dynamic range, and at a live music performance this range may be considerable (60 dB or more). If such a range occurred in recorded music, then at times the noise level would equal that of the signal and the noise would be very obtrusive. Thus the dynamic range of recorded music is almost always 'compressed' to about 30 dB. This allows satisfactory performance from amplifiers and associated equipment with relatively modest signal-to-noise ratios, and in practice a signal-to-noise ratio of 60 dB or greater is adequate in most domestic situations.

B   *Loudspeakers*

Consider now the characteristics of loudspeakers. The efficiency aspect has already been mentioned, and we shall not discuss it further. Just as was the case for an amplifier, the ideal loudspeaker would have a uniform or flat frequency response over the entire audible range; a constant electrical input would lead to a constant sound output, regardless of the frequency of the applied voltage. The degree to which the response of the loudspeaker differs from this ideal can be specified by using the output in response to a given midfrequency (often 1 kHz) as a reference level. The output at other frequencies can then be specified in relation to this level, and the overall response can be specified in terms of the range of frequencies over which the variations in output level fall within certain limits. Thus the frequency response for a good loudspeaker might be stated as 50–15 000 Hz ± 5 dB. This would mean that the sound level did not vary over more than a 10 dB range for any frequency from 50 Hz to 15 000 Hz. Notice that in this respect even a good loudspeaker will be much worse than an amplifier, which might have a frequency response of 20–20 000 Hz ± 1 dB. Many loudspeakers are so bad that the manufacturers do not specify decibel limits in quoting a 'frequency range' for their loudspeakers. A *frequency response without decibel limits is meaningless.* In practice it is only in recent years, with improvements in loudspeaker design, that manufacturers of the better loudspeakers have felt able to quote accurately specified frequency responses, and this is still not common practice for medium and low priced loudspeakers.

The frequency response of a loudspeaker is normally measured in an anechoic chamber, so that there is no reflected sound from walls, ceiling and floor which could affect the results. In domestic situations reflected sound will always be present and will influence the overall sound to some extent.

High frequencies are usually absorbed more than low frequencies, so that the effective level of the low frequencies is boosted, and this partially compensates for the falling frequency response which is found at low frequencies in most loudspeakers. A second but less desirable effect of reflected sound is that resonances may be set up at particular frequencies, so that when a piece of music is reproduced, those frequencies are more prominent, giving the music an unpleasant 'coloured' sound. The frequencies of the resonances depend upon the dimensions of the listening room; the larger the room the lower will be the frequencies of the resonances. In general, three major resonances will be produced, corresponding to the length, width and height of the room. Ideally none of these dimensions should coincide, otherwise a particularly strong resonance may be produced. The resonances may be 'broken up' by large pieces of furniture, so that their effect is reduced. Thus it is desirable that the listening room should not be too sparsely furnished, but should contain settees, armchairs, and so on.

Given that room acoustics are bound to have an influence on the 'effective' frequency response of a loudspeaker, one might think that the response of a loudspeaker measured in an anechoic chamber is not particularly relevant to how the loudspeaker will sound. This is not in fact the case, because peaks and dips in the 'anechoic' frequency response will combine with peaks and dips produced by room resonances to produce an overall response which is more irregular than either alone. To minimize this irregularity the 'anechoic' frequency response should be as flat as possible. In addition, listeners appear to compensate for the characteristics of a room in judging the nature of a sound source. This is shown by the everyday experience that the quality of the voice of a familiar person does not change markedly with changes in the room in which the person is heard. The effect is an example of perceptual constancy; the properties of an object (in this case a voice) as perceived by an observer vary little with quite large changes in the conditions of observation. It may be that something analogous to the precedence effect (Chapter 5, section 5) operates in judgements of sound quality as well as in the localization of sound. If this were the case, then the perceived quality of a sound would be determined by that part of the sound that reached the ears first, as direct sound from the loudspeaker rather than reflected sound. Thus changes in signals produced by loudspeaker imperfections would be noticed much more than changes produced by room reflections. This is not to deny that room acoustics have an effect, but their effect is less noticeable than might be predicted from physical measurements. As far as loudspeakers are concerned, a frequency response of 50–15 000 Hz ± 3 dB would be exceptionally good, and provided that other aspects of the performance were also good, a loudspeaker with this response would add little of its own quality to the reproduced sound; it would be an accurate transducer.

One aspect of loudspeaker performance which has been largely neglected until recently is the phase response. In order for a waveform to be reproduced accurately not only should all the frequency components be reproduced at the correct relative amplitudes, but also the relative phases of the components should be preserved. This is equivalent to saying that at the listener's ear the time delay of all frequency components should be equal. Changes in the relative phases of the components can produce marked changes in a waveform. Loudspeaker manufacturers have not paid much attention to this, because it has generally been assumed that the ear is insensitive to changes in relative phase. The statement that the ear is phase deaf is often ascribed to Helmholtz (1863), who experimented with harmonic complex tones containing eight successive harmonics, including the fundamental. In fact, Helmholtz did not exclude the possibility that phase changes were detectable for high harmonics, beyond the sixth to eighth, and more recent work has shown that phase changes produce both changes in timbre (Plomp and Steeneken, 1969) and changes in the clarity of pitch (Bilsen, 1973). The effects for steady tones are, however, rather small. This is not particularly surprising, since, for steady sounds, room reflections will produce marked alterations in the relative phases of components, and we have already seen that room acoustics have relatively little effect on the perceived quality of reproduced sounds.

The situation is rather different for transient or short-duration sounds, which are, of course, common in music. The results of a number of experiments have indicated that we can discriminate between sounds differing only in the relative phases of the components (and not in component amplitude), even when those sounds have durations as small as 2–3 ms (Patterson and Green, 1970). When such sounds are reproduced by loudspeakers, any given sound will be completed before any reflected sounds (echoes) reach the ears, provided that the head of the listener is more than 60–90 cm from any room surface. Thus room reflections will have little effect on our ability to discriminate between short-duration sounds differing in the relative phases of the components. This has been confirmed by Hansen and Madsen (1974).

What these results mean is that the phase response of a loudspeaker can be important in determining the subjective quality of the reproduced sound. Changes in the relative phases of components are much more noticeable when those components are close together in frequency than when they are widely separated, so that phase changes which occur abruptly as a function of frequency will have a larger subjective effect than phase changes which occur gradually over a wide frequency range. Unfortunately, the former is the more common situation. Most modern 'high fidelity' loudspeakers contain two or more transducers to deal with different parts of the frequency range. A 'woofer' is used for low frequencies and a 'tweeter' for high. The electronic input to the loudspeaker is split into high and low frequency bands by electronic filters known as crossover networks, and the transition frequency between a high and a low band is known as the crossover frequency. It is in the region of the crossover frequency that rapid phase changes occur, and thus the crossover network is a source of phase distortion. In addition, certain cabinet designs, such as the vented enclosure or reflex cabinet, introduce marked phase changes in particular frequency regions. It is noteworthy that loudspeakers which avoid rapid changes in phase as a function of frequency, such as the Quad electrostatic, tend to be judged as reproducing sounds with a greater clarity and realism than those which have a rapidly changing or irregular phase response. Unfortunately, it is difficult to isolate this aspect of performance from other differences between loudspeakers, so it has not yet been conclusively demonstrated that a given loudspeaker sounds better because of its superior phase response.

Recently Blauert and Laws (1978) investigated the audibility of phase distortion by taking a variety of complex sounds, including speech, music, noise and brief impulses, and delaying a group of frequency components with respect to the remainder. They found that the minimum detectable delay was about 400 microseconds (μs) when the frequencies delayed were in the range 1–4 kHz. They also measured the delays which actually occurred for several loudspeakers and headphones. For the headphones the worst case corresponded to a delay of 500 μs, which is only just above the threshold. For the loudspeakers delays up to 1500 μs were found. These are well above the threshold for detection, and might therefore have a significant effect on the perceived quality of the sound reproduced by the loudspeakers. It is to be hoped that in the future the aspects of phase response which are subjectively important will become more clearly defined.

A property of loudspeakers which is connected to the phase response is the transient response, which refers to the ability of a loudspeaker to reproduce rapidly changing or short-duration sounds. In theory a loudspeaker with a perfect frequency and phase response would also have a perfect transient response, but since the former are never perfect, some alteration of the temporal characteristics of sounds always occurs. Transient response is often measured with short tone bursts, with a rectangular envelope, which are gated on and off at zero-crossings so as to contain a whole number of periods. Most loudspeakers will not reproduce such a waveform exactly, one common effect being that the abrupt cessation of a tone burst is transformed into an oscillation decaying to zero over several periods. This is known as ringing, and its effect is to lengthen the apparent duration of short sounds and to 'blur' the overall sound quality. Thus excessive ringing in a loudspeaker is undesirable, producing a loss of clarity and definition. It is worth noting that most amplifiers have flat frequency and phase responses with the tone controls in the 'flat' or '12 o'clock' position. If the low frequencies are boosted using the bass control, so as to compensate for a poor low frequency response in a loudspeaker, then the phase response is markedly altered. If a large boost is required, then quite severe ringing may occur at low frequencies, so that the sound becomes 'boomy'. This again results in a loss of definition, so that it becomes difficult to tell a bowed string from a plucked string. Similar considerations apply to the use of treble controls or high frequency filters. Thus, while amplifier tone controls can be used to compensate for defects in loudspeaker performance, the corrections if excessive are accompanied by undesirable changes in phase and transient responses. If possible, it is better to use good loudspeakers so that the amplifier can be operated with the controls close to the 'flat' position.

The frequency response of a loudspeaker is usually measured with a microphone directly in front of the loudspeaker, a position known as 'on axis'. If the microphone is placed 'off axis', at some angle to the loudspeaker but at the same distance from it, the measured output will generally fall. This is because the sound is 'beamed' forward by the loudspeaker, rather than being propagated equally in all directions. A very narrow beam at any given frequency is undesirable, since the character of the reproduced sound would be strongly influenced by listening position. On the other hand the exceptionally wide beam in 'omnidirectional loudspeakers' also has undesirable effects. With such loudspeakers the perceived sound quality is relatively independent of listening position, but at the listener's ear the ratio of reflected sounds from wall and ceilings to direct sound will be much greater than for conventional loudspeakers. This makes sound localization very difficult, since the precedence effect (Chapter 5, section 5) may break down when this ratio is too high. A further result is that the room echoes will not be perceptually suppressed, as is normally the case when the precedence effect operates. Thus the changes in frequency and phase response produced by room reflections will become subjectively more noticeable, and the clarity of the sound will be impaired.

Although there is a paucity of research in this area, it is generally held that most listeners prefer a directional characteristic in which some beaming occurs, but where the response is reasonably uniform over an angle of about 45° on either side of the axis. In conventional loudspeakers the degree of beaming depends on the size of the transducer (the vibrating area) relative to the wavelength of the sound being reproduced. The smaller the transducer, and the lower the frequency, the wider is the beam. Thus for a single transducer the beam gets narrower as the frequency increases. Most manufacturers have dealt with this problem by using more than one unit (the woofers and tweeters mentioned above) each of which produces a reasonably wide beam over the range of frequencies it reproduces. However, because the angle of dispersion for each unit varies with frequency, the response off axis tends to be a lot less regular than the response on axis. It is difficult to determine how successful a manufacturer has been in dealing with this problem, since this aspect of performance is usually poorly specified. Sometimes it is possible to obtain polar diagrams which indicate the response as a function of angle at various selected frequencies. Ideally the polar diagrams at different frequencies should be as similar as possible.

An ingenious solution to the problem of achieving a uniform angle of dispersion over a wide range of frequencies is incorporated in the Quad ESL-63 loudspeaker. This has a plane radiating surface, but it is made to behave like a point source situated centrally behind the plane. For such a point source, a given wavefront will reach the centre of the plane surface before it reaches the edges. Thus the plane surface can be made to mimic the point source by introducing a progressive time delay between sounds radiated from the centre and sounds radiated from the edge. The amount of delay affects the distance of the 'virtual' source from the plane, and thus the angle of dispersion. Thus the delay can be chosen to optimize the angle of dispersion, and this angle will be maintained over a wide frequency range.

Finally, there is one old wives' tale about loudspeaker performance which should be laid to rest. Occasionally in technical and hi-fi magazines the phrase 'Doppler distortion' is used. This distortion arises because the cone in a given unit of a loudspeaker will be reproducing more than one frequency. Consider a high frequency tone together with a low one. When the phase of the low tone is such that the cone is moving towards the listener, this will produce an upward shift in the apparent frequency of the high tone. Conversely, when the phase of the low tone is such that the cone is moving away from the listener, the apparent frequency of the high tone is lowered. These Doppler shifts are similar to the shift in pitch of a train whistle as the train passes you at a station. In principle, therefore, the low frequency tone produces a slight frequency modulation of the high tone, which might be heard as a distortion. In fact Villchur and Allison (1980) have shown, both by listening tests and by a theoretical analysis, that Doppler distortion will be *completely inaudible* for any practical cone velocity.

C   Pickups

We have dealt at some length on the characteristics of loudspeakers, since loudspeakers are usually the 'weakest link' in a sound-reproducing chain, and so they will have the largest effect on how the system will sound. However, the signal source at the start of the chain (e.g. record player or tape recorder) may also have a significant effect on the overall sound. Many of the characteristics of pickups or cartridges in record players are defined in a similar way to those of loudspeakers, except that the input signal is a mechanical movement imposed by a record groove and the output is an electrical signal. Thus the same criteria as were used in evaluating loudspeakers can be applied to the evaluation of pickups. In general, topclass pickups are capable of excellent performance, superior to that of most loudspeakers, in terms of frequency response, transient response and phase response, but this is not always true of cheaper models. However, even high quality pickups produce non-negligible amounts of harmonic and inter-modulation distortion, the latter being typically 2–5%. The level of inter-modulation distortion may well contribute significantly to the overall sound quality of a pickup, high levels of distortion being accompanied by a loss of clarity and by a loss of the definition of individual instruments.

Several important aspects of performance are unique to pickups. One of these, called tracking, refers to the ability of the stylus to maintain contact with the record grooves in highly modulated (i.e. high amplitude) passages of the record. In modern recordings the stylus may be subject to accelera-tions 1000 times the acceleration due to gravity (g), so that it is something of a miracle that good groove contact can be maintained with downward forces on the stylus of one gram or less. When groove contact is partially lost, a condition known as mistracking, the sound may become fuzzy or distorted, or severe crackling may occur. The cure is usually to *increase* the playing weight, provided that it is within the range specified by the manufacturer. Pickups vary considerably in their tracking ability, and few manufacturers (except for Shure) give accurate specifications of this factor; the best that the prospective buyer can do is to rely on test reports. It is worth noting that the tracking ability of a pickup will only be fully realized if it is used with an arm of appropriate quality. A high quality pickup, tracking at one gram or less, requires an arm with very low pivot friction and very low mass.

When stereophonic, or two-channel, reproduction is required, the pickup must be capable of providing two sets of electrical signals, each one derived from the movement of just one wall of the groove. Two factors are of relevance here: the channel separation and the channel balance. Channel separation is usually measured using a signal recorded so that ideally it would be reproduced in one channel only. The ratio of the output in the desired channel to that in the unwanted channel, expressed in decibels, gives a measure of the extent to which the pickup can separate the two channels. A figure of 15–20 dB is generally considered adequate, and many pickups can easily exceed this. It is important, however, that the separation be main-tained over a wide frequency range.

Channel balance is measured by recording signals which should be repro-duced with equal amplitude on both channels. The ratio of the output levels of the two channels, expressed in decibels, is used as the measure of balance. A difference in level in the two channels which is independent of signal frequency is not important, since it can be corrected using the balance control on the amplifier. However, a difference in level which varies as a function of frequency is more serious. The subjective location of any given instrument in a stereo recording is determined by the relative levels at which the instrument is reproduced by the two loudspeakers. A sound produced equally by the two loudspeakers, and heard by a listener equally distant from them, will be located midway between the two loudspeakers. If the sound coming from the left-hand loudspeaker is slightly higher in level than that from the right, then the sound image will be displaced slightly to the left. If the sound from the left-hand loudspeaker is 10–15 dB higher in level than that from the right, the sound will be located entirely at the left-hand loudspeaker. Clearly, then, channel balance is important in determining the subjective location of individual instruments. If the balance varies as a function of frequency, then different frequency components produced by the same instrument will be subjectively located in different places. Thus there will not be a well-defined 'stereo image'. Instead the 'image' corresponding to any given instrument will be diffuse, and the separation of individual instruments will be reduced. Similar considerations apply to the two loudspeakers of a stereo pair; these should be matched as closely as possible in terms of frequency and phase response, otherwise the 'stereo image' will suffer.

D   *Turntables*

Finally, we will consider briefly the characteristics of turntables. These may affect sound quality in two ways. Firstly, mechanical vibrations in the turntable itself may be detected by the pickup and reproduced as a rumbling sound. Secondly, the fluctuations in the speed of the turntable produce corresponding fluctuations in the frequencies of the reproduced sounds. Slow fluctuations, called wow, produce pitch changes which are particularly noticeable on steady piano tones, while rapid fluctuations, called flutter, give the sound a 'rough' quality. Rumble is usually specified by measuring its level in relation to a tone recorded at a particular reference level, most often a 1 kHz pure tone at a groove velocity (in the lateral direction) of 10 cm/s. A good figure for a high quality turntable would be −45 dB. Although this does not look very good as a noise-to-signal ratio, it should be remembered that rumble is composed mainly of very low frequency components (usually below 100 Hz), and the ear is not very sensitive to these low frequencies (see Fig. 2.1). Some manufacturers have tried to take this into account by using a weighting characteristic which reduces the contribution of very low frequencies. The principle is similar to that used in the loudness level meters which were described in Chapter 2, section 3. This results in rumble-to-signal ratios which look very much more favourable; figures of −65 to −70 dB are not unusual. As yet there has been no systematic study to determine whether the weighted or the unweighted measure gives a closer correlation with the degree of annoyance produced by the rumble. The extent to which rumble is audible will, or course, depend on the ability of the loudspeakers to reproduce low frequencies. Consequently, high quality loudspeakers, with a good low frequency response, should be accompanied by a turntable with minimal rumble. Wow and flutter are not normally noticeable unless their level exceeds about 0.3%, although somewhat lower levels of wow may just be detectable in sustained tones. Levels of wow and flutter less than 0.1% would certainly not be detectable, and such levels are relatively common in modern turntables.

E   General conclusions

In summary, in the selection of components for a high fidelity system it is important that no component be selected in isolation. Rather each component must be chosen so as to be compatible in quality with the other components. If funds are limited, then the best performance will be obtained by buying efficient loudspeakers, which will produce sufficiently high sound levels using an amplifier of moderate power. However, many of the highest quality loudspeakers are relatively inefficient, and if such loudspeakers are to be used, a high power amplifier may be necessary. An inefficient loudspeaker may require 100 times the power of an efficient loudspeaker to produce the same sound level, so if a 1 W amplifier were sufficient for the former, a 100 W amplifier would be needed for the latter. The record playing equipment (turntable, arm and pickup) should be chosen after the loudspeakers. The better the quality of the loudspeakers, the more likely they will be to show up faults in the record player. The loudspeakers and pickup are by far the most critical components of a hi-fi system, but many of the factors which influence sound quality are not specified by manufacturers, or are specified in ways which are not easily related to subjective impressions. Thus it is difficult to determine from manufacturer's specifications how good a given pickup or loudspeaker will sound. If possible, the best way to choose these components is by listening to them, preferably using a familiar well-recorded record, and preferably in one's own home.

F   Multichannel reproduction

To conclude this section we shall briefly discuss multichannel sound reproduction. Stereophonic or two-channel reproduction, as was mentioned above, creates the impression of instruments located in different positions in space by varying the relative levels of different instruments in the two channels. For sounds which are emitted solely from one or the other loudspeaker there is no problem in subjectively locating the sound source, but for sounds which are intended to be heard as coming from between the two loudspeakers there is sometimes a problem. The sounds reaching the

250 Introduction to the psychology of hearing

listeners' ears are, in fact, quite different from those which would have been produced by a real sound source lying between the loudspeakers, and for many listeners the reproduced sound of a given instrument does not occupy any single position in space, but is broadened, or spread out, between the two loudspeakers. Thus stereophonic reproduction is limited both in its ability to create a precise impression of the location of different instruments and by the fact that the range of possible subjective locations is limited to a horizontal arc between (and sometimes slightly beyond) the two loudspeakers. However, for most listeners the main benefit of stereophonic reproduction over monophonic (single-channel) reproduction is not connected with localization *per se*, but rather with improved clarity and definition, so that individual instruments can be heard more precisely. This effect is probably related to the BMLD phenomenon, which was discussed in Chapter 5, sections 8–10.

In recent years various forms of multichannel reproduction have been introduced, the most common approach being to use four channels, but there is no clear consensus of opinion as to the object of such systems, or their expected advantages. It is worthwhile to distinguish between the number of separate channels of auditory information and the number of loudspeakers over which the sounds are reproduced. An ordinary stereo record can carry two effectively independent sets of auditory information, but these two sets can be processed and replayed via any number of loudspeakers. For example, the two conventional loudspeakers can be retained, but a third loudspeaker, receiving inputs equally from the two channels, can be placed between them. Many of the 'four-channel' systems currently in use, the so-called matrix systems, actually use only two independent sets of information, the outputs to the four loudspeakers being derived from these two channels. Thus conventional stereo records, or two-channel tape recorders, can be used, but the signals emitted by the four loudspeakers are not independent of one another. This is not necessarily a disadvantage. Other four-channel systems, those called discrete, do actually use four independent sets of information, but in order to do so they require either a four-channel tape recorder or a special kind of record on which a high frequency tone is recorded and used to decode the two stereo channels into four channels.

In most of the four-channel systems which are currently available 'quadraphonic' reproduction is really just an extension of stereophonic reproduction. The direction of sound sources is encoded by pairwise blending between loudspeakers associated with adjacent corner positions. As we saw above, conventional stereo systems are not very good in creating a precise impression of location, and the problems associated with this kind of approach become even more marked for pairs of loudspeakers lying to the side of, or behind, the listener. Thus, although quadraphonic systems can be

used to broaden the range of subjective locations associated with the reproduced instruments, the improvement in this respect is severely limited.

A phrase which is often used in conjunction with quadraphonics is 'surround-sound', although, as Fellgett (1974) has pointed out, the two are not
identical, and surround-sound can be achieved with fewer than four
channels. For Fellgett one of the most important factors in sound reproduction is connected with the reverberation or ambience of the concert hall in
which the performance takes place. He points out that each instrument, by
virtue of its location, will have associated with it a particular set of echoes.
Thus each section of the orchestra is "labelled with an acoustic ambience
characteristic of its place of origin". This leads Fellgett to conclude that

> . . . the highest fidelity in sound reproduction requires that the directionality of
> sound should mimic both the direct and the reverberant sound of the concert
> hall. This is not just a matter of a vague splash of delayed echoes, but of a
> relationship between directionality and time delay which gives specific informa-
> tion; this information is what we shall mean by ambience. Systems capable of
> reproducing it will be called "ambisonic".

As was mentioned at the beginning of this section, it is not possible to
mimic exactly in a normal room the sound field which a listener would have
experienced at a live concert. However, Fellgett has reported that with
suitable recording and processing techniques a reasonable approximation
can be obtained using a relatively small number of channels and loudspeakers. For a system in which only horizontal direction information is
preserved (Fellgett calls this a pantophonic system) two independent
channels and four loudspeakers seem to provide a subjectively satisfactory
approximation. Unfortunately, there has been no published work in which
subjects have judged the merits of this system as compared with other
systems under appropriately controlled listening conditions. The ambisonic
approach undoubtedly does have something to offer. Gerzon (1971) found
that correctly recorded reverberation did aid sound localization during
reproduction, while poor artificial reverberation made the sound image less
distinct. However, the technique is limited in the accuracy with which the
original sound field can be reproduced. The accuracy is least at high frequencies, where pinnae encoding effects become significant, and this means
that the localization information at high frequencies will conflict to some
extent with that at low frequencies. In addition, the acoustics of the listening
room will always influence the reproduced sound field in a largely uncon-
trolled way. Ambisonic recordings are made with a microphone array at
some distance from the instruments, usually at a position which would have
been occupied by the listener's head. This is necessary for the encoding of
the reverberation information. However, this approach is incompatible with
the close-microphone techniques which are commonly used in recording
studios and which contribute so much to the quality and clarity of modern

recordings. Thus the ambience information is gained at the expense of a possible loss of clarity, while at the same time the record producer has much less flexibility in terms of adjusting the balance of the various instruments and manipulating their sound qualities. The preferences of the listening audience will ultimately determine which approach is the more successful.

One sound-reproduction technique which has been developed in the past few years does appear to be remarkably successful in creating for the listener an impression similar to that which he would have obtained at a live concert. This technique uses a dummy head, whose acoustic properties are designed to mimic those of the human head and pinnae as closely as possible. The recording is made via microphones which are placed in positions corresponding to the eardrums of the dummy head. Thus the sound picked up by the microphones is very close to that which would have been heard by a listener. The recorded sounds are replayed via headphones and the result can be astonishingly realistic. According to Stahl (1975),

> . . sound sources are correctly localised outside the head; various distances from a few centimetres to more than 100 m are reproduced precisely; the timbre corresponds to the distance from the sound source; the impression of reverberation is natural; all directions of sound incidence, from the left, right, front, from behind, above and below can be distinguished.

The system, in addition, has the advantage of requiring only two channels, so that existing recording media can be used.

Experimental radio broadcasts of dummy head recordings, transmitted in West Germany and in the UK, have generally met with an enthusiastic response from the public, although it is not at the present time clear whether this enthusiasm is partly a response to the novelty of the effects. The system is certainly not without its drawbacks. Not all individuals are satisfied with the accuracy of subjective location produced, although the reasons for this are not entirely clear. One possible factor is that the signals essentially pass through an ear canal twice, which produces changes in phase and frequency response. (This can be corrected using appropriate filters.) A second factor is that pinnae differ slightly from person to person, so that the dummy head will not precisely mimic the head of any given listener. A more serious effect is that the cues to auditory localization which normally are produced by head movements are completely absent in dummy head recordings. Indeed, rather than producing additional cues, movements of the listener's head produce changes in the apparent orientation of the orchestra and concert hall, which is a disconcerting effect. It is likely that cues relating to head movements are normally of considerable importance in the location of sounds in the frontal plane, and in distinguishing front from back, and it is noteworthy that in dummy head recordings the least accurately defined positions tend to be at the front (Gerzon, 1975). Stahl (1975) has suggested that this problem could be at least partially eliminated by monitoring the movements of the listener's head and using these movements to introduce appropriate time and intensity differences between the two ears. This solution would be expensive, and probably impracticable in a domestic situation. One final criticism of the dummy head technique is similar to the one applied to ambisonics. The clarity and definition which is achieved on modern recordings is made possible by the separate recording of individual instruments or groups of instruments. This method also allows subsequent alterations in musical balance and corrections of the imperfections of individual instruments. A dummy head recording provides a means of reproducing the total orchestral sound at a particular seat in a particular concert hall, which generally does not allow such clear discrimination of individual instruments and which carries with it any limitations in musical balance and concert hall acoustics. Once again, the preferences of listeners must ultimately be the factor determining the future of these systems.

4   APPLICATIONS OF PSYCHOACOUSTIC RESEARCH IN THE ALLEVIATION OF DEAFNESS

A   *Psychoacoustics and audiology*

Audiology is the science of the evaluation of hearing, particularly in relation to the hearing-impaired. On the basis of an audiological examination, particular types of hearing disorders may be diagnosed and particular types of hearing aids recommended. Psychoacoustics is the scientific basis of audiology, and most tests in clinical audiology are based on the findings of psychoacoustic research and on changes in psychoacoustic phenomena which may occur in different disorders of the auditory pathways. Some of these have been discussed already in Chapter 2.

The basic difference between audiology and psychoacoustics lies in the methodology employed. A psychoacoustician may have a theoretical interest in quite small and subtle effects, and may be willing to test individual subjects for many hours and/or to average results across a large number of subjects, in order to investigate these effects. The audiologist, on the other hand, requires tests which can be applied quickly and simply to a particular patient, in order to determine the nature of the disorder and localize the site of the auditory lesion. This difference in approach, although it is quite obvious, has nevertheless considerably impeded the interchange of results and ideas between the two disciplines.

There are several areas in which psychoacoustics may be able to make useful contributions in the treatment of the hearing-impaired. One is in the development of new tests which can be used in clinical situations to investigate particular aspects of hearing disorders. The need for such tests is particularly evident in cases of sensorineural hearing loss, where at the present time there may be problems both in diagnosing the site of the lesion and in predicting the extent of the difficulties which the patient may encounter in everyday life. One test which might well prove to be useful is a measure of frequency selectivity. We discussed in Chapter 3 the finding that impairments in frequency selectivity are commonly associated with hearing losses of cochlear origin. The degree of impairment in frequency selectivity might well provide useful information about the nature and severity of the disorder, as well as being related to its effects in everyday life. One measure which has been applied already in the clinic is the psychophysical tuning curve (Chapter 3, section 2 and Fig. 3.3). However, the exact method of measurement has not yet been standardized. Further, the maskers used have most often been sinusoids, whereas narrowband noises might be preferable, since they prevent the listener using beats as a cue.

An alternative to the psychophysical tuning curve would be to measure the auditory filter shape using notch-noise maskers (Fig. 3.4 and 3.5, and Patterson, 1976). In a clinical test it would not be necessary to measure the entire filter shape. In fact, just two threshold measurements, one for a notch width of zero, and the other for a notch width of 80% of the centre frequency, would give a good indication of the degree of frequency selectivity. In a normal listener these two thresholds typically differ by 35–40 dB for a centre frequency of 1 kHz. In the impaired ear the difference may be much less, so that the normal and abnormal ears are easily and clearly distinguished.

B   *Hearing aid design and prescription*

An area in which there is scope for considerable improvement is in the choice of a particular hearing aid for a particular patient. At the present time there is a huge variety of hearing aids available (the list published by the Royal National Institute for the Deaf in February 1975 contained over 200 different aids), each of which has its own particular characteristics such as high or low gain, wide or narrow frequency response, a frequency response tailored to the subject's audiogram, directional or nondirectional microphones, and so on. Unfortunately, there is a paucity of systematic research on which type of aid is best for which type of hearing disorder, and the 'prescription' of a hearing aid is often made by inspired guesswork rather than on the basis of sound scientific evidence.

In order to evaluate an aid it is essential to maintain contact with the patient, to see that the patient is using the aid in the most appropriate way and to determine whether, in fact, the aid is of real benefit. It is in this area that there is scope for the application of psychoacoustic methods. In order to determine the benefits of any particular aid for a patient, it is necessary to conduct an extensive series of tests using a great variety of materials, and to allow the patient the opportunity of learning to make full use of the acoustic cues provided by the aid. It may be that a series of such studies would allow the formulation of general rules for determining the best type of aid for a particular type of disorder. It is the experience of clinical audiologists that some rules of this type are already known, but that the results of their application are not always predictable. A set of hearing aids which have very similar specifications on paper may nevertheless perform very differently when fitted to a patient. This provides some justification for trial-and-error methods, but it would clearly be more satisfactory if the reasons for the discrepancies were known. More research is needed into those aspects of hearing aid performance which are at present poorly specified but which may have important effects on an aid's usefulness to a patient. These include frequency response (which is usually measured via couplers or artificial ears, giving results which are known to be different from those obtained on real ears), harmonic distortion, intermodulation and transient distortion, and the effect of different ear mould fittings. Improvements in the performance of hearing aids and in their selection for particular patients will only be achieved by isolating those aspects of performance which are most important from the point of view of the patient, and this will require careful psychoacoustic testing.

A further application of psychoacoustic research comes in the design of new types of hearing aids to compensate for some of the abnormalities of perception which occur in the impaired ear. Psychoacoustics has two roles to play in this. The first is in the characterization of the perceptual abnormalities, so that the nature of the compensation can be defined. The second is in the testing of particular compensation schemes. An example of this approach is found in attempts to compensate for the loudness recruitment which commonly occurs in hearing losses of cochlear origin (see Chapter 2, section 8.A). In a recruiting ear the absolute threshold is elevated, but the level at which sounds become uncomfortably loud may be almost normal; the growth of loudness with increasing intensity is more rapid than normal. A hearing aid which amplifies all sounds equally is not satisfactory in such cases. If the gain of the aid is set so as to make faint sounds audible, then the more intense sounds will be overamplified, and will be painfully loud.

One method of compensating for recruitment is to use a hearing aid which compresses the dynamic range of the input, so that low-level sounds are amplified more than high-level sounds. This can be done in a crude way simply by peak-clipping the output above a certain level, but this introduces a considerable amount of distortion. Alternative methods include using amplifiers whose gain is adjusted according to the overall level of the input. While such aids have proved useful in some cases, they suffer from at least one drawback. The amount of recruitment is usually not constant as a function of frequency. For example, the rate of growth of loudness with intensity may be almost normal at low frequencies, but markedly abnormal at high frequencies, where the threshold elevation is usually greatest. Thus the compensation appropriate at one frequency will be inappropriate at other frequencies.

One way of getting round this problem is to split the input into a number of frequency bands, using a bank of bandpass filters, and to apply the appropriate amount of compression to the output of each filter. The compressed signals are then recombined. An evaluation of a computer based system of this type has been reported by Lippmann *et al.* (1981). They compared a 16-channel compression system with various linear systems which differed only in their gain as a function of frequency. They used five subjects with sensorineural hearing losses, all of whom showed recruitment. Subjects were required to identify monosyllables and sentences presented both in quiet/anechoic and noisy/reverberant conditions. They found that of the linear systems, those in which the high frequencies were emphasized gave better performance than the system with a flat frequency response. Disappointingly, performance with compression was slightly worse than with linear amplification. However, this worse performance was obtained using material presented at the most comfortable level for each listener. The compression system was superior to the linear amplification systems when speech materials with significant variations in level from item to item were used. This is more representative of real-life situations, and suggests that compression systems could provide benefits in a wearable hearing aid.

It is likely that in a wearable aid it would not be necessary to use as many as 16 channels. Adequate compensation for recruitment could probably be achieved with, say, three of four channels. Indeed, there may be a disadvantage in using a large number of channels, since the compression will tend to reduce spectral contrasts in complex stimuli. In a multichannel compression system the differences in level between peaks and dips in the spectrum of the input will be reduced. If the impaired ear has a reduced frequency selectivity, as will often be the case (Chapter 3, section 7), then the reduction in spectral contrast will compound the difficulties experienced in picking out the spectral features of complex sounds. For example, the formants in speech sounds (Chapter 7) may not be resolved, so that speech recognition is impaired. To avoid this problem, the channels in a compression aid should have bandwidths which are broad in comparison to the 'auditory filters' of the impaired listener.

A second way in which the preprocessing of sounds could be useful, is in reducing the amount of background noise or reverberation. We described in Chapter 3 the common experience of hearing-impaired people, that they can understand speech well in a quiet situation with one speaker, but that understanding is difficult when there is background noise or reverberation.

There are several computer based schemes for reducing background noise and/or reverberation, but they all have drawbacks and limitations, and none has been implemented, as yet, in a wearable aid.

C   *Cochlear implants*

One relatively new and exciting area of research aims to bring help to those people who are totally deaf through disorders of the sensory organ—the cochlea. The number of people in this category is not clearly known, but may be considerable. In the USA there are 200 000–300 000 people who are so deaf that they cannot hear anything using a conventional hearing aid. In a large proportion of these the disorder is in the sensory organ rather than in the central nervous system, and the auditory nerve is partially intact (but degenerated to some extent) in the majority of individuals. In such people it is possible to create a sensation of sound by direct electrical stimulation of the auditory nerve. This occurs because of the way in which the auditory nerve is connected to the central nervous system; nerve impulses in the auditory nerve lead to activity in those parts of the brain that are normally concerned with the analysis and perception of sounds, and are interpreted as having arisen from acoustic stimulation. Thus, as Merzenich *et al.* (1974) have put it:

> The reasoning behind current efforts to develop acoustic prostheses is that one can generate some facsimile of the normal input that the acoustic nerve receives when stimulated with normal sounds, and thereby generate sensation that constitutes a facsimile of normal sound sensation.

The extent to which a 'normal sound sensation' can be achieved is still in considerable doubt, and many fundamental questions remain to be answered. However, it has become clear that the problem requires a multi-disciplinary approach, with the cooperation of surgeons, neurophysiologists, audiologists, engineers, speech researchers and psychoacousticians. The early work in this field involved the implantation of single bipolar electrodes, which excited simultaneously a large proportion of neurones in the auditory nerve. For surgical reasons it has proved easiest to excite those neurones which would normally respond to high frequency sounds and would derive their input from the basal part of the cochlea (Simmons, 1966; Merzenich *et al.*, 1973b). Psychoacoustic experiments on patients with these electrodes have revealed that 'sounds' can be heard for a wide range of electrical frequencies of stimulation (25–10 000 Hz), but changes in sensation with changes in rate of stimulation only occur for rates below about 600 Hz. The apparent 'pitch' of electrical stimuli derived by scaling procedures (see Chapter 2) increases regularly with frequency for frequencies up to 500–600 Hz, but then flattens off. The smallest detectable change in frequency varies considerably from patient to patient. Some patients can detect changes of about 5% for frequencies up to a few hundred Hz, others require changes of around 30%, and a few appear to have hardly any ability to detect frequency changes (Merzenich *et al.*, 1973b; Fourcin *et al.*, 1979).

The interpretation of these results is somewhat controversial. Clearly, since the same population of neurones is excited by the electrode whatever the rate of stimulation, the changes in sensation with changing frequency must have been coded by changes in the time pattern of neural impulses. Thus these results provide some support for the temporal or periodicity theory of pitch perception which was discussed in Chapter 4. However, the upper frequency limit for which frequency changes could be detected was considerably lower than the limit for which temporal information is available in the normal auditory nerve (4–5 kHz), and the ability to detect changes in frequency was poorer than is found in normal subjects. This has led some workers to suggest that in normal listeners the place cues are the most important and that the use of temporal information is restricted to very low frequencies. It should be remembered, however, that the auditory nerve in these deaf patients was abnormal, and almost certainly had degenerated to some extent. Thus it would be wrong to conclude that the poor frequency discrimination of the patients in response to electrical stimulation indicates a general limitation of the usefulness of temporal information.

A second serious problem with this work is that no-one is quite sure what kind of electrical stimulation to use in order to mimic the patterns of neural activity which would be produced by an acoustic stimulus. The two most commonly used types of stimulation have been sinusoidal waves and periodic impulses, but it is clear that neither of these is entirely satisfactory. Unfortunately, the transduction process in the normal ear is not fully understood, so we do not know what the 'normal' input to the auditory nerve is like. More research in this area is clearly needed. At the present time the problem is being tackled by implanting stimulating electrodes in animals and by recording responses in the nervous systems of the animals in response to electrical stimulation. Usually the animals are treated with kanamycin, or some similar drug, which destroys the hair cells of the cochlea. This ensures that neural responses are the results of electrical stimulation and are not mediated by the cochlea. While it has not been possible to define the 'best' method of electrical stimulation, such experiments have provided useful information, both about the effects of stimulating waveform and about the site of stimulation.

The studies on human patients have demonstrated that substantial benefit can be gained by the totally deaf from a single stimulating electrode. The sound sensations, crude though they are, provide valuable contact with the environment and act as warning signals. It is also clear that it will not be possible, using a single electrode, to generate a neural input which would be sufficient for the coding of speech. This is because speech discrimination requires a simultaneous representation of several different frequency components of the stimulus. This can only be achieved by exploiting the place organization of the auditory nervous system, i.e. by exciting independently several different sets of neurones, each with its own characteristic frequency. Preliminary work on multichannel electrical stimulation has been done, using animal subjects, and the technique does appear to be feasible. Merzenich *et al.* (1974) have developed and tested an electrode suitable for implantation into the scala tympani in man. The scala tympani is one of the fluid-filled chambers of the cochlea, which is relatively easy to approach surgically, and which gives good access to the array of nerve fibres forming the auditory nerve. Merzenich *et al.* have pointed out that it might be possible to excite predetermined sectors of the auditory nerve from within the scala tympani if two conditions can be met. These conditions are: (1) the nerve must survive longterm cochlear implantation; (2) the resistance to current flow in the scala tympani must be sufficiently great to restrict stimulation to a reasonably small group of fibres. There has been considerable debate over both of these points, but preliminary results are favourable. The auditory nerve does appear to survive the implantation, for at least several months, and discrete stimulation of groups of fibres within the auditory nerve does appear to be possible.

An alternative approach to the cochlear implant has been described by Douek *et al.* (1977). They used a single stimulating electrode on the surface of the cochlea. This does not allow the discrete excitation of separate groups of nerve fibres, but it has the major advantages that the operation is very simple, and no damage is done to the cochlea or auditory nerve. Rather than trying to mimic the patterns of neural activity which would be evoked by acoustic stimuli in the normal ear, they attempted to find a form of stimulus which was matched both to the deaf patient's abilities and to his needs. They reasoned that since a single electrode was unlikely to transmit enough information to allow unaided speech comprehension, it would be best to isolate some element or feature of speech which could be used to enhance *lip reading*, and to apply that element to the electrode. Most deaf adults rely on lip reading for everyday communication, but it is often a slow and tiring process.

For a feature to be useful to the deaf lip reader, it should be invisible on the lips or face. A feature which fits the bill, and which carries important distinctions between different speech sounds, is that of *voicing* (see Chapter 7). Information about the activity of the vocal cords can help the deaf lip reader to distinguish between pairs of speech sounds which look identical (e.g. /f/ and /v/), and over longer time periods the intonation patterns associated with voice pitch can give important clues to the overall structure of sentences. Further, the range of fundamental frequencies in the human voice (i.e. the range of rates of vibration of the vocal cords) corresponds very well with the range over which changes in the rate of electrical stimulation are heard as changes in pitch.

Fourcin *et al.* (1979) have shown that electrically stimulated patients are able to make judgements about intonation on the basis of patterns of electrical stimulation. For example a rising frequency of stimulation is labelled as a question, and a falling frequency as a statement. Further, it does seem to be possible to combine lip read information with voicing information to enhance speech communication. Rosen *et al.* (1981) simulated in normal subjects the experience of electrically stimulated patients, by providing the normal subjects with an auditory signal derived directly from the vibration of the vocal cords of the speaker. The signal consisted of a pulse train which was only present when the vocal cords were vibrating, and whose repetition rate equalled the rate of vibration of the vocal cords. The pulse train was high-pass filtered so that only high harmonics were present. This reduced the discriminability of the pitch changes (Chapter 4, section 3.A) and made the normal subjects functionally like electrically stimulated deaf subjects. Rosen *et al.* found that, in comparison to lip reading alone, subjects could lip read connected discourse about twice as fast when they were provided with the voicing information. This bodes well for the success of cochlear implants based on this approach.

It will be many years before the full potential of the cochlear implant is realized, but the first important steps have been taken. We do not know if such implants will ever allow the deaf to discriminate speech efficiently in everyday conditions, but even if they do not they can be of substantial aid to the lip reader, and they can provide valuable contact with and awareness of the sounds and warning signals which occur in everyday life.

5   COCHLEAR ECHOES

In 1978 Kemp reported a most remarkable phenomenon. If a low-level click is applied to the ear, then it is possible to detect sound being reflected from the ear, using a microphone sealed into the ear canal. The early part of this reflected sound is attributable to activity in the middle ear, but some sound can be detected for delays from 5 to 60 ms following the instant of click presentation. These delays are far too long to be attributed to the middle ear, and thus they almost certainly result from activity in the cochlea itself. Hence the reflected sounds are known as cochlear echoes, although they have been dubbed by some as 'the Kemp echo'.

Since Kemp's original discovery, there has been a considerable amount of work studying this phenomenon. We do not have space to report in detail on this work, and we will restrict ourselves to certain aspects of it. Although the input click in Kemp's experiment contained energy over a wide range of frequencies, only certain frequencies were present in the reflected sound. Kemp suggested that the reflections are generated at points on the basilar membrane, or in the transduction mechanism, where there is a gradient or discontinuity in impedance. The response is nonlinear, in that the reflected sound does not have a level in direct proportion to the input level. In fact, the relative level of the reflection is greatest at low sound levels; the echo grows about 3 dB for each 10 dB increase in input level. This nonlinear behaviour can be used to distinguish the response arising from the cochlea from the middle ear response; the latter behaves in a linear manner.

Cochlear echoes can be very stable in a given individual, both in waveform and frequency content, but each ear gives its own characteristic response. Responses tend to be strongest between 500 and 2500 Hz, probably because transmission from the cochlea back through the middle ear is most efficient in this range.

Cochlear echoes can be measured for brief tone bursts as well as clicks, and it is even possible to detect a reflected component in response to continuous stimulation with pure tones. The echo response to a particular component in a stimulus can be suppressed if the ear is stimulated more strongly at a neighbouring frequency. By presenting neighbouring tones at a variety of frequencies, and adjusting their levels, it is possible to map out equal-suppression contours. These contours have the same general shape as neural tuning curves (Fig. 1.13) and psychophysical tuning curves (Fig. 3.3). This lends strong support to the notion that the echoes are generated within the cochlea.

Cochlear echoes are only observed in ears which are in good physiological condition. Thus human ears with even moderate pathology of cochlear origin show no detectable ecohes. The echo is also abolished in ears which have been exposed to intense sounds or ototoxic drugs. In the former case the echo may return after a period of recovery. The measurement of cochlear echoes may provide a sensitive way of monitoring the physiological state of the cochlea.

When the ear is stimulated with two tones, having frequencies f_1 and f_2, then an echo may be detected with frequency $2f_1 - f_2$ (Kim *et al.*, 1980). This corresponds to a combination tone which has been frequently observed in auditory research (Chapter 4, section 3). Its presence as a cochlear echo implies that it was present as a mechanical disturbance in the cochlea, probably as a travelling wave on the basilar membrane. The level of the combination tone, relative to the level of the primaries in the ear canal, could be as high as -30 dB. The level was reversibly reduced by exposing the ear to a fatiguing tone of 80–90 dB SPL at a frequency near or slightly below the primary frequencies. Again this indicates that the nonlinear aspect of cochlear function is physiologically vulnerable.

Sometimes the amount of energy reflected from the cochlea at a given frequency may exceed that which was present in the input click. This has led Kemp and others to suggest that the echo reflects an *active* process of biological amplification. Sometimes the transient stimulation induces a sustained oscillation at a particular frequency, and the subject may report hearing this oscillation as a tonal sensation. The phenomenon of hearing sound in the absence of external stimulation is known as *tinnitus*. It appears that tinnitus may arise from abnormal activity at several different points in the auditory system, but in some cases it corresponds to mechanical activity in the cochlea. This mechanical activity may result in sound which is detectable in the ear canal (Zurek, 1981).

In summary, the cochlear echo has many fascinating properties. While the exact mechanism by which it is generated is not understood, there is agreement that it is connected with processes occurring inside the cochlea. These processes have a strong nonlinear component, they may be biologically active, and they are physiologically vulnerable.

6   THE EVALUATION OF CONCERT HALL ACOUSTICS

This topic is one of great complexity, and it is beyond the scope of this book to cover it in any detail. The interested reader is referred to Beranek (1962) for further details. We shall content ourselves with a brief view of some recent techniques which go a considerable way towards solving the problems inherent in the comparison of concert hall acoustics.

Judgements of the acoustic quality of concert halls, and comparisons between different concert halls, are difficult because of two major factors. Firstly, the perceived quality at a given performance will depend as much on the manner of playing of the musicians and their seating arrangements as on the characteristics of the hall itself. Secondly, long-term acoustical memory is relatively poor, so that many of the subtleties of acoustical quality will not be recalled by the time a listener has travelled from one hall to another. Ultimately the consensus of opinion of a large number of listeners will determine whether a hall is 'good' or 'bad', but it is not easy to determine the crucial features which influence such judgements, or to derive general rules which could be applied in the design of new halls. Indeed, many new halls are simply modelled on other halls which have been judged as good. While this approach does have some validity, it is also very inflexible.

Schroeder *et al.* (1974) have developed recording and reproduction techniques which make possible instantaneous comparisons of the acoustic qualities of different halls under realistic free-field conditions on the basis of identical musical source material. The first step is to use as a source material a recording of an orchestra which is played from the stage. This ensures that the musical material is always identical. The orchestra is recorded in an anechoic chamber, so that the acoustics of the recording room are not superimposed on those of the hall being tested. Schroeder *et al.* used a two-channel recording, replayed via two loudspeakers on the stage of the hall, so as to simulate in a crude way the spatial extent of the orchestra. However, there is no reason why the technique should not be extended to multichannel recordings, which would mimic more accurately the sounds radiated by a live orchestra.

The second step is to record the signals using microphones at the 'eardrums' of a dummy head, as we described in section 3.F. Two different positions were used for each hall, both corresponding to places which would normally be occupied by a listener's head. Care was taken to ensure that the acoustic properties of the dummy head, including the ear canal and pinnae, were as accurate as possible.

The third step is to present the dummy head recordings to listeners for evaluation. One obvious way of doing this is to replay the signals via stereo headphones, but, as we discussed in section 3.F, this technique does have its limitations. One problem which Schroeder *et al.* mention is that ". . . listening over earphones does not properly recreate the perceived acoustic 'space' or the sense of being surrounded by sound, which is one of the important qualities that we wish to describe in an objective way". To overcome this problem the recordings were electronically processed so that, when played back over two selected loudspeakers in an anechoic chamber, the recorded signals were recreated at the eardrums of a human listener. Schroeder *et al.* explain the technique as follows:

> The sound radiated from each loudspeaker goes into *both* ears and not just the 'near' ear of the listener as would be desired. In other words, there is 'cross-talk' from each loudspeaker to the 'far' ear. However, by radiating properly mixed and filtered compensation signals from the loudspeakers, the unwanted 'cross-talk' can be cancelled out.

The appropriate filter responses in the compensation scheme are computed from measurements obtained by applying short electrical impulses to one of the two loudspeakers and recording the resulting microphone signals from the ears of a dummy head at some distance in front of the loudspeakers. For further details the reader is referred to the original article and to Schroeder and Atal (1963).

The result of this is that, when the original dummy head recording is replayed,

> . . . the signal from the dummy's right ear will go *only* to the listener's right ear and that from the dummy's left ear will go only to the listener's left ear, just as in earphone listening but with the proper free-field coupling of the ear canal and the desired invariance of the perceived acoustical space when the listener's head is rotated around a vertical axis.

Schroeder *et al.* report that for head movements up to about ± 10° the externalized sound image remains stationary with respect to the listening room, and does not turn with the head as in earphone listening.

Using this technique, Schroeder *et al.* asked subjects to indicate preferences for different concert halls presented in pairs. For a given pair the subject was allowed to switch back and forth between recordings made in the two halls as often as he liked. The score for a preferred hall was 1, and for the other −1. If there was no preference, both halls were given a score of 0. This was repeated for all subjects and all pairs of halls, and the resulting scores were accumulated in a preference matrix indicating how many times each hall was preferred by each listener.

The results were subjected to a factor analysis (Slater, 1960) which yielded the significant factors accounting for the variance in the data. There was one factor of overriding significance, accounting for 50% of the relative variance, which was called the consensus preference factor. All subjects showed positive weights on this factor. What this means is that if a given hall (say X) has a greater value on this factor than another hall (say Y), then hall X is preferred over hall Y by *all* listeners. The other factors isolated by the analysis seem to represent individual-difference preferences. The original recordings were made in unoccupied halls. This has little effect on the acoustics in modern halls, but in older halls with hard wooden seats it can result in excessively long reverberation times. When the analysis was limited to those halls having reverberation times less than 2.2 s, the consensus preference factor became even more important, accounting for 88% of the total variance, while individual preference factors became much less significant.

Schroeder *et al.* also made various physical measurements in the halls, in order to correlate the consensus preference factor with the geometrical and acoustical parameters of the halls. We will not detail all of the measures they considered, but will mention those that appeared to be most significant. For the halls with reverberation times less than 2.2 s reverberation time was highly correlated with preference. Thus the greater the reverberation time the greater was the preference. However, for the halls with reverberation times greater than 2 s the reverberation time is slightly negatively correlated with consensus preference, but shows a fairly large correlation with the first individual difference factor. Thus, in this range of reverberation times, some listeners prefer greater reverberation times and others smaller reverberation times.

One factor which showed a strong negative correlation with preference, for halls with both long and short reverberation times, was the interaural coherence. This is a measure of the correlation of the signals at the two ears. Thus listeners prefer halls which produce a low interaural coherence, so that the signals at the two ears are relatively independent of one another. Schroeder *et al.* suggested that "This effect might be mediated by a more pronounced feeling—of being immersed in the sound—that presumably occurs for less coherent ear signals". Interaural coherence can be manipulated by sound diffusers on the walls and ceiling of the concert hall.

Finally, for the halls with longer reverberation times, which also tended to be the larger halls, the volume of the halls showed a strong negative correlation with consensus preference. Thus, once a hall has reached a certain size, further increases in size result in a worsening of acoustic quality.

The work we have described is very much a beginning in this area, and there are a number of ways in which the techniques could be improved and extended. The number of channels and loudspeakers used in the reproduction of the original sound source on the stage of the concert hall could be increased, a greater variety of musical material could be used, and the dummy head could be positioned so as to sample a greater number of points within each hall. A further possibility, described by Schroeder *et al.*, is to transform all the recordings, using a computer, so that they have the same reverberation time! It is known that reverberation time plays a large part in preference judgements, and when there are large differences in reverberation times, this tends to obscure other factors which might affect preference. By working with the processed recordings, a set of halls with identical reverberation times can be obtained, so that other factors can be more easily isolated.

7   GENERAL DISCUSSION AND FUTURE OUTLOOK

The preceding sections have described a few of the ways in which studies of auditory perception have had, or may have in the future, practical applications. There are, of course, many other ways in which sounds may influence our lives. Miller (1974), in a review of the effect of noise on people, described the value of sound in the following way:

> Thus, sound is of great value to man. It warns him of danger and appropriately arouses and activates him. It allows him the immeasurable advantage of speech and language. It can calm, excite, and it can elicit joy or sorrow. The recent discovery that five-day-old infants will work to produce a variety of sounds (Butterfield and Siperstein, 1970) only reinforces the everyday observation that man enjoys hearing and making sounds.

It may be that future research will pay greater heed to the mood-influencing and aesthetic properties of sound. These properties are not, of course, independent of the purely perceptual aspects of sounds which have been emphasized in this book. In the future composers will no doubt exploit the increasing flexibility in the generation of novel sounds which is provided by modern electronic circuits and computers. This will free them from the limitations of conventional instruments, but will require that they have considerable insight into the perceptual effects of the novel sounds. Psycho-acoustics may have a great deal to offer in the development of new forms of music, and in generally increasing our understanding of musical appreciation. Unfortunately, sound can also have ugly, annoying or unpleasant effects. Miller (1974) has described many of these effects, and we shall content ourselves with a brief summary of his conclusions. Noise of sufficient intensity and duration can permanently damage the inner ear, with resulting hearing losses that can range from slight impairment to nearly total deafness. This was discussed briefly in Chapter 2, section 7. There is a clear need for increasing the monitoring of public noise exposure and audiometric monitoring of the population at risk. In this way individuals who are particularly susceptible to noise damage could be isolated before the damage becomes severe. There is also a need for education and information to create and enhance public awareness of noise as a hazard to hearing. In addition to actually damaging hearing, noise can have the following undesirable effects: it can interefere with speech communication and the perception of other auditory signals; it can disturb sleep; it can be a source of annoyance; it can interefere with the performance of complicated tasks, especially when speech communication or response to auditory signals is demanded; it can reduce the opportunity for privacy; it can adversely influence mood and disturb relaxation. It is to be hoped that an increasing awareness of these effects will lead to improved noise control in the design of buildings, vehicles, machinery and the environment as a whole.

8   GENERAL SUMMARY

In this chapter we have described several recent developments in auditory research, as well as some practical applications.

Studies of adaptation to tones which are modulated or swept in frequency indicate the presence of 'channels' tuned for detecting frequency changes. There may also be 'channels' tuned for the detection of particular features in speech sounds.

In the reproduction of sounds, particularly music, the transducers in the reproduction system, i.e. loudspeakers and pickups, are the most critical components. Unfortunately, the aspects of performance which determine how good a system will sound are often poorly specified. Sounds recorded via a dummy head, and reproduced via headphones, can give a realistic impression of the position of the sound sources in space.

Psychoacoustic tests may be of use in the differential diagnosis of hearing disorders, and in predicting the extent to which an impaired person will suffer in everyday life. Measures of frequency selectivity may be particularly useful in this respect. Hearing aids which preprocess sounds prior to delivery to an impaired ear, may be of benefit in some cases. In patients who are totally deaf, electrical stimulation of the auditory nerve may provide a means of restoring a limited, but useful form of hearing.

A microphone sealed into the ear canal can reveal the presence of sounds reflected back from the cochlea. These cochlear echoes have many fascinating properties, and their measurement may provide a noninvasive way of monitoring the condition of the cochlea.

Recordings made using dummy heads provide a way of comparing the acoustics of different concert halls. The factors correlating most strongly with preference are reverberation time, and interaural coherence.

Our knowledge of the processes involved in the perception of sound has advanced considerably since the pioneering work of Helmholtz (1863) yet the scientific study of hearing is still in its infancy. At the physiological level we now know a good deal about the coding of sounds in the auditory nerve, and the cochlear nucleus, but relatively little is known of how that basic neural information is processed at higher levels in the auditory system. At the perceptual level we know a good deal about people's abilities to detect changes in simple stimuli such as pure tones and bands of noise, but we are a long way from understanding how complex auditory patterns such as speech and music are perceived. Unfortunately, the elementary level of our understanding is not accompanied by simplicity in the concepts involved. Many students are deterred by the technical jargon which appears in scientific papers on auditory perception or the neurophysiology or anatomy of the auditory system. For students without a physics background even the nature of auditory stimuli, and their analysis in terms of Fourier components, may present considerable conceptual difficulties. It is my hope that readers who have reached this point in the book by working through the previous chapters will have overcome these initial difficulties, and that some real feeling will have been developed for the fascinating and complex processes that underlie our perception of sound.

FURTHER READING

Since many of the topics discussed in this chapter are recent developments, there are not yet review articles or books which cover them. However, a good many papers concerned with the cochlear echo may be found in:

Kemp, D. T. and Anderson, S. D. (1980). *Proceedings of the International Symposium on Nonlinear and Active Mechanical Processes in the Cochlea. Hearing Research*, 2, nos. 3 and 4.

References

Abeles, M. and Goldstein, M. H. (1972). Responses of single units in the primary auditory cortex of the cat to tones and to tone pairs. *Brain Res.* **42**, 337–352.

American Standards Association (1960). *Acoustical Terminology* SI. 1–1960, American Standards Association, New York.

Anderson, C. M. B. and Whittle, L. S. (1971). Physiological noise and the missing 6 dB. *Acustica* **24**, 261–272.

Arthur, R. M., Pfeiffer, R. R. and Suga, N. (1971). Properties of 'two-tone inhibition' in primary auditory neurones. *J. Physiol.* **212**, 593–609.

Attneave, F. and Olson, R. K. (1971). Pitch as a medium: a new approach to psychophysical scaling. *Am. J. Psychol.* **84**, 147–166.

Bailey, P. J. (1973). Perceptual adaptation for acoustic features in speech. *Speech Perception* ser. 2, no. **2**, 29–34 (Dept of Psychology, Queen's University of Belfast).

Bailey, P. J. (1974). Procedural variables in speech adaptation. *Speech Perception* ser. 2, no. **3**, 27–34 (Dept of Psychology, Queen's University of Belfast).

Batteau, D. W. (1967). The role of the pinna in human localization. *Proc. R. Soc. B* **168**, 158–180.

Batteau, D. W. (1968). Listening with the naked ear. In *Neuropsychology of Spatially Oriented Behavior* (ed. S. J. Freedman), Dorsey Press, Illinois.

Bauer, B. B., Torick, E. L. and Allen, R. G. (1971). The measurement of Loudness Level. *J. Acoust. Soc. Am.* **50**, 405–414.

Beckett, P. and Haggard, M. P. (1973). The psychoacoustical specification of 'tone deafness'. *Speech Perception* ser. 2, no. **2**, 17–22 (Dept of Psychology, Queen's University of Belfast).

Békésy, G. von (1928). Zur Theorie des Hörens; die Schwingungsform der Basilarmembran. *Phys. Z.* **29**, 793–810.

Békésy, G. von (1942). Über die Schwingungen der Schneckentrennwand beim Präparet und Ohrenmodell. *Akust. Z.* **7**, 173–186.

Békésy, G. von (1947). The variation of phase along the basilar membrane with sinusoidal vibrations. *J. Acoust. Soc. Am.* **19**, 452–460.

Békésy, G. von. (1960). *Experiments in Hearing* (trans. and ed. E. G. Wever), McGraw-Hill, New York.

Békésy, G. von (1961). Concerning the fundamental component of periodic pulse patterns and modulated vibrations observed on the cochlear model with nerve supply. *J. Acoust. Soc. Am.* **33**, 888–896.

Békésy, G. von (1963). Three experiments concerned with pitch perception. *J. Acoust. Soc. Am.* **35**, 602–606.

Békésy, G. von and Rosenblith, W. A. (1951). The mechanical properties of the ear. In *Handbook of Experimental Psychology* (ed. S. S. Stevens), Wiley, New York.

Beranek, L. L. (1962). *Music, Acoustics and Architecture*, Wiley, New York.

Bilger, R. C. and Feldman, R. M. (1968). Frequency dependence in temporal integration. *76th Meeting of the Acoustical Society of America*, paper A1.

Billone, M. and Raynor, S. (1973). Transmission of radial shear forces to cochlear hair cells. *J. Acoust. Soc. Am.* **54**, 1143–1156.

Bilsen, F. A. (1973). On the influence of the number and phase of harmonics on the perceptibility of the pitch of complex signals. *Acustica* **28**, 60–65.

Bilsen, F. A. and Goldstein, J. L. (1974). Pitch of dichotically delayed noise and its possible spectral basis. *J. Acoust. Soc. Am.* **55**, 292–296.

Bilsen, F. A. and Ritsma, R. J. (1967). Repetition pitch mediated by temporal fine structure at dominant spectral regions. *Acustica* **19**, 114–116.

Blauert, J. (1969/1970). Sound localization in the median plane. *Acustica* **22**, 206–213.

Blauert, J. and Laws, P. (1978). Group delay distortions in electroacoustical systems. *J. Acoust. Soc. Am.* **63**, 1478–1483.

Blumstein, S. E. and Stevens, K. N. (1979). Acoustic invariance in speech production: Evidence from measurements of the spectral characteristics of stop consonants. *J. Acoust. Soc. Am.* **66**, 1001–1017.

Blumstein, S. E. and Stevens, K. N. (1980). Perceptual invariance and onset spectra for stop consonants in different vowel environments. *J. Acoust. Soc. Am.* **67**, 648–662.

Boer, E. de (1969a). Reverse correlation. II. Initiation of nerve impulses in the inner ear. *Proc. K. Ned. Akad. Wet.* **72**, ser. C, 129–151.

Boer, E. de (1969b). Encoding of frequency information in the discharge pattern of auditory nerve fibres. *Int. Audiol.* **8**, 547–556.

Boomsliter, P. and Creel, W. (1961). The long pattern hypothesis in harmony and hearing. *J. Music Theory* **5**, 2–31.

Boomsliter, P. and Creel, W. (1963). Extended reference: an unrecognized dynamic in melody. *J. Music Theory* **7**, 2–22.

Boone, M. M. (1973). Loudness measurements on pure tone and broad band impulsive sounds. *Acustica* **29**, 198–204.

Bray, D. A., Dirks, D. D. and Morgan, D. E. (1973). Perstimulatory Loudness Adaptation. *J. Acoust. Soc. Am.* **53**, 1544–1548.

Bredberg, G. (1968). Cellular pattern and nerve supply of the human organ of Corti. *Acta Otolaryngol.* Suppl., **236**.

Bregman, A. S. (1978). The formation of auditory streams. In *Attention and Performance* Vol. 7 (ed. J. Requin), Lawrence Erlbaum Associates, New Jersey.

Bregman, A. S. and Campbell, J. (1971). Primary auditory stream segregation and perception of order in rapid sequences of tones. *J. Exp. Psychol.* **89**, 244–249.

Bregman, A. S. and Dannenbring, G. L. (1973). The effect of continuity on auditory stream segregation. *Percept. Psychophys.* **13**, 308–312.

Bregman, A. S. and Pinker, S. (1978). Auditory streaming and the building of timbre. *Can. J. Psychol.* **32**, 19–31.

Bregman, A. S. and Rudnicky, A. I. (1975). Auditory segregation: Stream or streams? *J. Exp. Psychol.: Human Percept. Perform.* **1**, 263–267.

Broadbent, D. E. (1958). *Perception and Communication*, Pergamon, London.

Broadbent, D. E. (1967). Word frequency and response bias. *Psychol. Rev.* **74**, 1–15.

Broadbent, D. E. and Gregory, M. (1964). Accuracy of recognition for speech presented to the right and left ears. *Q. J. Exp. Psychol.* **16**, 359–360.

Broadbent, D. E. and Ladefoged, P. C. (1957). On the fusion of sounds reaching different sense organs. *J. Acoust. Soc. Am.* **29**, 708–710.

Brugge, J. F. and Merzenich, M. M. (1973). Responses of neurones in auditory cortex of macaque monkey to monaural and binaural stimulation. *J. Neurophysiol.* **36**, 1138–1158.

Brugge, J. F., Anderson, D.J., Hind, J. E. and Rose, J. E. (1969). Time structure of discharges in single auditory nerve fibres of the Squirrel Monkey in response to complex periodic sounds. *J. Neurophysiol.* **32**, 386–401.

Butler, R. A. (1969). Monaural and binaural localization of noise bursts vertically in the median sagittal plane. *J. Aud. Res.* **3**, 230–235.

Butler, R. A. (1971). The monaural localisation of tonal stimuli. *Percept. Psychophys.* **9**, 99–101.

Butterfield, E. C. and Siperstein, G. N. (1970). Influence of contingent auditory stimulation upon non-nutritional suckle. Paper presented at *Third Symposium on Oral Sensation and Perception: The Mouth of the Infant*, C. C. Thomas, Springfield, Illinois.

Byrne, D. and Dermody, P. (1975). Localization of sound with binaural body-worn hearing aids. *Br. J. Audiol.* **9**, 107–115.

Carhart, R., Tillman, T. W. and Greetis. (1969). Release from multiple maskers: effects of interaural time disparities. *J. Acoust. Soc. Am.* **45**, 411–418.

Carter, N. L. (1972). Effects of rise time and repetition rate on the loudness of acoustic transients. *J. Sound Vib.* **21**, 227–239.

Carterette, E. C., Friedman, M. P. and Lovell, J. D. (1969). Mach bands in hearing. *J. Acoust. Soc. Am.* **45**, 986–998.

Christman, R. J. and Victor, G. (1955). The perception of direction as a function of binaural temporal and amplitude disparity. Rome Air Development Center ARDC, USAF, Tech. Note RADC-TH-55-302.

Clack, T. D., Erdreich, J. and Knighton, R. W. (1972). Aural harmonics: the monaural phase effects at 1500 Hz, 2000 Hz, and 2500 Hz observed in tone-on-tone masking when $f_1 = 1000$ Hz. *J. Acoust. Soc. Am.* **52**, 536–541.

Cole, R. A. and Scott, B. (1974). Towards a theory of speech perception. *Psychol. Rev.* **81**, 348–374.

Coleman, P. D. (1962). Failure to localize the source distance of an unfamiliar sound. *J. Acoust. Soc. Am.* **34**, 345–346.

Coleman, P. D. (1963). An analysis of cues to auditory depth perception in free space. *Psychol. Bull.* **60**, 302–315.

Cooper, W. E. (1974). Perceptuomotor adaptation to a speech feature. *Percept. Psychophys.* **16**, 229–234.

Corliss, E. L. R. (1967). Mechanistic aspects of hearing. *J. Acoust. Soc. Am.* **41**, 1500–1516.

Corliss, E. L. R. and Winzer, G. E. (1964). Study of methods of estimating loudness. *J. Acoust. Soc. Am.* **38**, 424–428.

Cotzin, M. and Dallenbach, K. M. (1950). 'Facial vision': The role of pitch and loudness in perception of obstacles by the blind. *Am. J. Psychol.* **63**, 485–515.

Cuddy, L. L. (1968). Practice effects in the absolute judgment of pitch. *J. Acoust. Soc. Am.* **43**, 1069–1076.

Dadson, R. S. and King, J. H. (1952). A determination of the normal threshold of hearing and its relation to the standardization of audiometers. *J. Laryngol. Otol.* **66**, 366–378.

Dallos, P., Billone, M. C., Durrant, J. D., Wang, C.-Y. and Raynor, S. (1972). Cochlear inner and outer hair cells: functional differences. *Science, N.Y.* **177**, 356–358.

Darwin, C. J. (1971). Dichotic backward masking of complex sounds. *Q. J. Exp. Psychol.* **23**, 386–392.

Darwin, C. J. and Baddeley, A. D. (1974). Acoustic memory and the perception of speech. *Cognitive Psychol.* **6**, 41–60.

Darwin, C. J. and Bethell-Fox, C. E. (1977). Pitch continuity and speech source attribution. *J. Exp. Psychol.: Human Percept. Perform.* **3**, 665–672.

Deatherage, B. H. and Evans, T. R. (1969). Binaural masking: backward, forward and simultaneous effects. *J. Acoust. Soc. Am.* **46**, 362–371.

Deatherage, B. H. and Hirsh, I. J. (1957). Auditory localization on clicks. *J. Acoust. Soc. Am.* **29**, 132–137.

Dirks, D. and Bower, D. (1970). Effects of forward and backward masking on speech intelligibility. *J. Acoust. Soc. Am.* **47**, 1003–1008.

Divenyi, P. L. and Hirsh, I. J. (1974). Identification of temporal order in three-tone sequences. *J. Acoust. Soc. Am.* **56**, 144–151.

Dix, M. R. and Hood, J. D. (1973). Symmetrical hearing loss in brain stem lesions. *Acta. Otolaryngol.* **75**, 165–177.

Djupesland, G. and Zwislocki, J. J. (1972). Sound pressure distribution in the outer ear. *Scand. Audiol.* **1**, 197–203.

Dolan, T. R. and Trahiotis, C. (1972). Binaural interaction in backward masking. *Percept. Psychophys.* **11**, 92–94.

Douek, E., Fourcin, A. J., Moore, B. C. J. and Clarke, G. P. (1977). A new approach to the cochlear implant. *Proc. R. Soc. Med.* **70**, 379–383.

Dowling, W. J. (1968). Rhythmic fission and perceptual organization. *J. Acoust. Soc. Am.* **44**, 369.

Dowling, W. J. (1973). The perception of interleaved melodies. *Cognitive Psychol.* **5**, 322–337.

Duifhuis, H. (1971). Audibility of high harmonics in a periodic pulse II. Time effect. *J. Acoust. Soc. Am.* **49**, 1155–1162.

Duifhuis, H. (1972). *Perceptual Analysis of Sound*, Doctoral dissertation, Eindhoven University of Technology.

Duifhuis, H. (1973). Consequences of peripheral frequency selectivity for non-simultaneous masking. *J. Acoust. Soc. Am.* **54**, 1471–1488.

Duifhuis, H. (1976). Cochlear nonlinearity and second filter: possible mechanism and implications. *J. Acoust. Soc. Am.* **59**, 408–423.

Durlach, N. I. (1963). Equalization and cancellation theory of binaural masking level differences. *J. Acoust. Soc. Am.* **35**, 1206–1218.

Durlach, N. I. (1972). Binaural signal detection: equalization and cancellation theory. In *Foundations of Modern Auditory Theory*, Vol. 2 (ed. J. V. Tobias), Academic Press, New York.

Egan, J. P. and Hake, H. W. (1950). On the masking pattern of a simple auditory stimulus. *J. Acoust. Soc. Am.* **22**, 622–630.

Eimas, P. D. and Corbit, J. D. (1973). Selective adaptation of linguistic feature detectors. *Cognitive Psychol.* **4**, 99–109.

Eimas, P. D., Cooper, W. E. and Corbit, J. D. (1973). Some properties of linguistic feature detectors. *Percept. Psychophys.* **13**, 247–252.

Elliot, D. N. and Fraser, W. R. (1970). Fatigue and adaptation. In *Foundations of Modern Auditory Theory*, Vol. 1 (ed. J. V. Tobias), Academic Press, New York.

Elliot, D. N., Stein, L. and Harrison, M. J. (1960). Determination of absolute-intensity thresholds and frequency-difference thresholds in cats. *J. Acoust. Soc. Am.* **32**, 380–384.

Elliot, L. L. (1962). Backward and forward masking of probe tones of different frequencies. *J. Acoust. Soc. Am.* **34**, 1116–1117.

Elliot, L. L. (1967). Development of auditory narrow-band frequency contours. *J. Acoust. Soc. Am.* **42**, 143–153.

Elliot, L. L. (1969). Masking of tones before, during, and after brief silent periods in noise. *J. Acoust. Soc. Am.* **45**, 1277–1279.

Elliot, L. L. (1971). Backward and forward masking. *Audiology* **10**, 65–76.

Evans, E. F. (1968). Cortical Representation. In *Hearing Mechanisms in Vertebrates* (eds A. V. S. de Reuck and J. Knight), Churchill, London.

Evans, E. F. (1975). The sharpening of cochlear frequency selectivity in the normal and abnormal cochlea. *Audiology* **14**, 419–442.

Evans, E. F. (1978). Place and time coding of frequency in the peripheral auditory system: some physiological pros and cons. *Audiology* **17**, 369–420.

Evans, E. F. (1980). Comment on "Two-tone suppression and intermodulation distortion in the cochlea: effects of outer hair-cell lesions". In *Psychophysical Physiological and Behavioural Studies in Hearing* (eds G. van den Brink and F. A. Bilsen), Delft UP, Delft.

Evans, E. F. and Palmer, A. R. (1975). Responses of units in the cochlear nerve and nucleus of the cat to signals in the presence of bandstop noise. *J. Physiol.* **252**, 60–62P.

Exner, S. (1876). Zur Lehre von den Gehörsempfindungen, *Pflügers Archiv* **13**, 228–253.

Fant, G. C. M. (1960). *Acoustic Theory of Speech Production*, Mouton, The Hague.

Fant, C. G. M. (1963). Comments on 'A motor theory of speech perception' by A. M. Liberman, F. S. Cooper, K. S. Harris and P. F. Macneilage, In *Proceedings of the Speech Communication Seminar*, Vol. 3 (ed. C. G. M. Fant), Royal Institute of Technology, Stockholm.

Fastl, H. and Schorn, K. (1981). Discrimination of level differences by hearing impaired patients. *Audiology*, **20**, 488–502.

Feldtkeller, R. and Zwicker, E. (1956). *Das Ohr als Nachrichtenempfänger*, S. Hirzel, Stuttgart.

Fellgett, P. B. (1974). Ambisonic reproduction of directionality in surround-sound systems. *Nature*, Lond. **252**, 534–538.

Feth, L. L. (1972). Combinations of amplitude and frequency difference in auditory discrimination. *Acustica* **26**, 67–77.

Fischer-Jørgensen, E. (1972). Tape cutting experiments with Danish stop consonants in initial position. Ann. Rep. VII, University of Copenhangen, Institute of Phonetics.

Fletcher, H. (1940). Auditory patterns. *Rev. Mod. Phys.* **12**, 47–65.

Florentine, M., Buus, S., Scharf, B. and Zwicker, E. (1980). Frequency selectivity in normally-hearing and hearing-impaired observers. *J. Speech Hear. Res.* **23**, 646–669.

Fourcin, A. J., Rosen, S. M., Moore, B. C. J., Douek, E. E., Clarke, G. P., Dodson, H. and Bannister, L. H. (1979). External electrical stimulation of the cochlea: clinical, psychophysical, speech-perceptual and histological findings. *Br. J. Audiol.* **13**, 85–107.

Fourcin, A. J. (1970). Central pitch and auditory lateralization. In *Frequency Analysis and Periodicity Detection in Hearing* (eds R. Plomp and G. F. Smoorenburg), A. W. Sijthoff, Leiden.

Fourcin, A. J. (1975). Speech perception in the absence of speech productive ability. In *Language, Cognitive Defects and Retardation* (ed. N. O'Conner), Butterworths, London.

Freedman, S. J. and Fisher, H. G. (1968). The role of the pinna in auditory localization. In *Neuropsychology of Spatially Oriented Behavior* (ed. S. J. Freedman), Dorsey Press, Illinois.

Freedman, S. J., Wilson, L. and Rekosh, J. H. (1967). Compensation for auditory re-arrangement in hand–ear coordination. *Percept. Motor Skills* **24**, 1207–1210.

Gardner, M. B. and Gardner, R. S. (1973). Problem of localization in the median plane: effect of pinnae cavity occlusion. *J. Acoust. Soc. Am.* **53**, 400–408.

Gardner, R. B. and Wilson, J. P. (1979). Evidence for direction-specific channels in the processing of frequency modulation. *J. Acoust. Soc. Am.* **66**, 704–709.

Garner, W. R. and Miller, G. A. (1974). The masked threshold of pure tones as a function of duration. *J. Exp. Psychol.* **37**, 293–303.

Gässler, G. (1954). Über die Hörschwelle für Schallereignisse mit verschieden breitem Frequenzspektrum. *Acustica* **4**, 408–414.

Gebhardt, C. J. and Goldstein, D. P. (1972). Frequency discrimination and the M.L.D. *J. Acoust. Soc. Am.* **51**, 1228–1232.

Gerzon, M. A. (1971). Synthetic stereo reverberation. *Studio Sound* **13**, 632–635.

Gerzon, M. A. (1975). Dummy head recording. *Studio Sound* **17**, 42–44.

Goldstein, J. L. (1967). Auditory nonlinearity. *J. Acoust. Soc. Am.* **41**, 676–689.

Goldstein, J. L. (1972). Evidence from aural combination tones and musical tones against classical periodicity theory. In *Hearing Theory 1972*, IPO, Eindhoven, The Netherlands.

Goldstein, J. L. (1973). An optimum processor theory for the central formation of the pitch of complex tones. *J. Acoust. Soc. Am.* **54**, 1496–1516.

Goldstein, J. L. and Srulovicz, P. (1977). Auditory-nerve spike intervals as an adequate basis for aural frequency measurement. In *Psychophysics and Physiology of Hearing* (eds E. F. Evans and J. P. Wilson), Academic Press, London and New York.

Green, D. M. (1973). Temporal acuity as a function of frequency. *J. Acoust. Soc. Am.* **54**, 373–379.

Green, D. M., Birdsall, T. G. and Tanner, W. P. (1957). Signal detection as a function of signal intensity and duration. *J. Acoust. Soc. Am.* **29**, 523–531.

Greenwood, D. D. (1961). Auditory masking and the critical band. *J. Acoust. Soc. Am.* **33**, 484–501.

Groen, J. J. (1964). Super- and subliminal binaural beats. *Acta Otolaryngol.* **57**, 224–230.

Gruber, J. and Boerger, G. (1971). Binaurale Verdeckungspegeldifferenzen (BMLD) und Vor- und Rückwärtsverdeckung. *Proc. 7th Int. Congr. on Acoustics, Budapest*, paper 23H5.

Hafter, E. R. and Carrier, S. C. (1972). Binaural interaction in low-frequency stimuli: the inability to trade time and intensity completely. *J. Acoust. Soc. Am.* **51**, 1852–1862.

Hafter, E. R. and Jeffress, L. A. (1968). Two-image lateralization of tones and clicks. *J. Acoust. Soc. Am.* **44**, 563–569.

Haggard, M. P. (1974). Feasibility of rapid critical bandwidth estimates. *J. Acoust. Soc. Am.* **55**, 304–308.

Haggard, M. P. and Bates, J. (1974). Changes in auditory perception in the menstrual cycle. *Speech Perception*, ser. 2, no. 3, 55–74. (Dept of Psychology, Queen's University of Belfast).

Hall, J. W. and Peters, R. W. (1981). Pitch for nonsimultaneous successive harmonics in quiet and noise. *J. Acoust. Soc. Am.* **69**, 509–513.

Hamilton, P. M. (1957). Noise masked threshold as a function of tonal duration and masking noise band width. *J. Acoust. Soc. Am.* **29**, 506–511.

Handel, S. (1973). Temporal segmentation of repeating auditory patterns. *J. Exp. Psychol.* **101**, 46–54.

Hansen, V. and Madsen, E. R. (1974). On aural phase detection. *J. Audio Engng. Soc.* **22**, 10–14.

Harris, G. G. (1960). Binaural interactions of impulsive stimuli and pure tones. *J. Acoust. Soc. Am.* **32**, 685–692.

Harris, J. D. (1963). Loudness discrimination. *J. Speech Hear. Dis. Monogr. Suppl.* **11**, 1–63.

Harris, J. D. (1972). Audition. *A. Rev. Psychol.* **23**, 313–346.

Harris, J. D. and Sergeant, R. L. (1971). Monaural/binaural minimum audible angles for a moving sound source. *J. Speech Hear. Res.* **14**, 618–629.

Hawkins, J. E. and Stevens, S. S. (1950). The masking of pure tones and of speech by white noise. *J. Acoust. Soc. Am.* **22**, 6–13.

Held, R. (1955). Shifts in binaural localization after prolonged exposures to atypical combinations of stimuli. *Am. J. Psychol.* **68**, 526–548.

Helmholtz, H. L. F. von (1863). *Die Lehre von den Tonempfindungen als physiologische Grundlage für die Theorie der Musik*, 1st edn, F. Vieweg, Braunschweig.

Henning, G. B. (1966). Frequency discrimination of random amplitude tones. *J. Acoust. Soc. Am.* **39**, 336–339.

Henning, G. B. (1967). A model for auditory discrimination and detection. *J. Acoust. Soc. Am.* **42**, 1325–1334.

Henning, G. B. (1974). Detectability of interaural delay with high-frequency complex waveforms. *J. Acoust. Soc. Am.* **55**, 84–90.

Heyes, A. D. and Ferris, A. J. (1975). Auditory localization using hearing aids. *Br. J. Audiol.* **9**, 102–106.

Hind, J. E. (1972). Physiological correlates of auditory stimulus periodicity. *Audiology* **11**, 42–57.

Hind, J. E., Rose, J. E., Brugge, J. F. and Anderson, D. J. (1967). Coding of information pertaining to paired low-frequency tones in single auditory nerve fibers of the squirrel monkey. *J. Neurophysiol.* **30**, 794–816.

Hirsh, I. J. (1950). The relation between localization and intelligibility. *J. Acoust. Soc. Am.* **22**, 196–200.

Hirsh, I. J. (1959). Auditory perception of temporal order. *J. Acoust. Soc. Am.* **31**, 759–767.

Hirsh, I. J. (1971). Masking of speech and auditory localization. *Audiology* **10**, 110–114.

Hirsh, I. J. and Bilger, R. C. (1955). Auditory-threshold recovery after exposures to pure tones. *J. Acoust. Soc. Am.* **27**, 1186–1194.

Hirsh, I. J. and Ward, W. D. (1952). Recovery of the auditory threshold after strong acoustic stimulation. *J. Acoust. Soc. Am.* **24**, 131–141.

Hood, J. D. (1950). Studies in auditory fatigue and adaptation. *Acta Otolaryngol. Suppl.* 92.

Hood, J. D. (1972). Fundamentals of identification of sensorineural hearing loss. *Sound* **6**, 21–26.

House, A. S., Stevens, K. N., Sandel, T. T. and Arnold, J. B. (1962). On the learning of speechlike vocabularies. *J. Verb. Learn. Verb. Behav.* **1**, 133–143.

Houtgast, T. (1972). Psychophysical evidence for lateral inhibition in hearing. *J. Acoust. Soc. Am.* **51**, 1885–1894.

Houtgast, T. (1973). Psychophysical experiments on 'tuning curves' and 'two-tone inhibition'. *Acustica* **29**, 168–179.

Houtgast, T. (1974). Lateral suppression in hearing. Thesis, Free University of Amsterdam, Academische Pers. BV, Amsterdam.

Houtgast, T. (1976). Subharmonic pitches of a pure tone at low S/N ratio. *J. Acoust. Soc. Am.* **60**, 405–409.

Houtsma, A. J. M. and Goldstein, J. L. (1972). The central origin of the pitch of complex tones: evidence from musical interval recognition. *J. Acoust. Soc. Am.* **51**, 520–529.

Howes, W. L. (1971). Loudness determined by power summation. *Acustica* **25**, 343–349.

Hubel, D. H. and Wiesel, T. N. (1968). Receptive fields and functional architecture of monkey striate cortex. *J. Physiol.* **195**, 215–243.

Huggins, W. H. and Cramer, E. M. (1958). Creation of pitch through binaural interaction. *J. Acoust. Soc. Am.* **30**, 413–417.

Huggins, W. H. and Licklider, J. C. R. (1951). Place mechanisms of auditory frequency analysis. *J. Acoust. Soc. Am.* **23**, 290–299.

Hughes, J. R. and Rosenblith, W. A. (1957). Electrophysiological evidence for auditory sensitization. *J. Acoust. Soc. Am.* **29**, 275–280.

Hughes, J. W. (1946). The threshold of audition for short periods of stimulation. *Proc. R. Soc.* B **133**, 486–490.

Hyde, S. R. (1972). Automatic speech recognition: a critical survey of the literature. In *Human Communication: A Unified View* (eds E. E. David and P. B. Denes), McGraw-Hill, New York.

Jacobs, J. E. and Wittman, P. (1964). Psychoacoustics, the determining factor in stereo disc recording. *J. Audio Engng. Soc.* **12**, 115–123.

Javel, E. (1980). Coding of AM tones in the chinchilla auditory nerve: implications for the pitch of complex tones. *J. Acoust. Soc. Am.* **68**, 133–146.

Jeffress, L. A. (1964). Stimulus-oriented approach to detection. *J. Acoust. Soc. Am.* **36**, 766–774.

Jeffress, L. A. (1971). Detection and lateralization of binaural signals. *Audiology* **10**, 77–84.

Jerger, J. F. (1957). Auditory adaptation. *J. Acoust. Soc. Am.* **29**, 357–363.

Johnson, D. L. and Gierke, H. von (1974). Audibility of infrasound. *J. Acoust. Soc. Am.* **56**, Suppl., S37.

Johnson-Davies, D. B. and Patterson, R. D. (1979). Psychophysical tuning curves: Restricting the listening band to the signal region. *J. Acoust. Soc. Am.* **65**, 765–770.

Johnstone, B. M. and Boyle, A. J. F. (1967). Basilar membrane vibration examined with the Mössbauer technique. *Science, N.Y.* **158**, 389–390.

Johnstone, B. M. and Sellick, P. M. (1972). The peripheral auditory apparatus. *Q. Rev. Biophys.* **5**, 1–57.

Johnstone, B. M., Taylor, K. J. and Boyle, A. J. (1970). Mechanics of guinea-pig cochlea. *J. Acoust. Soc. Am.* **47**, 504–509.

Kalil, R. and Freedman, S. J. (1967). Compensation for auditory rearrangement in the absence of observer movements. *Percept. Motor Skills* **24**, 475–478.

Karlan, M. S., Tonndorf, J. and Khanna, S. M. (1972). Dual origin of cochlear microphonics: inner and outer hair cells. *Ann. Otol. Rhinol. Laryngol.* **81**, 696–705.

Katz, S. J. and Berry, R. C. (1971). Speech modulated noise. Paper presented at the *81st Meeting of the Acoustical Society of America*.

Kay, L. (1966). Spectacles for the blind. In *Sensory Devices for the Blind*, St Dunstan's, London.

Kay, R. H. and Matthews, D. R. (1972). On the existence in human auditory pathways of channels selectively tuned to the modulation present in frequency modulated sounds. *J. Physiol.* **225**, 657–677.

Kellog, W. N. (1962). Sonar system of the blind. *Science, N.Y.* **137**, 399–404.

Kemp, D. T. (1978). Stimulated acoustic emissions from within the human auditory system. *J. Acoust. Soc. Am.* **64**, 1386–1391.

Kiang, N. Y.-S. (1968). A survey of recent developments in the study of auditory physiology. *Ann. Otol. Rhinol. Laryngol.* **77**, 656–675.

Kiang, N. Y.-S., Watanabe, T., Thomas, E. C. and Clark, L. F. (1965). *Discharge Patterns of Single Fibers in the Cat's Auditory Nerve*, MIT Press, Cambridge, Massachusetts.

Kim, D. O. and Molnar, C. E. (1979). A population study of cochlear nerve fibres: comparison of spatial distributions of average-rate and phase-locking measures of responses to single tones. *J. Neurophysiol.* **42**, 16–30.

Kim, D. O., Molnar, C. E. and Mathews, J. W. (1980). Cochlear mechanics: nonlinear behavior in two-tone responses as reflected in cochlear-nerve-fiber responses and in ear-canal sound pressure. *J. Acoust. Soc. Am.* **67**, 1704–1721.

Kimura, D. (1961). Some effects of temporal lobe damage on auditory perception. *Can. J. Psychol.* **15**, 156–165.

Kimura, D. (1964). Left–right differences in the perception of melodies. *Q. J. Exp. Psychol.* **16**, 355–358.

Klump, R. G. and Eady, H. R. (1956). Some measurements of interaural time difference thresholds. *J. Acoust. Soc. Am.* **28**, 859–860.

Koffka, K. (1935). *Principles of Gestalt Psychology*, Harcourt and Brace, New York.

Kohllöffel, L. U. E. (1972). A study of basilar membrane vibrations II. The vibratory amplitude and phase pattern along the basilar membrane (post-mortem). *Acustica* **27**, 66–81.

Kruskal, J. B. (1964). Nonmetric multidimensional scaling: a numerical method. *Psychometrika* **29**, 115–129.

Kubovy, M., Cutting, J. E. and McGuire, R. M. (1974). Hearing with the third ear: dichotic perception of a melody without monaural familiarity cues. *Science, N.Y.* **186**, 272–274.

Kuyper, P. (1972). The cocktail party effect. *Audiology* **11**, 277–282.

Kuyper, P. and de Boer, E. (1969). Evaluation of stereophonic fitting of hearing aids to hard-of-hearing children. *Int. Audiol.* **8**, 524–528.

Ladefoged, P. and Broadbent, D. E. (1960). Perception of sequence in auditory events. *Q. J. Exp. Psychol.* **12**, 162–170.

Lamore, P. J. J. (1972). Perception of two-tone octave complexes. *Acustica* **34**, 1–14.

Lamore, P. J. J. and Rodenburg, M. (1980). Significance of the SISI test and its relation to recruitment. *Audiology* **19**, 75–85.

Lane, H. L. (1965). The motor theory of speech perception: a critical review. *Psychol. Rev.* **72**, 275–309.

Legouix, P. J., Remond, M. C. and Greenbaum, H. B. (1973). Interference and two-tone inhibition. *J. Acoust. Soc. Am.* **53**, 409–419.

Lenneberg, E. (1962). Understanding language without ability to speak: a case report. *J. Abnorm. Soc. Psychol.* **65**, 419–425.

Liberman, A. M. (1957). Some results of research on speech perception. *J. Acoust. Soc. Am.* **28**, 117–123.

Liberman, A. M., Cooper, E. S., Harris, K. S. and Macneilage, P. F. (1963). A motor theory of speech perception. In *Proceedings of Speech Communication Seminar*, Vol. 3 (ed. C. G. M. Fant), Royal Institute of Technology, Stockholm.

Liberman, A. M., Cooper, F. S., Shankweiler, D. P. and Studdert-Kennedy, M. (1967). Perception of the speech code. *Psychol. Rev.* **74**, 431–461.

Liberman, M. C. (1978). Auditory-nerve response from cats raised in a low-noise chamber. *J. Acoust. Soc. Am.* **63**, 442–455.

Licklider, J. C. R. (1956). Auditory frequency analysis. In *Information Theory* (ed. C. Cherry), Academic Press, New York.

Licklider, J. C. R., Webster, J. C. and Hedlun, J. M. (1950). On the frequency limits of binaural beats. *J. Acoust. Soc. Am.* **22**, 468–473.

Lindqvist, J. and Sundberg, J. (1971). Perception of the octave interval. *7th Int. Congr. on Acoustics, Budapest*, paper 20 S 12.

Lippmann, R. P., Braida, L. D. and Durlach, N. I. (1981). Study of multichannel amplitude compression and linear amplification for persons with sensorineural hearing loss. *J. Acoust. Soc. Am.* **69**, 524–534.

Locke, S. and Kellar, L. (1973). Categorical perception in a nonlinguistic mode. *Cortex* **9**, 353–369.

McFadden, D., Jeffress, L. A. and Ermey, H. L. (1971). Differences of interaural phase and level in detection and lateralization: 250 Hz. *J. Acoust. Soc. Am.* **50**, 1484–1493.

McFadden, D., Jeffress, L. A. and Ermey, H. L. (1972). Differences of interaural phase and level in detection and lateralization: 1000 and 2000 Hz. *J. Acoust. Soc. Am.* **52**, 1197–1206.

McGill, W. J. and Goldberg, J. P. (1968a). A study of the near-miss involving Weber's law and pure-tone intensity discrimination. *Percept. Psychophys.* **4**, 105–109.

McGill, W. J. and Goldberg, J. P. (1968b). Pure-tone intensity discrimination and energy detection. *J. Acoust. Soc. Am.* **44**, 576–581.

Maiwald, D. (1967). Die Berechnung von Modulationsschwellen mit Hilfe eines Funktionsschemas. *Acustica* **18**, 193–207.

Mayer, A. M. (1894). Researches in acoustics. *Lond. Edinb. Dubl. Phil. Mag.* **37**, ser. 5, 259–288.

Mersenne, M. (1636). *Traite des Instrumens*, Book IV, Sebastian Cramoisy, Paris.

Merzenich, M. M., Knight, P. L. and Roth, G. L. (1973a). Cochleotopic organization of primary auditory cortex in the cat. *Brain Res.* **63**, 343–346.

Merzenich, M. M., Michelson, R. P., Schindler, R. A., Pettit, C. R. and Reid, M. (1973b). Neural encoding of sound sensation evoked by electrical stimulation of the acoustic nerve. *Ann. Otol.* **82**, 486–503.

Merzenich. M. M., Schindler, D. N. and White, M. W. (1974). Symposium on cochlear implants. II. Feasibility of multichannel scala tympani stimulation. *Laryngoscope* **84**, 1887–1893.

Meyer, M. (1898). Zur Theorie der Differenztöne und der Gehörsempfindungen überhaupt. *Beitr. Akust. Musikwiss.* **2**, 25–65.

Miller, G. A. (1947). Sensitivity to changes in the intensity of white noise and its relation to masking and loudness. *J. Acoust. Soc. Am.* **191**, 609–619.

Miller, G. A. and Taylor, W. (1948). The perception of repeated bursts of noise. *J. Acoust. Soc. Am.* **20**, 171–182.

Miller, G. A. and Licklider, J. C. R. (1950). The intelligibility of interrupted speech. *J. Acoust. Soc. Am.* **22**, 167–173.

Miller, J. D. (1974). Effects of noise on people. *J. Acoust. Soc. Am.* **56**, 729–764.

Miller, J. D., Wier, C. C., Pastore, R., Kelly, W. J. and Dooling, R. J. (1976). Discrimination and labelling of noise-buzz sequences with varying noise-lead times: An example of categorical perception. *J. Acoust. Soc. Am.* **60**, 410–417.

Mills, A. W. (1960). Lateralization of high-frequency tones. *J. Acoust. Soc. Am.* **32**, 132–134.

Mills, A. W. (1972). Auditory localization. In *Foundations of Modern Auditory Theory*, Vol. 2 (ed. J. V. Tobias), Academic Press, New York.

Møller, A. R. (1972). Coding of sounds in lower levels of the auditory system. *Q. Rev. Biophys.* **5**, 59–155.

Mollon, J. (1974). After-effects and the brain. *New Scientist* 21st Feb., 479–482.

Moore, B. C. J. (1972). Some experiments relating to the perception of pure tones: possible clinical applications. *Sound* **6**, 73–79.

Moore, B. C. J. (1973a). Frequency difference limens for short-duration tones. *J. Acoust. Soc. Am.* **54**, 610–619.

Moore, B. C. J. (1973b). Frequency difference limens for narrow bands of noise. *J. Acoust. Soc. Am.* **54**, 888–896.

Moore, B. C. J. (1973c). Some experiments relating to the perception of complex tones. *Q. J. Exp. Psychol.* **25**, 451–475.

Moore, B. C. J. (1974). Relation between the critical bandwidth and the frequency-difference limen. *J. Acoust. Soc. Am.* **55**, 359.

Moore, B. C. J. (1975). Mechanisms of masking. *J. Acoust. Soc. Am.* **57**, 391–399.

Moore, B. C. J. (1978). Psychophysical tuning curves measured in simultaneous and forward masking. *J. Acoust. Soc. Am.* **63**, 524–532.

Moore, B. C. J. and Glasberg, B. R. (1981). Auditory filter shapes derived in simultaneous and forward masking. *J. Acoust. Soc. Am.* in press.

Moore, B. C. J. and Raab, D. H. (1974). Pure-tone intensity discrimination: some experiments relating to the 'near-miss' to Weber's law. *J. Acoust. Soc. Am.* **55**, 1049–1054.

Moore, B. C. J. and Raab, D. H. (1975). Intensity discrimination for noise bursts in the presence of a continuous, bandstop background: effects of level, width of the bandstop, and duration. *J. Acoust. Soc. Am.* **57**, 400–405.

Moore, B. C. J. and Rosen, S. M. (1979). Tune recognition with reduced pitch and interval information. *Q.J. Exp. Psychol.* **31**, 229–240.

Moore, T. J. and Welsh, J. R. (1970). Forward and backward enhancement of sensitivity in the auditory system. *J. Acoust. Soc. Am.* **47**, 534–539.

Morton, J. (1964). A model for continuous language behaviour. *Language and Speech* **7**, 40–70.

Mulligan, B., Mulligan, M. and Stonecypher, J. F. (1967). Critical band in binaural detection. *J. Acoust. Soc. Am.* **41**, 7–12.

Neisser, U. (1967). *Cognitive Psychology*, Appleton-Century-Crofts, New York.

Newman, E. B. (1948). Chapter 14 in *Foundations of Psychology* (eds E. G. Boring, H. S. Langfeld and H. P. Weld), Wiley, New York.

Noorden, L. P. A. S. van (1971). Rhythmic fission as a function of tone rate. *IPO Annual Progress Rep.* **6**, 9–12, Eindhoven, The Netherlands.

Noorden, L.P.A.S. van (1975). Temporal coherence in the perception of tone sequences. Thesis, Technical University Eindhoven.

Nordmark, J. O. (1970). Time and frequency analysis. In *Foundations of Modern Auditory Theory*, Vol. 1 (ed. J. V. Tobias), Academic Press, New York.

Ohm, G. S. (1843). Über die Definition des Tones, nebst daran geknüpfter Theorie der Sirene und ähnlicher tonbildender Vorrichtungen. *Ann. Phys. Chem.* **59**, 513–565.

O'Loughlin, B. J. and Moore, B. C. J. (1981). Off-frequency listening: Effects on psychoacoustical tuning curves obtained in simultaneous and forward masking. *J. Acoust. Soc. Am.* **69**, 1119–1125.

Olsen, W. O. and Carhart, R. (1966). Integration of acoustic power at threshold by normal hearers. *J. Acoust. Soc. Am.* **40**, 591–599.

Palmer, A. R. and Evans, E. F. (1979). On the peripheral coding of the level of individual frequency components of complex sounds at high sound levels. In *Hearing Mechanisms and Speech* (eds O. Creutzfeldt, H. Scheich and C. Schreiner), Springer-Verlag, Berlin.

Patterson, J. H. (1971). Additivity of foward and backward masking as a function of signal frequency. *J. Acoust. Soc. Am.* **50**, 1123–1125.

Patterson, J. H. and Green, D. M. (1970). Discrimination of transient signals having identical energy spectra. *J. Acoust. Soc. Am.* **48**, 894–905.

Patterson, R. D. (1974). Auditory filter shape. *J. Acoust. Soc. Am.* **55**, 802–809.

Patterson, R. D. (1976). Auditory filter shapes derived with noise stimuli. *J. Acoust. Soc. Am.* **59**, 640–654.

Patterson, R. D. and Henning, G. B. (1977). Stimulus variability and auditory filter shape. *J. Acoust. Soc. Am.* **62**, 649–664.

Patterson, R. D. and Milroy, R. (1980). The appropriate sound level for auditory warnings on civil aircraft. *J. Acoust. Soc. Am.* **67**, S58.

Pfeiffer, R. R. and Kim, D. O. (1975). Cochlear nerve fiber responses: Distribution along the cochlear partition. *J. Acoust. Soc. Am.* **58**, 867–869.

Pick, G. F., Evans, E. F. and Wilson, J. P. (1977). Frequency resolution in patients with hearing loss of cochlear origin. In *Psychophysics and Physiology of Hearing* (eds E. F. Evans and J. P. Wilson), Academic Press, London and New York.

Pisoni, D. B. (1973). Auditory and phonetic memory codes in the discrimination of consonants and vowels. *Percept. Psychophys.* **13**, 253–260.

Plenge, G. (1972). Über das Problem der Im-Kopf-Lokalisation. *Acustica* **26**, 213–221.

Plenge, G. (1974). On the differences between localization and lateralization. *J. Acoust. Soc. Am.* **56**, 944–951.

Plomp, R. (1964). The ear as a frequency analyser. *J. Acoust. Soc. Am.* **36**, 1628–1636.

Plomp, R. (1965). Detectability threshold for combination tones. *J. Acoust. Soc. Am.* **37**, 1110–1123.

Plomp, R. (1967). Pitch of complex tones. *J. Acoust. Soc. Am.* **41**, 1526–1533.

Plomp, R. (1968). Pitch, timbre and hearing theory. *Int. Audiol.* **7**, 322–344.

Plomp, R. (1970). Timbre as a multidimensional attribute of complex tones. In *Frequency Analysis and Periodicity Detection in Hearing* (eds R. Plomp and G. F. Smoorenburg), Sijthoff, Leiden.

Plomp, R. and Bouman, M. A. (1959). Relation between hearing threshold and duration for tone pulses. *J. Acoust. Soc. Am.* **31**, 749–758.

Plomp, R. and Levelt, W. J. M. (1965). Tonal consonance and critical bandwidth. *J. Acoust. Soc. Am.* **38**, 548–560.

Plomp, R. and Steeneken, H. J. M. (1969). Effect of phase on the timbre of complex tones. *J. Acoust. Soc. Am.* **46**, 409–421.

Plomp, R., Pols, L. C. W. and Geer, J. P. van de (1967). Dimensional analysis of vowel spectra. *J. Acoust. Soc. Am.* **41**, 707–712.

Pollack, I. (1952). The information of elementary auditory displays. *J. Acoust. Soc. Am.* **24**, 745–749.

Pollack, I. (1969). Periodicity pitch for white noise—fact or artifact? *J. Acoust. Soc. Am.* **45**, 237–238.

Pols, L. C. W., Kamp, L. J. Th. van der and Plomp, R. (1969). Perceptual and physical space of vowel sounds. *J. Acoust. Soc. Am.* **46**, 458–467.

Port, E. (1963). Uber die Lautstärke einzelner kurzer Schallimpulse. *Acustica* **13**, 212–223.

Potter, R. K., Kopp, G. A. and Green, H. C. (1947). *Visible Speech*, Van Nostrand, New York.

Rabinowitz, W. M., Bilger, R. C., Trahiotis, C. and Neutzel, J. (1980). Two-tone masking in normal hearing listeners. *J. Acoust. Soc. Am.* **68**, 1096–1106.

Raiford, C. A. and Schubert, E. D. (1971). Recognition of phase changes in octave complexes. *J. Acoust. Soc. Am.* **50**, 559–567.

Rainbolt, H. and Small, A. M. (1972). Mach bands in auditory masking: an attempted replication. *J. Acoust. Soc. Am.* **51**, 567–574.

Rakowski, A. (1972). Direct comparison of absolute and relative pitch. In *Hearing Theory 1972*, IPO Eindhoven, The Netherlands.

Rasch, R. A. (1978). The perception of simultaneous notes such as in polyphonic music. *Acustica* **40**, 21–33.

Rhode, W. S. (1971). Observations of the vibration of the basilar membrane in squirrel monkeys using the Mössbauer technique. *J. Acoust. Soc. Am.* **49**, 1218–1231.

Rhode, W. S. and Robles, L. (1974). Evidence from Mössbauer experiments for non-linear vibration in the cochlea. *J. Acoust. Soc. Am.* **55**, 588–596.

Rice, C. E. (1967). Human echo perception. *Science, N.Y.* **155**, 656–664.

Riesz, R. R. (1928). Differential intensity sensitivity of the ear for pure tones. *Phys. Rev.* **31** (ser. 2), 867–875.

Ritsma, R. J. (1962). Existence region of the tonal residue. I. *J. Acoust. Soc. Am.* **34**, 1224–1229.

Ritsma, R. J. (1963). Existence region of the tonal residue. II. *J. Acoust. Soc. Am.* **35**, 1241–1245.

Ritsma, R. J. (1967a). Frequencies dominant in the perception of the pitch of complex sounds. *J. Acoust. Soc. Am.* **42**, 191–198.

Ritsma, R. J. (1967b). Frequencies dominant in the perception of periodic pulses of alternating polarity. *IPO Annual Prog. Rep.* Eindhoven, **2**, 14–24.

Ritsma, R. J. (1970). Periodicity detection. In *Frequency Analysis and Periodicity Detection in Hearing* (eds R. Plomp and G. F. Smoorenburg), Sijthoff, Leiden.

Robertson, D. (1976). Correspondence between sharp tuning and two-tone inhibition in primary auditory neurones. *Nature, Lond.* **259**, 477–478.

Robertson, D. and Manley, G. A. (1974). Manipulation of frequency analysis in the cochlear ganglion of the guinea-pig. *J. Comp. Physiol.* **91**, 363–375.

Robinson, D. W. and Dadson, R. S. (1956). A redetermination of the equal-loudness relations for pure tones. *Br. J. Appl. Phys.* **7**, 166–181.

Rodenburg, M. (1972). *Sensitivity of the Auditory System to Differences in Intensity*, Unpublished PhD Thesis, Medical Faculty, Rotterdam.

Rose, J. E., Brugge, J. F., Anderson, D. J. and Hind, J. E. (1967). Phase-locked response to low-frequency tones in single auditory nerve fibers of the squirrel monkey. *J. Neurophysiol.* **30**, 769–793.

Rose, J. E., Brugge, J. F., Anderson, D. J. and Hind, J. E. (1968). Patterns of activity in single auditory nerve fibers of the squirrel monkey. In *Hearing Mechanisms in Vertebrates* (eds A. V. S. de Reuck and J. Knight), Churchill, London.

Rose, J. E., Hind, J. E., Anderson, D. J. and Brugge, J. F. (1971). Some effects of stimulus intensity on response of auditory nerve fibers in the squirrel monkey. *J. Neurophysiol.* **34**, 685–699.

Rosen, S. M., Fourcin, A. J. and Moore, B. C. J. (1981). Voice pitch as an aid to lip-reading. *Nature, Lond.* **291**, 150–152.

Royer, F. L. and Garner, W. R. (1966). Response uncertainty and perceptual difficulty of auditory temporal patterns. *Percept. Psychophys.* **1**, 41–47.

Royer, F. L. and Garner, W. R. (1970). Perceptual organization of nine-element auditory temporal patterns. *Percept. Psychophys.* **7**, 115–120.

Ruggero, M. A. (1973). Response to noise of auditory nerve fibers in the squirrel monkey. *J. Neurophysiol.* **36**, 569–587.

Russell, I. J. and Sellick, P.M. (1978). Intracellular studies of hair cells in the mammalian cochlea. *J. Physiol. (Lond.)* **284**, 261–290.

Sachs, M. B. (1971). *Physiology of the Auditory System*, National Educational Consultants, Baltimore.

Sachs, M. B. and Abbas, P. J. (1974). Rate versus level functions for auditory-nerve fibers in cats: tone-burst stimuli. *J. Acoust. Soc. Am.* **56**, 1835–1847.

Sachs, M. B. and Kiang, N. Y.-S. (1968). Two-tone inhibition in auditory-nerve fibers. *J. Acoust. Soc. Am.* **43**, 1120–1128.

Sachs, M. B. and Young, E. D. (1980). Effects of nonlinearities on speech encoding in the auditory nerve. *J. Acoust. Soc. Am.* **68**, 858–875.

Sandel, T. T., Teas, D. C., Feddersen, W. E. and Jeffress, L. A. (1955). Localization of sound from single and paired sources. *J. Acoust. Soc. Am.* **27**, 842–852.

Schacknow, P. N. and Raab, D. H. (1973). Intensity discrimination of tone bursts and the form of the Weber function. *Percept. Psychophys.* **14**, 449–450.

Scharf, B. (1961). Complex sounds and critical bands. *Psychol. Bull.* **58**, 205–217.

Scharf, B. (1970). Critical bands. In *Foundations of Modern Auditory Theory*, Vol. 1 (ed. J. V. Tobias), Academic Press, New York.

Scharf, B. (1971). Fundamentals of auditory masking. *Audiology* **10**, 30–40.

Scharf, B. (1981). Loudness adaptation. In *Hearing Research and Theory* (eds J. V. Tobias and E. D. Schubert), Academic Press, New York.

Schouten, J. F. (1940). The residue and the mechanism of hearing. *Proc. K. Ned. Akad. Wet.* **43**, 991–999.

Schouten, J. F. (1968). The perception of timbre. In *Reports 6th International Congress on Acoustics, Tokyo, Japan*, Vol. 1, GP–6–2.

Schouten, J. F. (1970). The residue revisited. In *Frequency Analysis and Periodicity Detection in Hearing* (eds. R. Plomp and G. F. Smoorenburg), Sijthoff, Leiden.

Schouten, J. F., Ritsma, R. J. and Cardozo, B. L. (1962). Pitch of the residue. *J. Acoust. Soc. Am.* **34**, 1418–1424.

Schroeder, M. R. and Atal, B. S. (1963). Computer simulation of sound transmission in rooms. *IEEE Int. Conv. Rec.* **7**, 150–155.

Schroeder, M. R., Gottlob, D. and Siebrasse, K. F. (1974). Comparative study of European concert halls: correlation of subjective preference with geometric and acoustic parameters. *J. Acoust. Soc. Am.* **56**, 1195–1201.

Schubert, E. D. (1969). On estimating aural harmonics. *J. Acoust. Soc. Am.* **45**, 790–791.

Schuknecht, H. F. (1970). Functional manifestations of lesions of the sensorineural structures. In *Foundations of Modern Auditory Theory*, Vol. 1 (ed. J. V. Tobias), Academic Press, New York.

Sellick, P. M. and Russell, I. J. (1979). Two-tone suppression in cochlear hair cells. *Hearing Res.* **1**, 227–236.

Shannon, R. V. (1976). Two-tone unmasking and suppression in a forward-masking situation. *J. Acoust. Soc. Am.* **59**, 1460–1470.

Shaxby, J. H. and Gage, F. H. (1932). Studies in the localization of sound. Med. Res. Council Spec. Rept. Ser. No. 166, 1–32.

Sheeley, E. C. and Bilger, R. C. (1964). Temporal integration as a function of frequency. *J. Acoust. Soc. Am.* **36**, 1850–1857.

Shepard, R. N. (1962). The analysis of proximities: multidimensional scaling with an unknown distance function. *Psychometrika* **27**, 125–140.

Shower, E. G. and Biddulph, R. (1931). Differential pitch sensitivity of the ear. *J. Acoust. Soc. Am.* **2**, 275–287.

Siebert, W. M. (1968). Stimulus transformations in the peripheral auditory system.

In *Recognizing Patterns* (eds P. A. Kolers and M. Eden), MIT Press, Cambridge, Massachusetts.

Siebert, W. M. (1970). Frequency discrimination in the auditory system: place or periodicity mechanisms. *Proc. IEEE* **58**, 723–730.

Simmons, F. B. (1966). Electrical stimulation of the auditory nerve in man. *Arch. Otolaryngol.* **84**, 2–54.

Slater, P. (1960). The analysis of personal preferences. *Br. J. Stat. Psychol.* **8**, 119.

Small, A. M., Boggess, J., Klich, R., Kuehn, D., Thelin, J. and Wiley, T. (1972). MLD's in forward and backward masking. *J. Acoust. Soc. Am.* **51**, 1365–1367.

Smoorenburg, G. F. (1970). Pitch perception of two-frequency stimuli. *J. Acoust. Soc. Am.* **48**, 924–941.

Soderquist, D. R. (1970). Frequency analysis and the critical band. *Psychon. Sci.* **21**, 117–119.

Soderquist, D. R. and Lindsey, J. W. (1972). Physiological noise as a masker of low frequencies: the cardiac cycle. *J. Acoust. Soc. Am.* **52**, 1216–1220.

Spoendlin, H. (1970). Structural basis of peripheral frequency analysis. In *Frequency Analysis and Periodicity Detection in Hearing* (eds R. Plomp and G. F. Smoorenburg), Sijthoff, Leiden.

Srinivasan, R. (1971). Auditory critical bandwidth for short duration signals. *J. Acoust. Soc. Am.* **50**, 616–622.

Stahl, D. (1975). Artificial head stereophony—first application in broadcasting. *SERT Journal* **9**, 171–173.

Stephens, S. D. G. (1973). Auditory temporal integration as a function of intensity. *J. Sound Vib.* **30**, 109–126.

Stephens, S. D. G. (1974). Methodological factors influencing loudness of short duration sounds. *J. Sound Vib.* **37**, 235–246.

Stevens, K. N. (1968). On the relations between speech movements and speech perception. *Z. Phonetik Sprachwiss. Kommunikationsforsch.* **21**, 102–106.

Stevens, K. N. (1980). Acoustic correlates of some phonetic categories. *J. Acoust. Soc. Am.* **68**, 836–842.

Stevens, K. N. (1981). Constraints imposed by the auditory system on the properties used to classify speech sounds. In *The Cognitive Representation of Speech* (eds T. F. Myers, J. Laver and J. Anderson), North-Holland, Amsterdam.

Stevens, K. N. and House, A. S. (1972). Speech perception. In *Foundations of Modern Auditory Theory*, Vol. 2 (ed. J. V. Tobias), Academic Press, New York.

Stevens, S. S. (1957). On the psychophysical law. *Psychol. Rev.* **64**, 153–181.

Stevens, S. S. (1972). Perceived level of noise by Mark VII and decibels (E). *J. Acoust. Soc. Am.* **51**, 575–601.

Stevens, S. S. and Newman, E. B. (1936). The localization of actual sources of sound. *Am. J. Psychol.* **48**, 297–306.

Sturges, P. T. and Martin, J. F. (1974). Rhythmic structure in auditory temporal pattern perception and immediate memory. *J. Exp. Psychol.* **102**, 377–383.

Summerfield, Q., Foster, J., Gray, S. and Haggard, M. P. (1981). Perceiving vowels from 'flat spectra'. *J. Acoust. Soc. Am.* **69**, S116.

Supa, M., Cotzin, M. and Dallenbach, K. M. (1944). 'Facial vision': The perception of obstacles by the blind. *Am. J. Psychol.* **57**, 133–183.

Swets, J. A., Green, D. M. and Tanner, W. P., Jr (1962). On the width of critical bands. *J. Acoust. Soc. Am.* **34**, 108–113.

Tanner, W. P. and Sorkin, R. D. (1972). The theory of signal detectability. In *Foundations of Modern Auditory Theory*, Vol. 2 (ed. J. V. Tobias), Academic Press, London and New York.

Tasaki, I. (1954). Nerve impulses in individual auditory nerve fibres of guinea-pig. *J. Neurophysiol.* **17**, 97–122.

Terhardt, E. (1970). Frequency analysis and periodicity detection in the sensations of roughness and periodicity pitch. In *Frequency Analysis and Periodicity Detection in Hearing* (eds R. Plomp and G. F. Smoorenburg), Sijthoff, Leiden.

Terhardt, E. (1971). Die Tonhöhe harmonischer Klänge und das Oktavintervall. *Acustica* **24**, 126–136.

Terhardt, E. (1972a). Zur Tonhöhenwahrnehmung von Klängen. I. Psychoakustische Grundlagen. *Acustica* **26**, 173–186.

Terhardt, E. (1972b). Zur Tonhöhenwahrnehmung von Klängen. II. Ein Funktionsschema. *Acustica* **26**, 187–199.

Terhardt, E. (1972c). Frequency and time resolution of the ear in pitch perception of complex tones. In *Hearing Theory 1972*, IPO, Eindhoven, The Netherlands.

Terhardt, E. (1974). Pitch, consonance and harmony. *J. Acoust. Soc. Am.* **55**, 1061–1069.

Thurlow, W. R. (1963). Perception of low auditory pitch: a multicue mediation theory. *Psychol. Rev.* **70**, 515–519.

Thwing, E. J. (1955). Spread of perstimulatory fatigue of a pure tone to neighboring frequencies. *J. Acoust. Soc. Am.* **27**, 741–748.

Tobias, J. V. (1963). Application of a 'relative' procedure to a problem in binaural-beat perception. *J. Acoust. Soc. Am.* **35**, 1442–1447.

Tobias, J. V. (1965). Consistency of sex differences in binaural-beat perception. *Int. Audiol.* **4**, 179–182.

Tobias, J. V. (1972). Curious binaural phenomena. In *Foundations of Modern Auditory Theory*, Vol. 2 (ed. J. V. Tobias), Academic Press, New York.

Tobias, J. V. and Schubert, E. D. (1959). Effective onset duration of auditory stimuli. *J. Acoust. Soc. Am.* **31**, 1595–1605.

Tobias, J. V. and Zerlin, S. (1959). Lateralization threshold as a function of stimulus duration. *J. Acoust. Soc. Am.* **31**, 1591–1594.

Tonndorf, J. (1970). Cochlear mechanics and hydro-dynamics. In *Foundations of Modern Auditory Theory*, Vol. 1 (ed. J. V. Tobias), Academic Press, New York.

Treisman, M. (1964), Sensory scaling and the psychophysical law. *Q. J. Exp. Psychol.* **16**, 11–22.

Tumarkin, A. (1972). A biologist looks at psycho-acoustics. *J. Sound Vib.* **21**, 115–126.

Verschuure, J. (1978). Auditory excitation patterns. Thesis, Erasmus University Rotterdam, W. D. Meinema B.V, Delft.

Viemeister, N. F. (1972). Intensity discrimination of pulsed sinusoids: the effects of filtered noise. *J. Acoust. Soc. Am.* **51**, 1265–1269.

Viemeister, N. F. (1974). Intensity discrimination of noise in the presence of band reject noise. *J. Acoust. Soc. Am.* **56**, 1594–1600.

Villchur, E. and Allison, R. F. (1980). The audibility of Doppler distortion in loudspeakers. *J. Acoust. Soc. Am.* **68**, 1561–1569.

Vogten, L. L. M. (1974). Pure tone masking; a new result from a new method. In *Facts and Models in Hearing* (eds E. Zwicker and E. Terhardt), Springer-Verlag, Berlin.

Wallach, H. (1940). The role of head movements and vestibular and visual cues in sound localization. *J. Exp. Psychol.* **27**, 339–368.

Wallach, H., Newman, E. B. and Rosenzweig, M. R. (1949). The precedence effect in sound localization. *Am. J. Psychol.* **62**, 315–336.

Walliser, K. (1968). *Zusammenwirken von Hüllkurvenperiode und Tonheit bei der*

Bildung der Periodentonhöhe, Doctoral dissertation. Technische Hochschule, München.

Walliser, K. (1969a). Zusammenhänge zwischen dem Schallreiz und der Periodentonhöhe. *Acustica* **21**, 319–328.

Walliser, K. (1969b). Zur Unterschiedsschwelle der Periodentonhöhe. *Acustica* **21**, 329–336.

Walliser, K. (1969c). Über ein Funktionsschema für die Bildung der Periodentonhöhe aus dem Schallreiz. *Kybernetik* **6**, 65–72.

Ward, W. D. (1954). Subjective musical pitch. *J. Acoust. Soc. Am.* **26**, 369–380.

Ward, W. D. (1963). Auditory fatigue and masking. In *Modern Developments in Audiology* (ed. J. F. Jerger), Academic Press, New York.

Ward, W. D. (1963a). Absolute pitch. Part I. *Sound* **2**, 14–21.

Ward, W. D. (1963b). Absolute pitch. Part II. *Sound* **2**, 33–41.

Ward, W. D. (1970). Musical perception. In *Foundations of Modern Auditory Theory*, Vol. 1 (ed. J. V. Tobias), Academic Press, New York.

Ward, W. D., Glorig, A. and Sklar, D. L. (1958). Dependence of temporary threshold shift at 4 kc on intensity and time. *J. Acoust. Soc. Am.* **30**, 944–954.

Warren, R. M. (1970a). Elimination of biases in loudness judgments for tones. *J. Acoust. Soc. Am.* **48**, 1397–1403.

Warren, R. M. (1970b). Perceptual restoration of missing speech sounds. *Science*, *N.Y.* **167**, 392–393.

Warren, R. M. (1974). Auditory temporal discrimination by trained listeners. *Cognitive Psychol.* **6**, 237–256.

Warren, R. M. (1976). Auditory perception and speech evolution. *Ann. N.Y. Acad. Sci.* **280**, 708–717.

Warren, R. M. (1981). Measurement of sensory intensity. *Behav. Brain Sci.* in press.

Warren, R. M., Obusek, C. J., Farmer, R. M. and Warren, R. P. (1969). Auditory sequence: confusion of patterns other than speech or music. *Science*, *N.Y.* **164**, 586–587.

Watson, C. S. and Gengel, R. W. (1968). Time-intensity trading relations as a function of signal frequency. *76th Meeting of the Acoustical Society of America*, paper A7.

Webster, F. A. (1951). Influence of interaural phase on masked thresholds. *J. Acoust. Soc. Am.* **23**, 452–462.

Weerts, T. C. and Thurlow, W. R. (1971). The effects of eye position and expectation on sound localization. *Percept. Psychophys.* **9**, 35–39.

Wegel, R. L. and Lane, C. E. (1924). The auditory masking of one sound by another and its probable relation to the dynamics of the inner ear. *Phys. Rev.* **23**, 266–285.

Weiler, M. and Friedman, L. (1973). Monaural heterophonic auditory adaptation. *J. Acoust. Soc. Am.* **54**, Suppl., 23.

Welford, A. T. (1968). *Fundamentals of Skill*, Methuen, London.

Whitfield, I. C. (1967). *The Auditory Pathway*, Arnold, London.

Whitfield, I. C. (1970). Central nervous processing in relation to spatio-temporal discrimination of auditory patterns. In *Frequency Analysis and Periodicity Detection in Hearing* (ed. R. Plomp and G. F. Smoorenburg), Sijthoff, Leiden.

Whitfield, I. C. and Evans, E. F. (1965). Responses of auditory cortical neurones to stimuli of changing frequency. *J. Neurophysiol.* **28**, 655–672.

Whittle, L. S., Collins, S. J. and Robinson, D. W. (1972). The audibility of low-frequency sounds. *J. Sound Vib.* **21**, 431–448.

Whitworth, R. H. and Jeffress, L. A. (1961). Time vs intensity in the localization of tones. *J. Acoust. Soc. Am.* **33**, 925–929.

Wiener, F. M. and Ross, D. A. (1946). The pressure distribution in the auditory canal in a progressive sound field. *J. Acoust. Soc. Am.* **18**, 401–408.

Willey, C. F., Inglis, E. and Pearce, C. H. (1937). Reversal of auditory localization. *J. Exp. Psychol.* **20**, 114–130.

Wilson, J. P. (1967). Psychoacoustics of obstacle detection using ambient or self generated noise. In *Animal Sonar Systems* (ed. R. G. Busnel), Gap, Hautes-Alpes, France.

Wilson, J. P. and Johnstone, J. R. (1972). Capacitive probe measures of basilar membrane vibrations. In *Hearing Theory*, IPO, Eindhoven.

Winckel, F. (1967). *Music, Sound and Sensation*, Dover, New York.

Wollberg, Z. and Newman, J. D. (1972). Auditory cortex of squirrel monkey: response patterns of single cells to species-specific vocalizations. *Science, N.Y.* **175**, 212–214.

Yost, W. A., Wightman, F. L. and Green, D. M. (1971). Lateralization of filtered clicks. *J. Acoust. Soc. Am.* **50**, 1526–1531.

Young, P. T. (1928). Auditory localization with acoustical transposition of the ears. *J. Exp. Psychol.* **11**, 399–429.

Zwicker, E. (1952). Die Grenzen der Hörbarkeit der Amplitudenmodulation und der Frequenzmodulation eines Tones. *Acustica* **2**, 125–133.

Zwicker, E. (1954). Die Verdeckung von Schmalbandgeräuschen durch Sinustöne. *Acustica* **4**, 415–420.

Zwicker E. (1956). Die elementaren Grundlagen zur Bestimmung der Informationskapazität des Gehörs. *Acustica* **6**, 365–381.

Zwicker, E. (1958). Über psychologische und methodische Grundlagen der Lautheit. *Acustica* **8** (Beih. 1), 237–258.

Zwicker, E. (1964). 'Negative afterimage' in hearing. *J. Acoust. Soc. Am.* **36**, 2413–2415.

Zwicker, E. (1965a). Temporal effects in simultaneous masking by white-noise bursts. *J. Acoust. Soc. Am.* **37**, 653–663.

Zwicker, E. (1965b). Temporal effects in simultaneous masking and loudness. *J. Acoust. Soc. Am.* **38**, 132–141.

Zwicker, E. (1970). Masking and psychological excitation as consequences of the ear's frequency analysis. In *Frequency Analysis and Periodicity Detection in Hearing* (eds R. Plomp and G. F. Smoorenburg), Sijthoff, Leiden.

Zwicker, E. and Fastl, H. (1972). On the development of the critical band. *J. Acoust. Soc. Am.* **52**, 699–702.

Zwicker, E. and Scharf, B. (1965). A model of loudness summation. *Psychol. Rev.* **72**, 3–26.

Zwicker, E. and Schorn, K. (1978). Psychoacoustical tuning curves in audiology. *Audiology* **17**, 120–140.

Zwicker, E. and Schutte, H. (1973). On the time-pattern of the threshold of tone impulses masked by narrow band noise. *Acustica* **29**, 343–347.

Zwicker, E., Flottorp, G. and Stevens, S. S. (1957). Critical bandwidth in loudness summation. *J. Acoust. Soc. Am.* **29**, 548–557.

Zwislocki, J. J. (1965). Analysis of some auditory characteristics. In *Handbook of Mathematical Psychology*, Vol. 3 (eds R. D. Luce, R. R. Bush and E. Galanter), Wiley, New York.

Zwislocki, J. J. (1971). Central masking and neural activity in the cochlear nucleus. *Audiology* **10**, 48–59.

Glossary

This glossary defines most of the technical terms which appear several times in the text but which are defined only once. Sometimes the definitions are specific to the context of the book and do not apply to everyday usage of the terms.

Absolute threshold The minimum detectable level of a sound in the absence of any other external sounds. The manner of presentation of the sound and the method of determining detectability must be specified.

Amplitude The instantaneous amplitude of an oscillating quantity (e.g. sound pressure) is its value at any instant, while the peak amplitude is the maximum value that the quantity attains. Sometimes the word peak is omitted when the meaning is clear from the context.

Audiogram A graph showing absolute threshold for pure tones as a function of frequency. It is often plotted as hearing loss (deviation from the average threshold) in dB as a function of frequency.

Aural harmonic A harmonic generated in the auditory mechanism.

Bandwidth A term used to refer to a range of frequencies. The bandwidth of a bandpass filter is often defined as the difference between the two frequencies at which the response of the filter has fallen by 3 dB (i.e. to half power).

Basilar membrane A membrane inside the cochlea which vibrates in response to sound and whose vibrations lead to activity in the auditory pathways. See Chapter 1.

Beats Periodic fluctuations which are heard when sounds of slightly different frequencies are superimposed.

Bel A unit for expressing the ratio of two powers. The number of bels is the logarithm to the base 10 of the power ratio.

Binaural A situation involving listening with two ears.

Binaural masking level difference (BMLD or MLD) This is a measure of the improvement in detectability of a signal which can occur under binaural listening conditions. It is the difference in threshold of the signal (in dB) for the case where the signal and masker have the same phase and level relationships at the two ears and the case where the interaural phase and/or level relationships of the signal and masker are different.

Characteristic frequency (CF) The frequency at which the threshold of a given single neurone is lowest, i.e. the frequency at which it is most sensitive.

Combination tone A tone perceived as a component of a complex stimulus which is not present in the sensations produced by the constituent components of the complex when they are presented alone.

Complex tone A tone composed of a number of simple tones of different frequencies.

Component One of the simple tones composing a complex sound. Also called a frequency component.

Cycle That portion of a periodic function that occurs in one period.

Decibel One-tenth of a bel, abbreviated dB.

Dichotic A situation in which the sounds reaching the two ears are not the same.

Difference limen (DL) Also called the just-noticeable difference (JND) or the differential threshold. The smallest detectable change in a stimulus. The method of determining detectability must be specified.

Diotic A situation in which the sounds reaching the two ears are the same.

Diplacusis Binaural diplacusis describes the case when a tone of fixed frequency evokes different pitches in the left and right ear.

Envelope The envelope of any function is the smooth curve joining the peaks of the function.

Equal-loudness contours Curves plotted as a function of frequency showing the sound pressure level required to produce a given loudness level for a typical listener.

Excitation pattern A term used to describe the pattern of neural activity evoked by a given sound as a function of the characteristic frequency (CF) of the neurones being excited. Sometimes the term is used to describe the effective level of excitation (in dB) at each CF.

Filter A device which modifies the frequency spectrum of a signal, usually while it is in electrical form.

Formant A peak in the spectral envelope of a sound. The term is used particularly in describing speech sounds.

Free field A field or system of waves free from the effects of boundaries.

Frequency For a sine wave the frequency is the number of periods occurring in one second. The unit is cycles per second, or Hz. For a complex periodic sound the term 'repetition rate' is used to describe the number of periods per second (p.p.s.).

Fundamental frequency The fundamental frequency of a periodic sound is that sinusoidal component of the sound that has the same period as the periodic sound.

Harmonic A harmonic is a component of a complex tone whose frequency is an integral multiple of the fundamental frequency of the complex.

Hz See Frequency.

Intensity Intensity is the sound power transmitted through a given area in a sound field. Units such as watts per square centimetre are used. The term is also used as a generic name for any quantity relating to amount of sound, such as amplitude, level, pressure, power, etc.

Level The level of a sound is specified in dB in relation to some reference level. See sensation level and sound pressure level.

Linear A linear system is a system which satisfies the conditions of superposition and homogeneity. See Chapter 1, section 3.

Loudness This is the intensive attribute of an auditory sensation, in terms of which sounds may be ordered on a scale extending from quiet to loud.

Loudness level The loudness level, in phons, of a sound is the sound pressure level in dB of a pure tone of frequency 1 kHz which is judged by the listener to be equivalent in loudness.

Masked audiogram This is a graph of the amount of masking (in dB) produced by a given sound as a function of the frequency of the masked sound.

Masking Masking is the amount (or the process) by which the threshold of audibility for one sound is raised by the presence of another (masking) sound.

Masking level difference (MLD) See Binaural masking level difference.

Modulation Modulation refers to a periodic change in a particular dimension of a stimulus. Thus a sinusoid may be modulated in frequency or in amplitude.

Monaural The situation in which sounds are presented to one ear only.

Noise Noise in general refers to any unwanted sound. White noise is a sound whose energy per unit bandwidth is constant, on average, over the range of audible frequencies. It usually has a normal (Gaussian) distribution of instantaneous amplitudes.

Octave An octave is the interval between two tones when their frequencies are in the ratio 2:1.

Partial A partial is any sinusoid frequency component in a complex tone.

Period The period of a periodic function is the smallest time interval over which the function repeats itself.

Periodic sound A periodic sound is one whose waveform repeats itself regularly as a function of time.

Phase The phase of a periodic waveform is the fractional part of a period through which the waveform has advanced, measured from some arbitrary point in time.

Phase-locking This is the tendency for nerve firings to occur at a particular phase of the stimulating waveform.

Phon The unit of loudness level.

Pitch Pitch is that attribute of auditory sensation in terms of which sounds may be ordered on a musical scale.

Pure tone a sound wave whose instantaneous pressure variation as a function of time is a sinusoidal function. Also called a simple tone.

Recruitment This refers to a more rapid than usual growth of loudness with increase in stimulus level, which occurs in certain types of hearing disorder.

Sensation level This is the level of a sound in decibels relative to the threshold level for that sound for the individual listener.

Simple tone See Pure tone.

Sine wave, Sinusoidal vibration A waveform whose pressure variation as a function of time is a sine function. This is the function relating the sine of an angle to the size of the angle.

Sound pressure level This is the level of a sound in decibels relative to an internationally defined reference level. The latter corresponds to an intensity of 10^{-16} W/cm^2, which is equivalent to a sound pressure of 2×10^{-5} N/m^2.

Spectrum The spectrum of a sound wave is the distribution in frequency of the magnitudes (and sometimes the phases) of the components of the wave. It can be represented by plotting power, or amplitude, or level as a function of frequency.

Spike A single nerve impulse or action potential.

Timbre Timbre is that attribute of auditory sensation in terms of which a listener can judge that two sounds similarly presented and having the same loudness and pitch are dissimilar. Put more simply, it relates to the quality of a sound.

Tone A tone is a sound wave capable of exciting an auditory sensation having pitch.

Tuning curve For a single nerve fibre this is a graph of the lowest sound level at which the fibre will respond, plotted as a function of frequency. Also called a frequency threshold curve (FTC).

Waveform Waveform is a term used to describe the form or shape of a wave. It may be represented graphically by plotting instantaneous amplitude, pressure or intensity as a function of time

Subject index

ABLB test, 68
Absolute pitch, 146–147, 186
Absolute thresholds, 41–44, 286
  of complex sounds, 85–86
Acoustic reflex, *see* Middle ear reflex
Adaptation, 60–66
  pathological, 69–70
Adaptation effects, 191–192, 232–236
Ambisonic reproduction, 251–252
Amplifiers, 238–241
Amplitude modulation, 53–54, 87–88,
  124–5, 156–7, 192–193, 200
Analysis by synthesis, 219–222
Anatomy of the auditory system, 13–25
Articulation tests, 227–228
Attention, 82–83, 129, 136–137, 141,
  150, 169–170, 201, 202–203
Audiogram, 42–44, 286, *see also*
  Masking
Audiology, 67–70, 253–254
Auditory filter, 76–84, 90–92, 104,
  106–108, *see also* Critical band
  origin of, 90–92, 105–106
  shape of, 80–82
Aural harmonics, 57, 286

Backward masking, *see* Masking, nonsimultaneous
Basilar membrane, 15–24, 76–77,
  90–91, 99–100, 105–106, 115–117,
  127–130, 135, 156, 166, 261, 286
Beats, 75, 79, 144–145, 153–154, 286,
  see also Binaural beats
  and intensity discrimination, 53
Belongingness, principle of, 201
Best frequency, *see* Tuning curve,
  neural
Binaural beats, 153–154
Binaural masking level difference,
  168–176, 193, 250, 286
  models of, 172–176

Binaural processing, *see* Localization,
  Binaural masking level difference,
  Pitch, binaural interaction in
BMLD, *see* Binaural masking level
  difference

Categorical perception, 215–216,
  220–221, 234
Cerebral asymmetry, 217
Change detection, 191–192, 199–200,
  203
Characteristic frequency (CF), *see*
  Tuning curve, neural
Clinical applications, *see* Audiology,
  Deafness
Closure, principle of, 201–202
Cochlea, 15–25, 260–262, *see also*
  Basilar membrane
Cochlear echoes, 260–262
Cochlear implants, 257–260
Cocktail party phenomenon, 170,
  202–203
Combination tones, 86, 132–133, 134,
  143, 261, 286
Common fate, principle of, 200
Concert hall acoustics, 262–265
Conductive deafness, *see* Deafness
Cone of confusion, 157–158
Consonance, 144–146
Consonants, 199–200, 208–216,
  223–226
Continuation, principle of, 199–200
Continuity effect, 101–104, 190,
  201–202, 207
Contrast, *see* Change detection
Cortex, *see* Neural responses at higher
  levels, Cerebral asymmetry
Cortical responses, *see* Neural re-
  sponses at higher levels
Critical band, 75–97, 117, 140–144
  in hearing impaired, 106–107